Genetics of Cardiomyopathy and Heart Failure

Guest Editor

CALUM A. MACRAE, MD, PhD

HEART FAILURE CLINICS

www.heartfailure.theclinics.com

Consulting Editors

RAGAVENDRA R. BALIGA, MD, MBA, FRCP, FACC, FRS (Med)

JAMES B. YOUNG, MD, FACC

Founding Editor

JAGAT NARULA, MD, PhD

April 2010 • Volume 6 • Number 2

SAUNDERS an imprint of ELSEVIER, Inc.

W.B. SAUNDERS COMPANY
A Division of Elsevier Inc.

1600 John F. Kennedy Boulevard • Suite 1800 • Philadelphia, Pennsylvania 19103-2899

http://www.theclinics.com

HEART FAILURE CLINICS Volume 6, Number 2
April 2010 ISSN 1551-7136, ISBN-13: 978-1-4377-1827-0

Editor: Barbara Cohen-Kligerman
Developmental Editor: Theresa Collier

Heart Failure Clinics (ISSN 1551-7136) is published quarterly by Elsevier Inc., 360 Park Avenue South, New York, NY 10010-1710. Months of publication are January, April, July, and October. Business and editorial offices: 1600 John F. Kennedy Boulevard, Suite 1800, Philadelphia, PA 19103-2899. Periodicals postage paid at New York, NY, and additional mailing offices. Subscription prices are USD 193.00 per year for US individuals, USD 326.00 per year for US institutions, USD 67.00 per year for US students and residents, USD 232.00 per year for Canadian individuals, USD 374.00 per year for Canadian institutions, USD 247.00 per year for international individuals, USD 374.00 per year for international institutions, and USD 85.00 per year for Canadian and foreign students/residents. To receive student and resident rate, orders must be accompanied by name of affiliated institution, date of term, and the *signature* of program/residency coordinator on institution letterhead. Orders will be billed at individual rate until proof of status is received. Foreign air speed delivery is included in all *Clinics* subscription prices. All prices are subject to change without notice. **POSTMASTER:** Send address changes to *Heart Failure Clinics*, Elsevier Health Sciences Division, Subscription Customer Service, 3251 Riverport Lane, Maryland Heights, MO 63043. **Customer Service: 1-800-654-2452 (US and Canada). From outside of the US and Canada, call 314-447-8871. Fax: 314-447-8029. For print support, e-mail: JournalsCustomerService-usa@elsevier.com. For online support, e-mail: JournalsOnlineSupport-usa@elsevier.com.**

Reprints. For copies of 100 or more of articles in this publication, please contact the Commercial Reprints Department, Elsevier Inc., 360 Park Avenue South, New York, NY 10010-1710. Tel.: 212-633-3812; Fax: 212-462-1935; E-mail: reprints@elsevier.com.

Heart Failure Clinics is covered in *MEDLINE/PubMed (Index Medicus).*

Printed and bound in the United Kingdom
Transferred to Digital Print on Demand 2011

Cover artwork courtesy of Umberto M. Jezek.

Contributors

CONSULTING EDITORS

RAGAVENDRA R. BALIGA, MD, MBA, FRCP, FACC, FRS (Med)
Professor of Internal Medicine, OSU Heart Center and Ross Heart Hospital, The Ohio State University Medical Center, Columbus, Ohio

JAMES B. YOUNG, MD, FACC
Executive Dean, Lerner College of Medicine and Professor of Internal Medicine, Division of Medicine, Cleveland Clinic, Cleveland, Ohio

GUEST EDITOR

CALUM A. MACRAE, MD, PhD
Cardiovascular Division, Brigham and Women's Hospital and Harvard Medical School, Boston, Massachusetts

AUTHORS

ROY BEINART, MD
Massachusetts General Hospital, Boston, Massachusetts

EMELIA J. BENJAMIN, MD, ScM
Professor, Section of Cardiology, Preventive Medicine, Whitaker Cardiovascular Institute, Boston University School of Medicine, Boston, Massachusetts; Department of Epidemiology, Boston University Schools of Medicine and Public Health, Framingham Heart Study; National Heart, Lung and Blood Institute's Framingham Heart Study, Framingham, Massachusetts

TIM BOUSSY, MD
Heart Rhythm Management Institute, University Hospital Brussels, Laarbeeklaan, Brussels, Belgium

JOSEP BRUGADA, MD, PhD
Thorax Institute, Hospital Clinic, University of Barcelona, Barcelona, Spain

PEDRO BRUGADA, MD, PhD
Heart Rhythm Management Institute, University Hospital Brussels, Laarbeeklaan, Brussels, Belgium

RAMON BRUGADA, MD, PhD
Montreal Heart Institute, Montreal, Quebec, Canada

GIAN BATTISTA CHIERCHIA, MD
Heart Rhythm Management Institute, University Hospital Brussels, Laarbeeklaan, Brussels, Belgium

CARLO DE ASMUNDIS, MD
Heart Rhythm Management Institute, University Hospital Brussels, Laarbeeklaan, Brussels, Belgium

RAHUL C. DEO, MD, PhD
Cardiology Division, Massachusetts General Hospital, Boston, Massachusetts

PATRICK T. ELLINOR, MD, PhD
Associate Professor, Cardiovascular Research Center and Cardiology Division, Massachusetts General Hospital, Charlestown, Massachusetts

DIANE FATKIN, MD
Associate Professor, Molecular Cardiology Division, Victor Chang Cardiac Research Institute, Darlinghurst; Cardiology Department, St Vincent's Hospital, Darlinghurst; St Vincent's Clinical School, Faculty of Medicine, University of New South Wales, Kensington, New South Wales, Australia

CAROLYN Y. HO, MD
Assistant Professor of Medicine and Medical Director, Cardiovascular Division, Brigham and Women's Hospital, Boston, Massachusetts

STEVEN A. LUBITZ, MD
Research Fellow, Cardiovascular Research Center, Massachusetts General Hospital, Charlestown Division of Preventive Medicine, Center for Cardiovascular Disease Prevention, Brigham and Women's Hospital, Boston, Massachusetts

CALUM A. MACRAE, MD, PhD
Cardiovascular Division, Brigham and Women's Hospital and Harvard Medical School, Boston, Massachusetts

WILLIAM J. McKENNA, MD, DSc, FRCP
Professor of Cardiology, Inherited Cardiovascular Disease Group, University College London, London, United Kingdom

DAVID MILAN, MD
Massachusetts General Hospital, Boston, Massachusetts

ROBYN OTWAY, PhD
Postdoctoral Fellow, Molecular Cardiology Division, Victor Chang Cardiac Research Institute, Darlinghurst, New South Wales, Australia

GAETANO PAPARELLA, MD
Heart Rhythm Management Institute, University Hospital Brussels, Laarbeeklaan, Brussels, Belgium

ZARA RICHMOND, BSc
Genetics Counselor, Molecular Cardiology Division, Victor Chang Cardiac Research Institute, Darlinghurst, New South Wales, Australia

JEREMY RUSKIN, MD
Massachusetts General Hospital, Boston, Massachusetts

ANDREA SARKOZY, MD
Heart Rhythm Management Institute, University Hospital Brussels, Laarbeeklaan, Brussels, Belgium

MARC J. SEMIGRAN, MD
Medical Director, Heart Failure and Transplantation, Cardiology Division, Department of Medicine, Massachusetts General Hospital; Associate Professor, Harvard Medical School, Boston, Massachusetts

SRIJITA SEN-CHOWDHRY, MBBS, MD (Cantab.), MRCP
Walport Clinical Lecturer, Faculty of Medicine, Imperial College, London, United Kingdom

JORDAN T. SHIN, MD, PhD
Assistant Physician, Cardiovascular Research Center, Department of Medicine, Massachusetts General Hospital; Instructor in Medicine, Harvard Medical School, Charlestown, Massachusetts

PETROS SYRRIS, PhD
Director of Cardiovascular Genetics Laboratory, Inherited Cardiovascular Disease Group, University College London, London, United Kingdom

LUDWIG THIERFELDER, MD
Associate Professor, Department of Cardiology, Max-Delbrueck Center for Molecular Medicine; Franz-Volhard Clinic, Charité, Campus Buch, Helios Clinic, Berlin, Germany

B. ALEXANDER YI, MD, PhD
Cardiology Division, Massachusetts General Hospital and Harvard Medical School, Boston, Massachusetts

Contents

Dilated cardiomyopathy (DCM) is a myocardial disorder defined by ventricular chamber enlargement and systolic dysfunction. DCM can result in progressive heart failure, arrhythmias, thromboembolism, and premature death, and contributes significantly to health care costs. In many cases, DCM results from acquired factors that affect cardiomyocyte function or survival. Inherited genetic variants are also now recognized to have an important role in the etiology of DCM. Despite substantial progress over the past decade, our understanding of familial DCM remains incomplete. Current concepts of the molecular pathogenesis, clinical presentation, natural history, and management of familial DCM are outlined in this review.

Important insights into the molecular basis of hypertrophic cardiomyopathy and related diseases have been gained by studying families with inherited cardiac hypertrophy. Integrated clinical and genetic investigations have demonstrated that different genetic defects can give rise to the common phenotype of cardiac hypertrophy. Diverse pathways have been identified, implicating perturbations in force generation, force transmission, intracellular calcium homeostasis, myocardial energetics, and cardiac metabolism in causing disease. Although not fully elucidated, the fundamental mechanisms linking gene mutations to clinical disease are being characterized. Further advances will allow a better understanding of pathogenesis, diagnosis, and treatment, not just of relatively rare inherited cardiomyopathies, but potentially also of relevance to more common acquired forms of hypertrophic remodeling.

Arrhythmogenic right ventricular cardiomyopathy (ARVC) originally emerged as a pathologic diagnosis based on distinctive autopsy findings in cases of premature sudden death. Subsequently these characteristic pathologic features were associated with ventricular tachycardia of right ventricular origin and syncope. ARVC is a rare condition and our understanding of the disorder has been confounded by multiple small, highly selected series. Driven by both family studies and improved non-invasive imaging tools the clinical diagnosis of ARVC has broadened, in some instances extending far beyond the original limits of the syndrome. In recent years false-positive diagnoses have increased, thus stimulating investigators to move toward

Newer clinical strategies to preferentially lower pulmonary pressures and pulmonary vascular tone improve functional performance and symptoms of heart failure by targeting the nitric oxide signal transduction pathways, as with PDE5 inhibition. Additional studies are needed to determine if these therapies will impact long-term patient outcomes and elucidate the specific mechanisms whereby these treatments are effective. Furthermore, the recent finding that mutations in *BMPR2* cause familial forms of pulmonary arterial hypertension and that *BMPR2* expression is decreased in secondary forms of PH strongly implicate BMP signaling in the underlying pathophysiology of PH. Translation of emerging basic science insights in the vascular biology of PH and BMP signaling will provide novel therapeutic strategies for the spectrum of pulmonary hypertensive diseases.

Integrating Current Knowledge for Common Forms of Heart Failure

The Genetics of Congestive Heart Failure **223**

Calum A. MacRae

The heart failure syndrome is known to represent a final common pathway for a broad range of etiologies, but there is tremendous variation in the propensity to develop congestive heart failure after a given insult. This variation is thought to result in part from inherited differences in myocardial, vascular or systemic responses, but the nature of the underlying traits responsible ultimately for the development of heart failure has remained elusive. There has been limited progress in the genetic exploration of the key clinical phenotype itself: heart failure. In this article, the author attempts to place the results of genetic studies of cardiomyopathy in the broader context of the clinical syndrome of heart failure, highlighting some of the key questions for future study.

Clinical Screening and Genetic Testing **231**

Rahul C. Deo and Calum A. MacRae

Clinical screening is most effective in diseases in which the disease in its earliest form and may not have symptoms or signs but can be readily diagnosed with an inexpensive, noninvasive test. This article discusses the general principles of genetic disease architecture that can guide screening and diagnostic approaches for all of the cardiomyopathies and inherited diseases. It addresses how the genetic architecture of the trait guides, and how clinical characteristics of the disease influence, a clinical screening approach.

Special Articles

Genetics of Atrial Fibrillation **239**

Steven A. Lubitz, B. Alexander Yi, and Patrick T. Ellinor

Recent studies of atrial fibrillation (AF) have identified mutations in a series of ion channels; however, these mutations appear to be relatively rare causes of AF. A genome-wide association study has identified novel variants on chromosome 4 associated with AF, although the mechanism of action for these variants remains unknown. Ultimately, a greater understanding of the genetics of AF should yield insights into novel pathways, therapeutic targets, and diagnostic testing for this common arrhythmia.

Sudden cardiac death caused by malignant ventricular arrhythmias is the most important cause of death in the industrialized world. Most of these lethal arrhythmias occur in the setting of ischemic heart disease. A significant number of sudden deaths, especially in young individuals, are caused by inherited ventricular arrhythmic disorders, however. Genetically induced ventricular arrhythmias can be divided in two subgroups: the primary electrical disorders or channelopathies, and the secondary arrhythmogenic cardiomyopathies. This article focuses on the genetic background of these electrical disorders and the current knowledge of genotype-phenotype interactions.

Heart Failure Clinics

FORTHCOMING ISSUES

July 2010

Anemia and Heart Failure
Stuart Katz, MD, Ajay Singh, MB, and Anil Agarwal, MD, *Guest Editors*

October 2010

Heart Failure in Children
Jeffrey A. Towbin, MD, *Guest Editor*

January 2011

Depression and Heart Failure
Philip F. Binkley, MD, MPH, and Stephen Gottlieb, MD, *Guest Editors*

RECENT ISSUES

January 2010

Pharmacogenetics in Heart Failure: How It Will Shape the Future
Dennis M. McNamara, MD, *Guest Editor*

October 2009

Biomarkers in Heart Failure
Eugene Braunwald, MD, *Guest Editor*

July 2009

MRI in Heart Failure
Raymond J. Kim, MD, and Dudley Pennell, MD, FRCP, FACC, *Guest Editors*

ISSUES OF RELATED INTEREST

Cardiac Electrophysiology Clinics March 2010 (Volume 2, Issue 1)
Epicardial Interventions in Electrophysiology
Kalyanam Shivkumar, MD, PhD, FHRS, and Noel G. Boyle, MD, PhD, FHRS, *Guest Editors*
Available at: http://www.cardiacep.theclinics.com/

Cardiology Clinics February 2010 (Volume 28, Issue 1)
Advanced Applied Interventional Cardiology
Samin K. Sharma, MD, FSCAI, FACC, and Annapoorna S. Kini, MD, MRCP, FACC, *Guest Editors*
Available at: http://www.cardiology.theclinics.com/

Editorial

Unleashing Our Healthy Avatars Using Cardiovascular Genetics

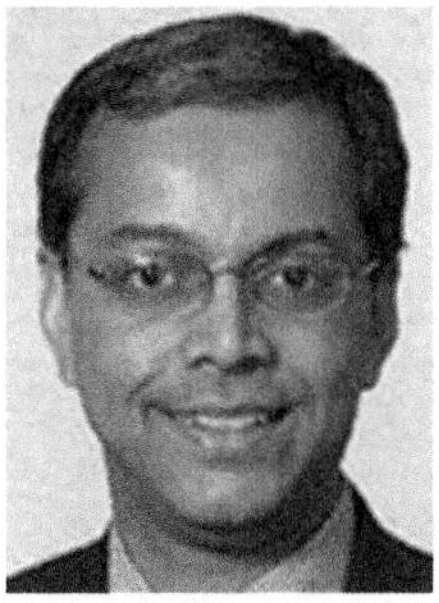

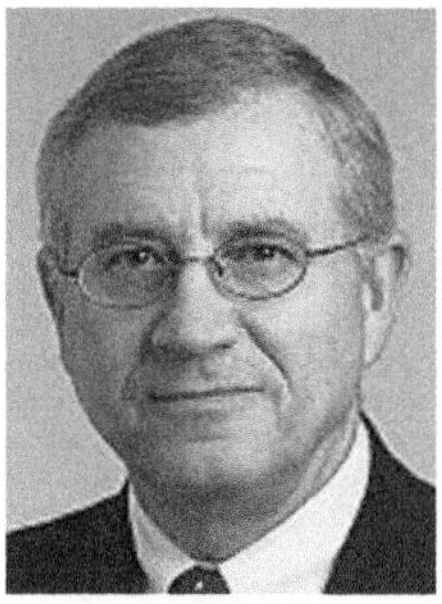

Ragavendra R. Baliga, MD, MBA, FRCP, FACC, FRS (Med)
James B. Young, MD, FACC
Consulting Editors

The field of genetics recently has witnessed quantum leaps of progress. In 1996, Megan and Morag, two lambs, were cloned from embryonic cells and the same team created Dolly the lamb from adult undifferentiated cells.[1] Subsequently mice, calves, piglets, kittens, horses, rats, and dogs all have been cloned (**Fig. 1**). The push for personalized medicine (the ability to tailor medical care to an individual's genes) also resulted in major efforts to better understand the human genetic make-up. These include the Human Genome Project,[2] The Single Nucleotide Polymorphism database,[3] the HapMap Project,[4,5] the 1000 Genome Project,[6] and the Genome 10K Initiative.[7] The Human Genome Project was successfully completed in 2003 in that it identified all of the approximately 25,000 genes in the human DNA and determined the sequence of 3 billion chemical base pairs that make up the human DNA. The Single Nucleotide Polymorphism database and International HapMap Project (unveiled in 2005) aim to provide essential data for research into single nucleotide polymorphisms, which are markers of genetic diversity. By comparing these data with single nucleotide polymorphisms from patients with specific diseases, researchers hope to determine the genetic "glitches" that underlie those disorders.

These innovative efforts have generated both political and ethical concerns. Several new regulatory measures have been announced to better harness these developments. On September 18, 2008, the US Food and Drug Administration published a document outlining how it proposes to regulate genetically engineered animals.[8] The proposed regulations effectively treat such animals as drugs to provide grounds for Food and Drug Administration oversight and control. The United States Senate outlawed genetic discrimination.[9] The Genetic Information Nondiscrimination Act bans the use of genetic information in hiring, firing, promotion, and compensation decisions, and prohibits collecting genetic information from employees by employers. This bill also prevents health plans and insurers from denying coverage or boosting premium prices based on a person's genetic data, such as whether they have gene variants known to increase disease risk. It also forbids them from requesting or requiring people to take genetic tests. More recently, in November 2009, the United States government issued draft guidelines for how synthetic-biology companies should screen customers and their gene orders to protect against bioterrorism. Additionally, several for-profit companies offer relatively inexpensive and quick-to-report personal genomic characterization for anyone willing to send a cotton swab of their cheek along with a check to the laboratory.

In the interim a virtual map of the expression of 20,000 genes in the mouse brain was completed in 2006,[10] and the first data to map the spinal cord have been released.[11] When completed, the freely accessible atlas will chart the expression patterns of at least 18,500 genes throughout the spinal cord of juvenile and adult mice. Although similar strides have not yet been made with the cardiovascular system, Dr Calum MacRae, from Harvard

Heart Failure Clin 6 (2010) xi–xiii
doi:10.1016/j.hfc.2010.01.001
1551-7136/10/$ – see front matter

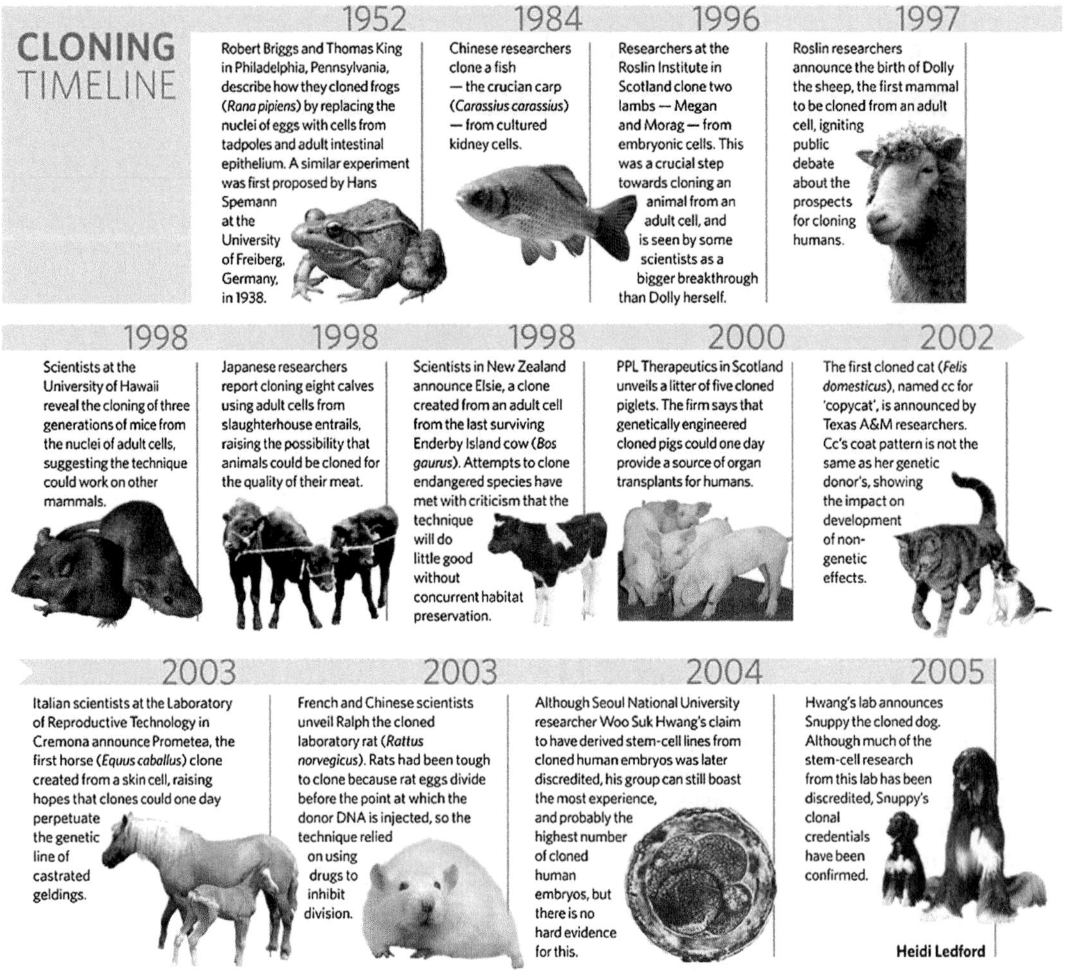

Fig. 1. Cloning timeline. (*From* Wadman M. Cloning special: Dolly: a decade on. Nature 2007;445:800–11; with permission.)

Medical School, has assembled a world-class team of genetic specialists with an interest in the genetics of cardiomyopathy and heart failure. These diseases cannot always be attributed to mutations in a single gene or genetic pathway, and teasing out each genetic contribution from the tangled knot of environmental and genetic factors is challenging. Despite these barriers, in this issue of *Heart Failure Clinics*, these contributors have helped us better understand the rapidly changing and dynamic field of cardiovascular genetics. It is hoped that this understanding of cardiovascular genetics provides impetus for the development of more powerful and safer therapeutic agents that should be more effective while allowing for more accurate determination of dosages, better compliance, promotion of advanced screening of heart failure patients, and development of better preventive strategies[12] by figuring out how to unleash our healthy genetic avatars.

Ragavendra R. Baliga, MD, MBA, FRCP, FACC, FRS (Med)
OSU Heart Center and Ross Heart Hospital
The Ohio State University Medical Center
Columbus, OH, USA

James B. Young, MD, FACC
Division of Medicine and Lerner
College of Medicine, Cleveland Clinic
Cleveland, OH, USA

E-mail addresses:
Ragavendra.Baliga@osumc.edu (R.R. Baliga)
youngj@ccf.org (J.B. Young)

REFERENCES

1. Wadman M. Cloning special: Dolly: a decade on. Nature 2007;445(7130):800–1.
2. McPherson JD, Marra M, Hillier L, et al. A physical map of the human genome. Nature 2001;409(6822): 934–41.
3. Sherry ST, Ward M, Sirotkin K. dbSNP-database for single nucleotide polymorphisms and other classes of minor genetic variation. Genome Res 1999;9(8): 677–9.
4. Phimister EG. Genomic cartography: presenting the HapMap. N Engl J Med 2005;353(17):1766–8.
5. Thorisson GA, Smith AV, Krishnan L, et al. The International HapMap project web site. Genome Res 2005;15(11):1592–3.
6. Kuehn BM. 1000 Genomes Project promises closer look at variation in human genome. JAMA 2008; 300(23):2715.
7. Genome 10K Community of Scientists. Genome 10K: a proposal to obtain whole-genome sequence for 10,000 vertebrate species. J Hered 2009; 100(6):659–74.
8. Gluck JP, Holdsworth MT. FDA releases draft guidance on regulation of genetically engineered animals. Kennedy Inst Ethics J 2008;18(4):393–402.
9. Tanne JH. US Senate outlaws genetic discrimination. BMJ 2008;336(7652):1038.
10. Lein ES, Hawrylycz MJ, Ao N, et al. Genome-wide atlas of gene expression in the adult mouse brain. Nature 2007;445(7124):168–76.
11. Wadman M. Spinal cord revealed in free gene map. Nature 2008;454(7203):373.
12. Baliga RR, Young JB. Pharmacogenomics transforming medicine to create a world of immortal Struldbruggs or even a Methuselah? So be it! Heart Fail Clin 2010;6(1):xi–xiii.

Preface

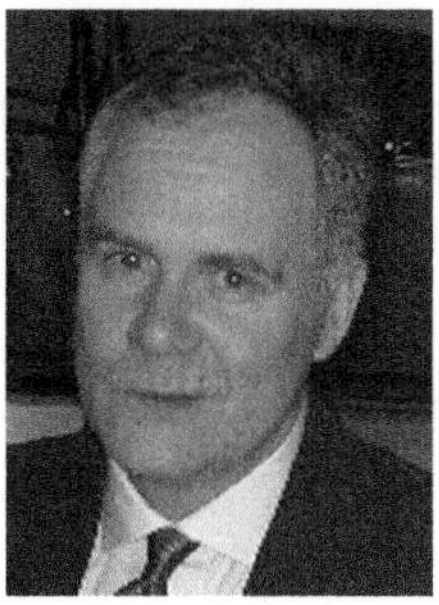

Calum A. MacRae, MD, PhD
Guest Editor

Heart failure remains the single most common cause of death in the developed world and is fast becoming a major problem in the developing world. Tremendous advances have been made over the last two decades in the treatment of the antecedent forms of heart disease, improving survival in the context of myocardial injury that would previously have been fatal, so that the prevalence of heart failure continues to increase. While progress has been made in the treatment of heart failure with substantial effects on morbidity and mortality, in many instances the progressive decline in function that accompanies the syndrome is only delayed. It is clear that new advances in the understanding of heart failure require much deeper insight into the earliest mechanisms underlying this complex syndrome, and in particular the pathophysiologic determinants of maladaptation as opposed to homeostatic compensation. In this effort genetics have already played a major role and will continue to do so.

Genetic studies of primary forms of heart failure have uncovered genes responsible for many of the key components of the final decompensated state. In this issue each of these relatively rare cardiomyopathies are reviewed with a focus on their contribution to heart failure pathophysiology at different levels. Perhaps the most obvious link between typical forms of acquired heart failure and is seen in dilated cardiomyopathy. Some of the genes underlying hypertrophic cardiomyopathy are now also recognized to cause dilated cardiomyopathy in certain contexts, and families exist in which these two apparently distinctive responses are seen in different individuals with the same genetic cause. Similar overlap syndromes exist between dilated cardiomyopathy and arrhythmogenic right ventricular cardiomyopathy, and between hypertrophic cardiomyopathy and inherited cases of restrictive physiology. In the first section of this issue each of these is discussed in turn by leading investigators in the field.

Recent epidemiologic data have identified links between several other cardiovascular phenotypes and the eventual emergence of decompensated heart failure. Atrial fibrillation and conduction system disease likely represent cardiomyopathies preferentially affecting specific cell subtypes within the heart: atrial or pulmonary venous excitable cells, or the fibers of the conduction system. Genetic variation in pulmonary vascular responses is now known to underlie the pathophysiology of pulmonary hypertension, but these same pathways are increasingly thought also to play a role in the progression of more common forms of heart failure. In the second section, these "cross-cutting" phenotypes seen in conjunction with heart failure, each with substantial inherited contributions, are dissected, offering insight into the complexity of the composite syndrome.

The role of these same genes in common forms of heart failure is far from clear. Only as the pathways downstream of the primary mutations are understood is it possible to define the contribution, if any, that these mechanisms make to common disease. Nevertheless, the experiments of nature represented in monogenic disease offer inroads into the key regulatory hubs that may be disrupted in cardiac physiology. In the final section there are two articles designed to offer an integrative overview and some future directions. In the first of these the relationship between large mendelian effects and the smaller common

Heart Failure Clin 6 (2010) xv–xvi
doi:10.1016/j.hfc.2009.12.006

effects thought prevalent in typical heart failure is outlined. Potential ways in which the comprehensive genetic architecture of heart failure might be explored are elaborated. The last article focuses on the practical aspects of genotype-phenotype correlation in the mendelian syndromes, highlighting the difficulties present even in the context of very large effect sizes, and emphasizing the role of improved phenotypes in moving the field forward.

Heart failure remains a challenging and exciting field. It is hoped that the perspectives gained from this issue stimulate future basic, clinical, and translational work in this arena.

Calum A. MacRae, MD, PhD
Cardiovascular Division
Brigham and Women's Hospital
Thorn 11
75 Francis Street
Boston, MA 02115, USA

E-mail address:
camacrae@bics.bwh.harvard.edu

Genetics of Dilated Cardiomyopathy

Diane Fatkin, MD[a,b,c,*], Robyn Otway, PhD[a], Zara Richmond, BSc[a]

KEYWORDS

• Genetics • Dilated cardiomyopathy
• Heart failure

Dilated cardiomyopathy (DCM) is a myocardial disorder defined by ventricular chamber enlargement and systolic dysfunction that can result in progressive heart failure, supraventricular and ventricular arrhythmias, and thromboembolism. Consequently, DCM is a major cause of morbidity and mortality and contributes significantly to health care costs. DCM develops frequently as a result of acquired factors that affect myocyte function or survival, such as ischemia, infectious agents, autoimmune disorders, alcohol excess, chemotherapeutic drugs, or nutritional deficiencies. DCM can occur as a primary manifestation of disease or as part of a multisystem disorder.[1] Inherited genetic variants have increasingly been recognized as having an important role in the etiology of DCM. Families in which DCM segregates as a mendelian trait have been instrumental in elucidation of diverse molecular defects that result in cardiac contractile dysfunction.[2] Despite substantial progress in this field over the past decade, several challenges for the diagnosis and treatment of familial DCM remain. Current concepts of the molecular pathogenesis, clinical presentation, natural history, and management of familial DCM are outlined in this review.

CHROMOSOMAL LOCI AND DISEASE GENES ASSOCIATED WITH DILATED CARDIOMYOPATHY

Genetic linkage and candidate gene screening studies performed in families and in cohorts of unrelated patients with adult-onset DCM have resulted in identification of nearly 40 chromosomal loci and disease genes (**Table 1**).[3–90] Several criteria are traditionally used to support an argument for a DNA sequence variant that is found in an index case to be disease-causing. These include segregation of the variant with affection status within a family, absence in a control population, location at a conserved amino acid residue, and relevant functional consequences. For many variants there are robust genetic data showing an association with DCM in large kindreds. For some variants, segregation with disease has been difficult to ascertain because there are few affected individuals in a family or several key individuals have declined genetic testing. In other cases, the demonstration of negative parental genotypes has indicated that DNA sequence variants have arisen de novo in individual probands. The case for a link between the gene in question and disease is strengthened if different variants

This work is supported by a Program Grant (354400) and a Senior Research Fellowship (404808 [D. Fatkin]) from the National Health and Medical Research Council of Australia
[a] Molecular Cardiology Division, Victor Chang Cardiac Research Institute, Lowy Packer Building, 405 Liverpool Street, PO Box 699, Darlinghurst, NSW 2010, Australia
[b] Cardiology Department, St Vincent's Hospital, Victoria Street, Darlinghurst, NSW 2010, Australia
[c] St Vincent's Clinical School, Faculty of Medicine, University of New South Wales, Kensington, NSW 2052, Australia
* Corresponding author. Molecular Cardiology Division, Victor Chang Cardiac Research Institute, Lowy Packer Building, 405 Liverpool Street, PO Box 699, Darlinghurst, NSW 2010, Australia.
E-mail address: d.fatkin@victorchang.edu.au

Heart Failure Clin 6 (2010) 129–140
doi:10.1016/j.hfc.2009.11.003
1551-7136/10/$ – see front matter

Table 1
Chromosomal loci and disease genes associated with adult-onset dilated cardiomyopathy[a]

Locus	Gene	Protein	No. Variants	Inheritance[b]	Phenotype	References
1q21	*LMNA*	Lamin A/C	43	Familial	DCM ± CD, SD, SkM	3–25
1q31-q42	*PSEN2*	Presenilin2	1	Familial	DCM	26
1q32	*TNNT2*	Cardiac troponin T	6	Familial; single case; sporadic	DCM ± SD	27–30
1q42-q43	*ACTN2*	α-Actinin 2	1	Single case	DCM	31
2q12-q14	*FHL2*	Four-and-a-half LIM protein 2	1	Single case	DCM	32
2q14-q22	?	?	0	Familial	DCM ± CD	33
2q31	*TTN*	Titin	7	Familial; single cases	DCM	34–36
2q35	*DES*	Desmin	8	Familial; single case	DCM ± CD, SkM	37–40
3p21	*SCN5A*	Cardiac sodium channel	5	Familial; sporadic	DCM ± CD	41,42
3p21-p14	*TNNC1*	Cardiac troponin C	3[c]	Familial; single case	DCM	29,43
5q33	*SGCD*	δ-Sarcoglycan	3	Familial; sporadic	DCM ± SD	44,45
6q12-q16	?	?	0	Familial	DCM	46
6q21	*LAMA4*	Laminin-α4	2	Single cases	DCM	47
6q22	*PLB*	Phospholamban	3	Familial	DCM	48–50
6q23	?	?	0	Familial	DCM ± CD, SkM	51
6q23	*EYA4*	Eya4	1	Familial	DCM + SHL	52
7q22-q31	?	?	0	Familial	DCM	53
7q35	*CHRM2*	M2 muscarinic receptor	1	Familial	DCM ± CD, SD	54
9q13-q22	?	?	0	Familial	DCM	55
10q21	*MYPN*	Myopallidin	4	Familial; single cases	DCM	56
10q21-q23	?	?	0	Familial	DCM ± MVP	57
10q22-q23	*VCL*	Metavinculin	2	Familial; single case	DCM	58
10q22-q23	*LDB3*	Cypher/ZASP	6	Familial; sporadic	DCM ± CD, LVNC	59,60
10q25-q26	?	?	0	Familial	DCM ± SD	61
11p11	*MYBPC3*	Cardiac myosin binding protein 3	1	Single case	DCM	62

11p15	*CSRP3*	Muscle LIM protein	1	Familial; single cases	DCM	63
11p15	*ILK*	Integrin-linked kinase	1	Single case	DCM	47
11q22-q23	*CRYAB*	αβ-Crystallin	1	Single case	DCM	64
12p12	*SUR2*	Sulphonylurea receptor 2	2	Single cases	DCM	65
12q22	*TMPO*	Thymopoeitin	1	Familial	DCM	66
14q12	*MYH6*	α-Myosin heavy chain	3	Single cases	DCM	67
14q12	*MYH7*	β-Myosin heavy chain	12	Familial; single cases	DCM	27,62,68,69
14q24	*PSEN1*	Presenilin 1	1	Familial	DCM	26
15q14	*ACTC*	Cardiac actin	2	Familial	DCM	70
15q22	*TPMI*	α-Tropomyosin	2	Familial; single case	DCM	71
17q12	*TCAP*	Telethonin	2	Single cases	DCM	63,72
19q13	*TNNI3*	Cardiac troponin I	1	Familial[d]	DCM	73
Xp21	*DMD*	Dystrophin	34	Familial[e]; single cases; sporadic	DCM ± SkM	74–89
Xq24	*LAMP2*	LAMP2	1	Familial[e]	DCM ± CD, SkM[f]	90

Abbreviations: CD, conduction system abnormalities; LVNC, left ventricular noncompaction; MVP, mitral valve prolapse; SD, sudden death; SHL, sensorineural hearing loss; SkM, skeletal myopathy; ?, unknown.

[a] Mutations included are those in which DCM is the prominent presenting phenotypic feature.

[b] Inheritance patterns defined as familial (clinically affected and genotype-positive first-degree family members), single case (proband with/without family history but no genotype data reported for other family members), or sporadic (clinically unaffected and genotype-negative first-degree family members). Autosomal dominant inheritance has been observed in the majority of familial cases, except where indicated.

[c] Two variants in the same gene present in one single case.

[d] Autosomal recessive inheritance.

[e] X-linked inheritance.

[f] Complex phenotype with varying expression, including hypertrophic cardiomyopathy and ocular abnormalities.

can be identified in several unrelated families. DNA sequence variants that segregate with the clinical phenotype are more likely to be mutations rather than benign polymorphisms if they are not present in a population of healthy control subjects. Although there is no consensus for the number of control chromosomes that should be studied, evaluation of variants in at least several hundred individuals is generally required to differentiate potential mutations from rare polymorphisms. To demonstrate altered function of mutant protein, a variety of in vitro studies have been employed. Although valuable data can be gained, these types of studies are limited by experimental conditions that do not replicate the physiologic milieu. The most compelling evidence that a DNA sequence variant is likely to be pathogenic is obtained from in vivo models in which cardiac contraction can be directly assessed. Taken together, current data demonstrate that familial DCM is genetically heterogeneous. The extent to which each of the reported mutations meets the criteria for disease causation is variable, and further evaluation of many of these variants is warranted.

The majority of mutations are "private" variants that are unique to a single family. There are several examples of recurrent variants (eg, Arg190Trp *LMNA*,[8] Trp4Arg *CSRP3*,[63] and δLys210 *CNNT2*[27]) that may be located at unstable residues (hot spots) or represent rare functional polymorphisms or founder effects. Although DCM in most families has been attributed to a single mutation, the presence of two potentially pathogenic variants in one gene has been reported.[43] Mutations in the *LMNA* and *DMD* genes have been identified most frequently. In the majority of genes, however, only a few mutations have been found. Although comprehensive mutation screening studies have yet to be performed, studies in which selected genes have been evaluated in cohorts of DCM patients indicate that mutations in the known disease genes are likely to account for a small proportion of cases. In summary, despite a long list of familial DCM disease genes, current data suggest that additional disease genes have yet to be discovered. Because mutation screening is usually limited to the evaluation of coding sequences, an alternative possibility is that some disease-causing variants in the known genes may be located in regulatory domains in introns or in regions remote from the gene and have been missed.

New methods for linkage analysis, identification of candidate genes, and sequence analysis should greatly facilitate the process of gene discovery and mutation detection in the future. The traditional approach to mapping a disease gene in large kindreds has been to perform genome-wide linkage analysis using a panel of polymorphic microsatellite markers. The availability of single nucleotide polymorphism (SNP) microarrays in combination with HapMap data has enabled fine mapping and further genetic narrowing of these intervals to be undertaken. Once a minimum disease interval has been defined, mutation screening of promising candidate genes is subsequently performed. In small families that are unsuitable for linkage studies, candidate genes can be directly evaluated. These candidate genes have been generally selected on the basis of having a known important role in cardiac structure and function, a relationship with known disease-causing genes, or high levels of expression in the heart. Novel bioinformatics approaches to candidate gene prediction have recently been developed that use domain-based comparative sequence analysis, protein pathway, and protein-protein interaction databases.[91] New insights into molecules that have important roles in the heart have also been gained from studies of various transgenic and knockout mouse models, and mutagenesis screens in mice, zebrafish, and *Drosophila*.[47,52,92,93] DNA sequence analysis has been the gold standard method for mutation detection in candidate genes. The development of long-range sequencing platforms and alternative technologies that detect differences in DNA melting properties between samples should increase throughput and reduce the time and costs of mutation screening.[94,95]

PATHOPHYSIOLOGIC MECHANISMS

A variety of types of gene mutations have been reported, including missense changes at a single amino acid residue, insertions, deletions, and splice site variants. These sequence changes may result in mutant proteins of normal size but altered function that exert a dominant negative effect on wild-type proteins. Alternatively, mutant proteins may be truncated or reduced in amount and act by haploinsufficiency. The "dose" of mutant protein may be a critical determinant of phenotype. For example, in one family with a Lys39stop variant in the *PLB* gene, heterozygous individuals show left ventricular hypertrophy, whereas homozygous family members develop DCM.[49]

Although a unifying paradigm for the pathogenesis of familial DCM has been sought, it is apparent that gene mutations have diverse and interacting downstream effects that culminate in left ventricular systolic dysfunction (**Fig. 1**). Mutations in nuclear, sarcomeric, cytoskeletal, and surface

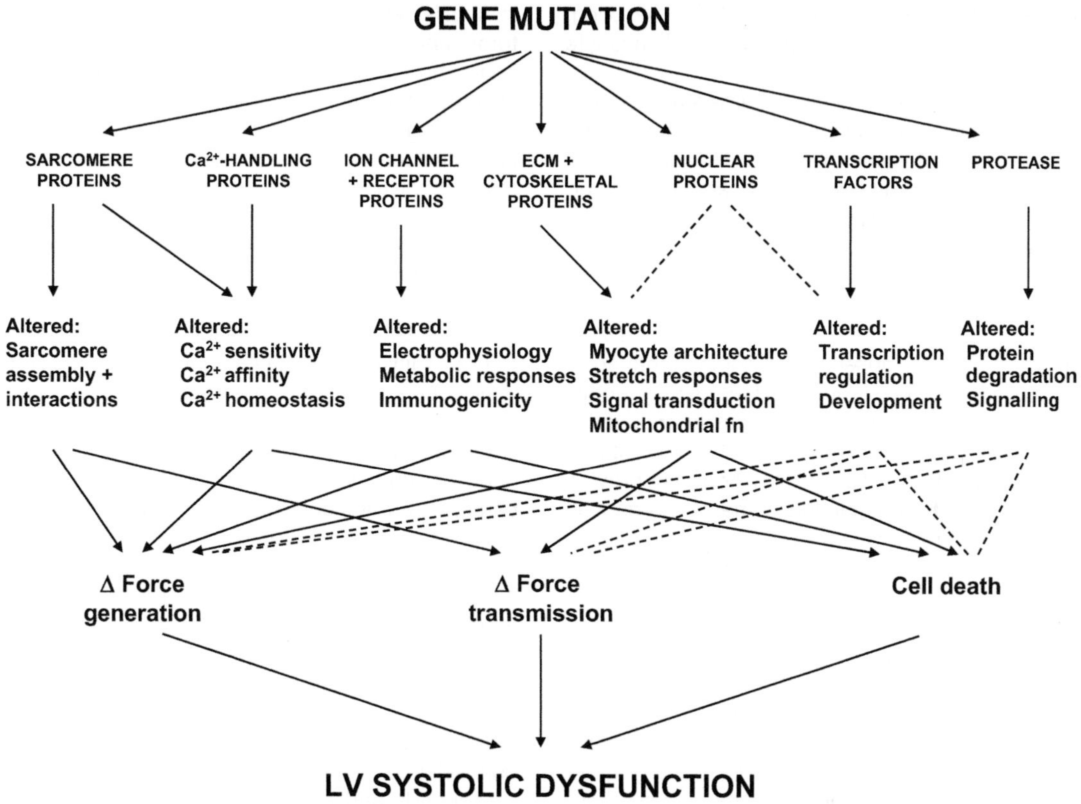

Fig. 1. Schematic of pathophysiologic pathways that have been proposed to link gene mutations to left ventricular (LV) systolic dysfunction. Pathways for which there is experimental evidence or strong support based on known gene functions are shown by solid arrows; pathways that are mainly speculative are shown by dashed lines.

membrane proteins have been identified that have several structural and functional consequences that impair myocardial force generation, force transmission, or cell survival. Force generation in cardiomyocytes is determined by cyclic interactions between actin and myosin in the thin and thick filaments. These interactions are dependent not only on the properties of actin and myosin but also on the regulatory effects of the Ca^{2+}-sensitive troponin-tropomyosin complex, the intrasarcomeric cytoskeletal scaffolding, and cardiac energy metabolism. Gene mutations that result in perturbation of any of these factors can result in impaired force generation. Mechanical force is transmitted from the sarcomere to the extracellular matrix through the network of cardiomyocyte cytoskeletal proteins. Gene mutations that alter the structural characteristics of the cytoskeleton or that affect signal transduction can impair myocardial mechanics and force transmission. Myocardial performance is also determined by the number of functional myocytes and by changes in Ca^{2+} homeostasis, metabolism, mitochondrial activity, and gene expression profiles that can accelerate cell death. The molecular defects that result from mutations in genes encoding nuclear proteins, cardiac transcription factors, and γ-secretase are incompletely understood but are likely to involve several nuclear and cytoskeletal functions.[3,26,52] Further studies to elucidate the pathophysiologic consequences of the broad range of DCM mutations should reveal fascinating insights into cardiomyocyte biology and disease mechanisms.

Although inherited gene mutations are present from birth, the phenotypic manifestations of DCM are not apparent until later adult life. This age-related penetrance of familial DCM suggests that disease processes may have cumulative effects that reach a critical threshold level of cellular dysfunction or that additional precipitating factors may be involved. Once DCM is established, a suite of secondary responses occurs that promote chamber remodeling and further functional impairment. These changes include activation of neurohumoral factors, re-induction of embryonic gene expression patterns, altered Ca^{2+} handling, apoptosis, deposition of collagen, and myocyte slippage.[96]

Familial DCM is generally regarded as a monogenic disorder in which single inherited gene defects are sufficient to cause disease. Clinical manifestations may vary significantly, however, within families or between families that carry the same variant. For example, individuals with the Arg377His or nt959 deletion *LMNA* mutations may have variable combinations of DCM, conduction system abnormalities, and skeletal myopathy.[4,10,11] These observations suggest that additional genetic or environmental factors may modify the disease phenotype. Quantitative trait locus mapping in mouse models that show strain-specific variation in cardiac function may provide a useful tool for pinpointing some of the genetic factors that are involved.[97]

IMPLICATIONS FOR MORE COMMONLY OCCURRING COMPLEX FORMS OF DILATED CARDIOMYOPATHY

Families in which DCM segregates as a mendelian trait due to a single inherited gene mutation represent one end of a spectrum. Like many other common diseases, it is predicted that in a substantial proportion of cases DCM is a complex disorder in which the collective effects of one or more SNPs or comorbid conditions predispose to disease development. Identification of the gene mutations that cause DCM in families provides clues for selecting SNPs for further analysis in case-control association studies in large cohorts of patients with complex forms of DCM. A better understanding of the genetic factors that promote DCM in families and in isolated cases may point to key genetic triggers or common downstream pathways that constitute novel targets for therapy. Studies of population risk due to SNPs might also provide a useful guide for prediction of drug responses and patient outcomes.

CLINICAL PRESENTATION

Families with DCM most commonly show an autosomal dominant mode of inheritance although autosomal recessive and X-linked inheritance can also be observed. The finding of a maternal inheritance pattern raises the possibility that DCM may be part of a multisystem mitochondrial disorder. Pedigree analysis is not necessarily straightforward and several factors may affect the recognition and classification of familial disease. Family size is important, as inheritance patterns may be more difficult to determine in smaller kindreds. The age of onset of symptoms and signs of DCM varies with different gene mutations and families. Phenotypic variability within family members may be a feature of a shared gene mutation or may be attributable to unrelated comorbidities. In most families, the penetrance of disease is high, but a minority of individuals who are genotype positive but who remain phenotype negative throughout life can be found. The absence of disease in younger adult family members does not necessarily implicate a negative genotype status but may reflect age-related penetrance. X-linked inheritance should be considered in all young male family members with apparently sporadic disease, because there may be significant implications for the development of DCM in female relatives and their offspring. Although female carriers are traditionally thought to remain phenotypically normal, the authors have observed that this is not necessarily the case, and X-linked inheritance can be missed if there are varying manifestations of disease in these individuals. Accurate ascertainment of inheritance is important for identifying at risk individuals who require cardiac screening, for selection of candidate genes for mutation screening, and for relevant genetics counseling.

Probands and all first-degree family members should undergo clinical evaluation with medical history, physical examination, 12-lead electrocardiography, and transthoracic echocardiography. Affected family members may present with symptoms and signs of congestive heart failure, including dyspnea, fatigue, palpitations, or peripheral edema. The diagnosis of DCM is based on the echocardiographic findings of left ventricular dilatation and reduced systolic function. Apart from family history, there are no specific clinical features that reliably differentiate between genetic and acquired causes of DCM.[98] Some families have a phenotype that is characterized predominantly by DCM, whereas in others, there may be associated cardiac features, such as conduction system abnormalities, atrial fibrillation, and mitral valve prolapse, or extracardiac features, including skeletal myopathy and sensorineural hearing loss. The clinical phenotype can give important clues about the underlying genotype (see **Table 1**). For example, families with *LMNA* gene mutations typically have a prodrome of progressive conduction abnormalities and supraventricular arrhythmias, with subsequent development of DCM. Conduction system abnormalities are also frequently present in families with *SCN5A* and *DES* gene mutations. Skeletal muscle involvement may be found with *LMNA*, *DES*, or *DMD* mutations.

NATURAL HISTORY

The natural history of familial DCM varies considerably with some individuals responding well to medical management and others experiencing progressive heart failure that may necessitate cardiac transplantation. Individuals in whom DCM is associated with conduction system abnormalities may develop high-grade atrioventricular conduction block and require pacemaker implantation. Sudden death is a devastating complication that can occur in DCM due to any cause but may be particularly prevalent in families with *LMNA*, *TNNT2*, *SGCD*, and *CHRM2* mutations. Although various clinical parameters have been evaluated for risk stratification in heart failure populations, it is likely that genotype will prove a major determinant of outcome in familial DCM. Reliable genotype-phenotype correlations have yet to be established, however, and will require longitudinal evaluation of large populations of genotyped individuals.

ROLE OF GENETIC TESTING

Because gene mutations are generally unique to a single family, the coding sequence of all known disease genes needs to be analyzed in each new proband. This process is time consuming and expensive. Moreover, given the large number of genes involved and low prevalence of mutations, systematic evaluation of the reported disease genes has a low yield. Mutation screening of specific genes that are associated with distinct phenotypes is more productive. For example, *LMNA* gene variants are found in less than 10% of unselected familial DCM populations but may be present in up to 45% families with DCM and conduction system abnormalities.[3,8,11,18,23] Similarly, *DMD* mutation screening is indicated in families with definite or suspected X-linked DCM.[83,87] Further gene discovery studies to compile a more comprehensive list of disease genes together with the refinement of high through-put mutation detection strategies will be required before genetic testing can become a routine diagnostic tool in clinical practice.

ROLE OF CLINICAL SCREENING

Approximately one in three patients with idiopathic DCM is likely to have a genetic etiology.[99] Hence, it is currently recommended that cardiac screening of first-degree relatives is performed in all newly diagnosed cases to identify kindreds with familial disease. In individuals who have a positive family history at presentation, ECG and echocardiographic screening of first-degree relatives is also indicated to detect asymptomatic DCM and early disease. In individuals at risk of developing DCM, due to having an affected parent or positive genotype, ongoing periodic follow-up is required. It is important that family members and clinicians alike appreciate that an initial finding of normal heart function, especially in younger family member, does not preclude the development of disease at a later age.

EARLY DISEASE IN FAMILIAL DILATED CARDIOMYOPATHY

As a direct consequence of implementation of clinical screening strategies, a substantial number of asymptomatic family members who have abnormal echocardiograms can be identified.[100–104] In 3% to 5% of asymptomatic family members, there is evidence of DCM. Additionally, a previously unrecognized subgroup of individuals who have left ventricular echocardiographic abnormalities that do not fulfill standard criteria for a diagnosis of DCM can be identified. Isolated left ventricular enlargement is the most frequent finding, occurring in 14% to 20% cases. Depression of left ventricular function with normal chamber size is seen less frequently, in 3% to 6% cases. The clinical significance of these findings has yet to be established but several observations suggest that, at least in some individuals, they represent early stages of disease. Several studies have shown that individuals with left ventricular enlargement have subclinical changes in myocardial structure and function, including altered myocardial histopathology and reductions in maximal oxygen consumption and systolic tissue Doppler velocity, that are intermediate in extent between normal control subjects and family members with DCM.[105–108] Levels of cardiac autoantibodies may also be elevated and predictive of progression to symptomatic DCM.[104] Longitudinal data in cohorts of individuals with asymptomatic echocardiographic changes are limited. In the largest series to date, Mahon and colleagues[103] found that 13 of 124 individuals (10%) with left ventricular enlargement or reduced fractional shortening progressed to DCM over a median 57-month follow-up period. Identification of clinical parameters that can better predict those individuals at greatest risk of progression and determination of optimal management strategies remain challenges for further research. In the interim, close medical surveillance of all family members with suspected early disease is indicated.

GENETIC COUNSELING

Genetic counseling is an essential component of the genetic screening process and encompasses patient education, establishing or verifying a diagnosis, risk assessment, and psychosocial counseling. Traditionally, DCM genetic screening is sought by affected individuals wanting to pinpoint a cause for their diagnosis and at-risk healthy individuals who wish to learn their genotype to enable informed personal and medical decisions. A multitude of genetic and psychosocial issues revolve around helping these individuals consider testing and with interpreting and coping with the test results. Pretest counseling should emphasize the key components of informed consent, including information about the screening process itself, possible limitations and benefits of testing, and the potential for unforeseen results or no result at all. The potential effects of a positive genetic result on personal coping mechanisms, family dynamics, and the ability to acquire insurance are of particular importance. A positive result may be emotionally traumatic, generating feelings of anxiety, anger, fear, and guilt. Of particular concern may be the fear of having passed on the genetic change to offspring. Benefits of a positive result include the ability to provide risk information for family members and guide the frequency of clinical follow-up assessment. Furthermore, a positive predictive result makes possible the choice for prophylactic treatment and lifestyle modification. The greatest challenge of DCM genetic counseling of genotype-positive patients is providing accurate information about how physical symptoms may manifest and the expected age of onset in their particular case. Additionally, due to the heterogeneity associated with familial DCM, a negative result for a particular familial mutation does not preclude the possibility of a subsequent positive finding for a second disease-associated genetic variant. Lastly, in the majority of cases, a result is never given, leading to continued anxiety and uncertainty over an impending prognosis. It is anticipated that future advances in understanding of the genetic causes of DCM and automated cost-effective methods for mutation screening will greatly increase the number of families in which disease-causing variants are identified.

SUMMARY

Familial DCM is genetically heterogeneous and there is a long and growing list of disease genes. Mutations in the majority of known disease genes are infrequent, however, and collectively account for a minority of all familial DCM cases. Genetic testing has yet to gain a role in routine patient care but may be indicated for subgroups of families with distinct phenotypes. Echocardiographic screening of relatives of probands with DCM is recommended to identify familial cases and asymptomatic early disease. Genetic counseling informs affected individuals and their relatives about the inheritance risks associated with familial DCM and the emotional, legal, and ethical implications of genetic testing and provides an important adjunct to medical management.

REFERENCES

1. Maron BJ, Towbin JA, Thiene G, et al. Contemporary definitions and classification of the cardiomyopathies. Circulation 2006;113(14):1807–16.
2. Fatkin D, Graham RM. Molecular mechanisms of inherited cardiomyopathies. Physiol Rev 2002; 82(4):945–80.
3. Fatkin D, MacRae C, Sasaki T, et al. Missense mutations in the rod domain of the lamin A/C gene as causes of dilated cardiomyopathy and conduction-system disease. N Engl J Med 1999; 341(23):1715–24.
4. Brodsky GL, Muntoni F, Miocic S, et al. Lamin A/C gene mutation associated with dilated cardiomyopathy with variable skeletal muscle involvement. Circulation 2000;101(5):473–6.
5. Genschel J, Baier P, Kuepferling S, et al. A new frameshift mutation at codon 466 (1397delA) within the LMNA gene. Hum Mutat 2000;16(3):278.
6. Genschel J, Bochow B, Kuepferling S, et al. A R644C mutation within lamin A extends the mutations causing dilated cardiomyopathy. Hum Mutat 2001;17(2):154.
7. Jakobs PM, Hanson EL, Crispell KA, et al. Novel lamin A/C mutations in two families with dilated cardiomyopathy and conduction system disease. J Card Fail 2001;7(3):249–56.
8. Arbustini E, Pilotto A, Repetto A, et al. Autosomal dominant dilated cardiomyopathy with atrioventricular block: a lamin A/C defect-related disease. J Am Coll Cardiol 2002;39(6):981–90.
9. Hershberger RE, Hanson EL, Jakobs PM, et al. A novel lamin A/C mutation in a family with dilated cardiomyopathy, prominent conduction system disease, and need for a permanent pacemaker. Am Heart J 2002;144(6):1081–6.
10. Taylor MRG, Fain PR, Sinagra G, et al. Natural history of dilated cardiomyopathy due to lamin A/C gene mutations. J Am Coll Cardiol 2003; 41(5):771–80.
11. Sebillon P, Bouchier C, Bidot LD, et al. Expanding the phenotype of *LMNA* mutations in dilated cardiomyopathy and functional consequences of these mutations. J Med Genet 2003;40(8):560–7.
12. MacLeod HM, Culley MR, Huber JM, et al. Lamin A/C truncation in dilated cardiomyopathy with conduction disease. BMC Med Genet 2003;4:4.

13. Verga L, Concardi M, Pilotto A, et al. Loss of lamin A/C expression revealed by immuno-electron microscopy in dilated cardiomyopathy with atrioventricular block caused by *LMNA* gene defects. Virchows Arch 2003;443(5):664–71.
14. Vytopil M, Benedetti S, Ricci E, et al. Mutation analysis of the lamin A/C gene (*LMNA*) among patients with different cardiomuscular phenotypes. J Med Genet 2003;40(12):e132.
15. Hermida-Prieto M, Monserrat L, Castro-Beiras A, et al. Familial dilated cardiomyopathy and isolated left ventricular noncompaction associated with lamin A/C gene mutations. Am J Cardiol 2004; 94(1):50–4.
16. Pethig K, Genschel J, Peters T, et al. *LMNA* mutations in cardiac transplant recipients. Cardiology 2005;103(2):57–62.
17. Otomo J, Kure S, Shiba T, et al. Electrophysiological and histopathological characteristics of progressive atrioventricular block accompanied by familial dilated cardiomyopathy caused by a novel mutation of lamin A/C gene. J Cardiovasc Electrophysiol 2005;16(2):137–45.
18. Sylvius N, Bilinska ZT, Veinot JP, et al. In vivo and in vitro examination of the functional significances of novel lamin gene mutations in heart failure patients. J Med Genet 2005;42(8):639–47.
19. Karkkainen S, Reissell E, Helio T, et al. Novel mutations in the lamin A/C gene in heart transplant recipients with end stage dilated cardiomyopathy. Heart 2006;92(4):524–6.
20. Wang H, Wang J, Zheng W, et al. Mutation Glu82Lys in lamin A/C gene is associated with cardiomyopathy and conduction defect. Biochem Biophys Res Commun 2006;344(1):17–24.
21. Perrot A, Sigusch HH, Nagele H, et al. Genetic and phenotypic analysis of dilated cardiomyopathy with conduction-system disease: demand for strategies in the management of presymptomatic lamin A/C mutant carriers. Eur J Heart Fail 2006;8(5): 484–93.
22. Song K, Dube MP, Lim J, et al. Lamin A/C mutations associated with familial and sporadic cases of dilated cardiomyopathy. Exp Mol Med 2007; 39(1):114–20.
23. Van Tintelen JP, Hofstra RMW, Katerberg H, et al. High yield of *LMNA* mutations in patients with dilated cardiomyopathy and/or conduction disease referred to cardiogenetics outpatient clinics. Am Heart J 2007;154(6):1130–9.
24. Geiger SK, Bar H, Ehlermann P, et al. Incomplete nonsense-mediated decay of mutant lamin A/C RNA provokes dilated cardiomyopathy and ventricular tachycardia. J Mol Med 2008;86(3): 281–9.
25. Fujimori Y, Okimatsu H, Kashiwagi T, et al. Molecular defects associated with antithrombin deficiency and dilated cardiomyopathy in a Japanese patient. Intern Med 2008;47(10):925–31.
26. Li D, Parks SB, Kushner JD, et al. Mutations of presenilin genes in dilated cardiomyopathy and heart failure. Am J Hum Genet 2006;79(6):1030–9.
27. Kamisago M, Sharma SD, DePalma SR, et al. Mutations in sarcomere protein genes as a cause of dilated cardiomyopathy. N Engl J Med 2000; 343(23):1688–96.
28. Li D, Czernuszewicz GZ, Gonzalez O, et al. Novel cardiac troponin T mutations as a cause of familial dilated cardiomyopathy. Circulation 2001;104(18): 2188–93.
29. Mogensen J, Murphy RT, Shaw T, et al. Severe disease expression of cardiac troponin C and T mutations in patients with idiopathic dilated cardiomyopathy. J Am Coll Cardiol 2004;44(10):2033–40.
30. Stefanelli CB, Rosenthal A, Borisov AB, et al. Novel troponin T mutation in familial dilated cardiomyopathy with gender-dependent severity. Mol Genet Metab 2004;83(1–2):188–96.
31. Mohapatra B, Jimenez S, Lin JH, et al. Mutations in the muscle LIM protein and α-actinin-2 genes in dilated cardiomyopathy and endocardial fibroelastosis. Mol Genet Metab 2003;80(1–2):207–15.
32. Arimura T, Hayashi T, Matsumoto Y, et al. Structural analysis of four and half LIM protein-2 in dilated cardiomyopathy. Biochem Biophys Res Commun 2007;357(1):162–7.
33. Jung M, Poepping I, Perrot A, et al. Investigation of a family with autosomal dominant dilated cardiomyopathy defines a novel locus on chromosome 2q14-q22. Am J Hum Genet 1999;65(4):1068–77.
34. Gerull B, Gramlich M, Atherton J, et al. Mutations of *TTN*, encoding the giant muscle filament titin, cause familial dilated cardiomyopathy. Nat Genet 2002;30(2):201–4.
35. Itoh-Satoh M, Hayashi T, Nishi H, et al. Titin mutations as the molecular basis for dilated cardiomyopathy. Biochem Biophys Res Commun 2002; 291(2):385–93.
36. Gerull B, Atherton J, Geupel A, et al. Identification of a novel frameshift mutation in the giant muscle filament titin in a large Australian family with dilated cardiomyopathy. J Mol Med 2006;84(6):478–83.
37. Li D, Tapscoft T, Gonzalez O, et al. Desmin mutation responsible for idiopathic dilated cardiomyopathy. Circulation 1999;100(5):461–6.
38. Kostareva A, Gudkova A, Sjoberg G, et al. Desmin mutations in a St Petersburg cohort of cardiomyopathies. Acta Myol 2006;25(3):109–15.
39. Taylor MRG, Slavov D, Ku L, et al. Prevalence of desmin mutations in dilated cardiomyopathy. Circulation 2007;115(10):1244–51.
40. Bergman JE, Veenstra-Knol HE, Van Essen AJ, et al. Two related Dutch families with a clinically variable presentation of cardioskeletal myopathy

caused by a novel S13F mutation in the desmin gene. Eur J Med Genet 2007;50(5):355–66.
41. McNair WP, Ku L, Taylor MRG, et al. *SCN5A* mutation associated with dilated cardiomyopathy, conduction disorder, and arrhythmia. Circulation 2004;110(15):2163–7.
42. Olson TM, Michels VV, Ballew JD, et al. Sodium channel mutations and susceptibility to heart failure and atrial fibrillation. JAMA 2005;293(4): 447–54.
43. Lim CC, Yang H, Yang M, et al. A novel mutant cardiac troponin C disrupts molecular motions critical for calcium binding affinity and cardiomyocyte contractility. Biophys J 2008;94(9):3577–89.
44. Tsubata S, Bowles KR, Vatta M, et al. Mutations in the human δ-sarcoglycan gene in familial and sporadic dilated cardiomyopathy. J Clin Invest 2000;106(5):655–62.
45. Karkkainen S, Miettinen R, Tuomainen P, et al. A novel mutation, Arg71Thr, in the δ-sarcoglycan gene is associated with dilated cardiomyopathy. J Mol Med 2003;81(12):795–800.
46. Sylvius N, Tesson F, Gayet C, et al. A new locus for autosomal dominant dilated cardiomyopathy identified on chromosome 6q12-q16. Am J Hum Genet 2001;68(1):241–6.
47. Knoll R, Postel R, Wang J, et al. Laminin-α4 and integrin-linked kinase mutations cause human cardiomyopathy via simultaneous defects in cardiomyocytes and endothelial cells. Circulation 2007; 116(5):515–25.
48. Schmidt JP, Kamisago M, Asahi M, et al. Dilated cardiomyopathy and heart failure caused by a mutation in phospholamban. Science 2003; 299(5611):1410–3.
49. Haghighi K, Kolokathis F, Pater L, et al. Human phospholamban null results in lethal dilated cardiomyopathy revealing a critical difference between mouse and human. J Clin Invest 2003;111(6):869–76.
50. Haghighi K, Kolokathis F, Gramolini AO, et al. A mutation in the human phospholamban gene, deleting arginine 14, results in lethal, hereditary cardiomyopathy. Proc Natl Acad Sci U S A 2006; 103(5):1388–93.
51. Messina DN, Speer MC, Pericak-Vance MA, et al. Linkage of familial dilated cardiomyopathy with conduction defect and muscular dystrophy to chromosome 6q23. Am J Hum Genet 1997;61(4): 909–17.
52. Schonberger J, Wang L, Shin JT, et al. Mutation in the transcriptional coactivator *EYA4* causes dilated cardiomyopathy and sensorineural hearing loss. Nat Genet 2005;37(4):418–22.
53. Schonberger J, Kuhler L, Martins E, et al. A novel locus for autosomal dominant dilated cardiomyopathy maps to chromosome 7q22.3-31.1. Hum Genet 2005;118(3–4):451–7.
54. Zhang L, Hu A, Yuan H, et al. A missense mutation in the CHRM2 gene is associated with familial dilated cardiomyopathy. Circulation 2008;102(11): 1426–32.
55. Krajinovic M, Pinamonti B, Sinagra G, et al. Linkage of familial dilated cardiomyopathy to chromosome 9. Am J Hum Genet 1995;57(4):846–52.
56. Duboscq-Bidot L, Xu P, Charron P, et al. Mutations in the Z-band protein myopalladin gene and idiopathic dilated cardiomyopathy. Cardiovasc Res 2008;77(1):118–25.
57. Bowles KR, Gajarski R, Porter P, et al. Gene mapping of familial autosomal dominant dilated cardiomyopathy to chromosome 10q21-23. J Clin Invest 1996;98(6):1355–60.
58. Olson TM, Illenberger S, Kishimoto NY, et al. Metavinculin mutations alter actin interaction in dilated cardiomyopathy. Circulation 2002;105(4):431–7.
59. Vatta M, Mohapatra B, Jimenez S, et al. Mutations in *Cypher/ZASP* in patients with dilated cardiomyopathy and left ventricular non-compaction. J Am Coll Cardiol 2003;42(11):2014–27.
60. Arimura T, Hayashi T, Terada H, et al. A *Cypher/ZASP* mutation associated with dilated cardiomyopathy alters the binding affinity to protein kinase C. J Biol Chem 2004;279(8):6746–52.
61. Ellinor PT, Sasse-Klaassen S, Probst S, et al. A novel locus for dilated cardiomyopathy, diffuse myocardial fibrosis, and sudden death on chromosome 10q25-26. J Am Coll Cardiol 2006;48(1): 106–11.
62. Daehmlow S, Erdmann J, Knueppel T, et al. Novel mutations in sarcomeric protein genes in dilated cardiomyopathy. Biochem Biophys Res Commun 2002;298(1):116–20.
63. Knoll R, Hoshijima M, Hoffman HM, et al. The cardiac mechanical stretch sensor machinery involves a Z disc complex that is defective in a subset of human dilated cardiomyopathy. Cell 2002;111(7):943–55.
64. Inagaki N, Hayashi T, Arimura T, et al. αβ-Crystallin mutation in dilated cardiomyopathy. Biochem Biophys Res Commun 2006;342(2):379–86.
65. Bienengraeber M, Olson TM, Selivanov VA, et al. *ABCC9* mutations identified in human dilated cardiomyopathy disrupt catalytic K_{ATP} channel gating. Nat Genet 2004;36(4):382–7.
66. Taylor MRG, Slavov D, Gajewski A, et al. Thymopoietin (lamina-associated polypeptide 2) gene mutation associated with dilated cardiomyopathy. Hum Mutat 2005;26(6):566–74.
67. Carniel E, Taylor MRG, Sinagra G, et al. α-myosin heavy chain. A sarcomeric gene associated with dilated and hypertrophic phenotypes of cardiomyopathy. Circulation 2005;112(1):54–9.
68. Karkkainen S, Helio T, Jaaskelainen P, et al. Two novel mutations in the beta-myosin heavy chain

gene associated with dilated cardiomyopathy. Eur J Heart Fail 2004;6(7):861–8.
69. Villard E, Duboscq-Bidot L, Charron P, et al. Mutation screening in dilated cardiomyopathy: prominent role of the beta myosin heavy chain gene. Eur Heart J 2005;26(8):794–803.
70. Olson TM, Michels VV, Thibodeau SN, et al. Actin mutations in dilated cardiomyopathy, a heritable form of heart failure. Science 1998;280(5364):750–2.
71. Olson TM, Kishimoto NY, Whitby FG, et al. Mutations that alter the surface charge of alpha-tropomyosin are associated with dilated cardiomyopathy. J Mol Cell Cardiol 2001;33(4):723–32.
72. Hayashi T, Arimura T, Itoh-Satoh M, et al. Tcap gene mutations in hypertrophic cardiomyopathy and dilated cardiomyopathy. J Am Coll Cardiol 2004;44(11):2191–201.
73. Murphy RT, Mogensen J, Shaw A, et al. Novel mutation in cardiac troponin I in recessive idiopathic dilated cardiomyopathy. Lancet 2004; 363(9406):371–2.
74. Gold R, Kress W, Meurers B, et al. Becker muscular dystrophy: detection of unusual disease courses by combined approach to dystrophin analysis. Muscle Nerve 1992;15(2):214–8.
75. Muntoni F, Cau M, Ganau A, et al. Deletion of the dystrophin muscle-promoter region associated with X-linked dilated cardiomyopathy. N Engl J Med 1993;329(13):921–5.
76. Piccolo G, Azan G, Tonin P, et al. Dilated cardiomyopathy requiring cardiac transplantation as initial manifestation of Xp21 Becker type muscular dystrophy. Neuromuscul Disord 1994;4(2):143–6.
77. Milasin J, Muntoni F, Severini GM, et al. A point mutation in the 5′ splice site of the dystrophin gene first intron responsible for X-linked dilated cardiomyopathy. Hum Mol Genet 1996;5(1):73–9.
78. Bies RD, Maeda M, Roberds SL, et al. A 5′ dystrophin duplication mutation causes membrane deficiency of alpha-dystroglycan in a family with X-linked cardiomyopathy. J Mol Cell Cardiol 1997; 29(12):3175–88.
79. Muntoni F, Di Lenarda A, Porcu M, et al. Dystrophin gene abnormalities in two patients with idiopathic dilated cardiomyopathy. Heart 1997;78(6):608–12.
80. Ortiz-Lopez R, Li H, Su J, et al. Evidence for a dystrophin missense mutation as a cause of X-linked dilated cardiomyopathy. Circulation 1997;95(10): 2434–40.
81. Ferlini A, Galie N, Merlini L, et al. A novel Alu-like element rearranged in the dystrophin gene causes a splicing mutation in a family with X-linked dilated cardiomyopathy. Am J Hum Genet 1998;63(2): 436–46.
82. Yoshida K, Nakamura A, Yazaki M, et al. Insertional mutation by transposable element, L1, in the *DMD* gene results in X-linked dilated cardiomyopathy. Hum Mol Genet 1998;7(7):1129–32.
83. Arbustini E, Diegoli M, Morbini P, et al. Prevalence and characteristics of dystrophin defects in adult male patients with dilated cardiomyopathy. J Am Coll Cardiol 2000;35(7):1760–8.
84. Franz WM, Muller M, Muller OJ, et al. Association of nonsense mutation of dystrophin gene with disruption of sarcoglycan complex in X-linked dilated cardiomyopathy. Lancet 2000;355(9217):1781–5.
85. Bastianutto C, Bestard JA, Lahnakoski K, et al. Dystrophin muscle enhancer 1 is implicated in the activation of non-muscle isoforms in the skeletal muscle of patients with X-linked dilated cardiomyopathy. Hum Mol Genet 2001;10(23):2627–35.
86. Tasaki N, Yoshida K, Haruta SI, et al. X-linked dilated cardiomyopathy with a large hot-spot deletion in the dystrophin gene. Intern Med 2001; 40(12):1215–21.
87. Feng J, Yan J, Buzin CH, et al. Comprehensive mutation screening of the dystrophin gene in patients with nonsyndromic X-linked dilated cardiomyopathy. J Am Coll Cardiol 2002;40(6):1120–4.
88. Feng J, Yan J, Buzin CH, et al. Mutations in the dystrophin gene are associated with sporadic dilated cardiomyopathy. Mol Genet Metab 2002; 77(1–2):119–26.
89. Kimura S, Ikezawa M, Ozasa S, et al. Novel mutation in splicing donor of dystrophin gene first exon in a patient with dilated cardiomyopathy but no clinical signs of skeletal myopathy. J Child Neurol 2007;22(7):901–6.
90. Taylor MRG, Ku L, Slavov D, et al. Danon disease presenting with dilated cardiomyopathy and a complex phenotype. J Hum Genet 2007;52:830–5.
91. George RA, Liu JY, Feng LL, et al. Analysis of protein sequence and interaction data for candidate disease gene prediction. Nucleic Acids Res 2006;34(19):e130.
92. Wolf MJ, Amrein H, Izatt JA, et al. Drosophila as a model for the identification of genes causing adult human heart disease. Proc Natl Acad Sci U S A 2006;103(5):1394–9.
93. Taghli-Lamallem O, Akasaka T, Hogg G, et al. Dystrophin deficiency in Drosophila reduces lifespan and causes a dilated cardiomyopathy phenotype. Aging Cell 2008;7(2):237–49.
94. Hodges E, Xuan Z, Balija V, et al. Genome-wide in situ exon capture for selective resequencing. Nat Genet 2007;39(12):1522–7.
95. Reed GH, Kent JO, Wittwer CT. High-resolution DNA melting analysis for simple and efficient molecular diagnostics. Pharmacogenomics 2007; 8(6):597–608.
96. Francis GS, Tang WH. Pathophysiology of congestive heart failure. Rev Cardiovasc Med 2003; 4(Suppl 2):S14–20.

97. Le Corvoisier P, Park HY, Carlson KM, et al. Multiple quantitative trait loci modify the heart failure phenotype in murine cardiomyopathy. Hum Mol Genet 2003;12(23):3097–107.
98. Kushner JD, Nauman D, Burgess D, et al. Clinical characteristics of 304 kindreds evaluated for familial dilated cardiomyopathy. J Card Fail 2006; 12(6):422–9.
99. Burkett EL, Hershberger RE. Clinical and genetic issues in familial dilated cardiomyopathy. J Am Coll Cardiol 2005;45(7):969–81.
100. Baig MK, Goldman JH, Caforio ALP, et al. Familial dilated cardiomyopathy: cardiac abnormalities are common in asymptomatic relatives and may represent early disease. J Am Coll Cardiol 1998; 31(1):195–201.
101. Crispell KA, Wray A, Ni H, et al. Clinical profiles of four large pedigrees with familial dilated cardiomyopathy. J Am Coll Cardiol 1999;34(3):837–47.
102. Michels VV, Olson TM, Miller FA, et al. Frequency of development of idiopathic dilated cardiomyopathy among relatives of patients with idiopathic dilated cardiomyopathy. Am J Cardiol 2003;91(1): 1389–92.
103. Mahon NG, Murphy RT, MacRae CA, et al. Echocardiographic evaluation in asymptomatic relatives of patients with dilated cardiomyopathy reveals preclinical disease. Ann Intern Med 2005;143(2):108–15.
104. Caforio ALP, Mahon NG, Baig MK, et al. Prospective familial assessment in dilated cardiomyopathy. Cardiac autoantibodies predict disease development in asymptomatic relatives. Circulation 2007; 115(1):76–83.
105. McKenna CJ, Sugrue DD, Kwon HM, et al. Histopathologic changes in asymptomatic relatives of patients with idiopathic dilated cardiomyopathy. Am J Cardiol 1999;83(1):281–3.
106. Mahon NG, Sharma S, Elliott PM, et al. Abnormal cardiopulmonary exercise variables in asymptomatic relatives of patients with dilated cardiomyopathy who have left ventricular enlargement. Heart 2000;83(5):511–7.
107. Mahon NG, Madden BP, Caforio ALP, et al. Immunohistologic evidence of myocardial disease in apparently healthy relatives of patients with dilated cardiomyopathy. J Am Coll Cardiol 2002;39(3): 455–62.
108. Matsumura Y, Elliott PM, Mahon NG, et al. Familial dilated cardiomyopathy: assessment of left ventricular systolic and diastolic function using Doppler tissue imaging in asymptomatic relatives with left ventricular enlargement. Heart 2006;92(3):405–6.

Hypertrophic Cardiomyopathy

Carolyn Y. Ho, MD

KEYWORDS

• Genetics • Hypertrophy • Cardiomyopathy

Important insights into the molecular basis of hypertrophic cardiomyopathy (HCM) and related diseases have been gained by studying families with inherited cardiac hypertrophy. Integrated clinical and genetic investigations have demonstrated that different genetic defects can give rise to the common phenotype of cardiac hypertrophy. Diverse pathways have been identified, implicating perturbations in force generation, force transmission, intracellular calcium homeostasis, myocardial energetics, and cardiac metabolism in causing disease. Although not fully elucidated, the fundamental mechanisms linking gene mutations to clinical disease are being characterized. Further advances will allow a better understanding of pathogenesis, diagnosis, and treatment, not just of relatively rare inherited cardiomyopathies, but potentially also of relevance to more common acquired forms of hypertrophic remodeling.

CLINICAL PHENOTYPE OF HCM

Natural History and Clinical Manifestations

Unexplained left ventricular hypertrophy (LVH), which develops in the absence of other inciting factors, including increased hemodynamic load (systemic hypertension, valvular heart disease), infiltrative or storage disorders, is a defining feature of HCM. Myocyte hypertrophy with disarray and fibrosis are pathognomonic histologic characteristics (**Fig. 1**). A diagnosis of HCM is typically made by identifying unexplained LVH on cardiac imaging studies, as illustrated in the echocardiographic images in **Fig. 2**. Clinical evaluation may be triggered in response to symptoms, in asymptomatic individuals in the course of family screening, or after detection of a systolic murmur or an abnormal EKG. The degree and distribution of LVH vary markedly. Asymmetric septal hypertrophy is the most common morphologic pattern; however, any configuration, including concentric, apical, and isolated segmental hypertrophy, can be seen (**Fig. 3**).[1] The morphologic pattern of LVH is not closely predictive of the severity of symptoms or prognosis.[2,3]

HCM is a complex and heterogeneous disease that demonstrates remarkable diversity in disease course, age of onset, severity of symptoms, left ventricular outflow obstruction, and risk for sudden cardiac death (SCD).[4] Although some individuals experience no or only minor symptoms, others may develop refractory symptoms or end-stage heart failure requiring cardiac transplantation. Shortness of breath, particularly exertional, is the most common symptom of HCM, and occurs in up to 90% of patients. Other manifestations include chest pain, palpitations, atrial and ventricular arrhythmias, orthostatic lightheadedness, presyncope and syncope, volume overload, and fatigue.[3,5] Atrial fibrillation develops in approximately 20% to 25% of patients and is associated with an increased risk of stroke and thromboembolic complications.

Left ventricular outflow tract obstruction is one of the most highly visible features of disease; however, its clinical significance has been debated. Obstructive physiology is likely an important contributor to symptomatology, particularly exertional dyspnea, pulmonary congestion, and orthostasis; however, large gradients may be asymptomatic and tolerated for long periods of time. Approximately 25% to 30% of patients have evidence of obstruction at rest, but most patients may develop obstruction in response to exercise or maneuvers that decrease preload or afterload or increase contractility or heart rate.[6]

Cardiovascular Division, Brigham and Women's Hospital, 75 Francis Street, Boston, MA 02115, USA
E-mail address: cho@partners.org

Heart Failure Clin 6 (2010) 141–159
doi:10.1016/j.hfc.2009.12.001
1551-7136/10/$ – see front matter

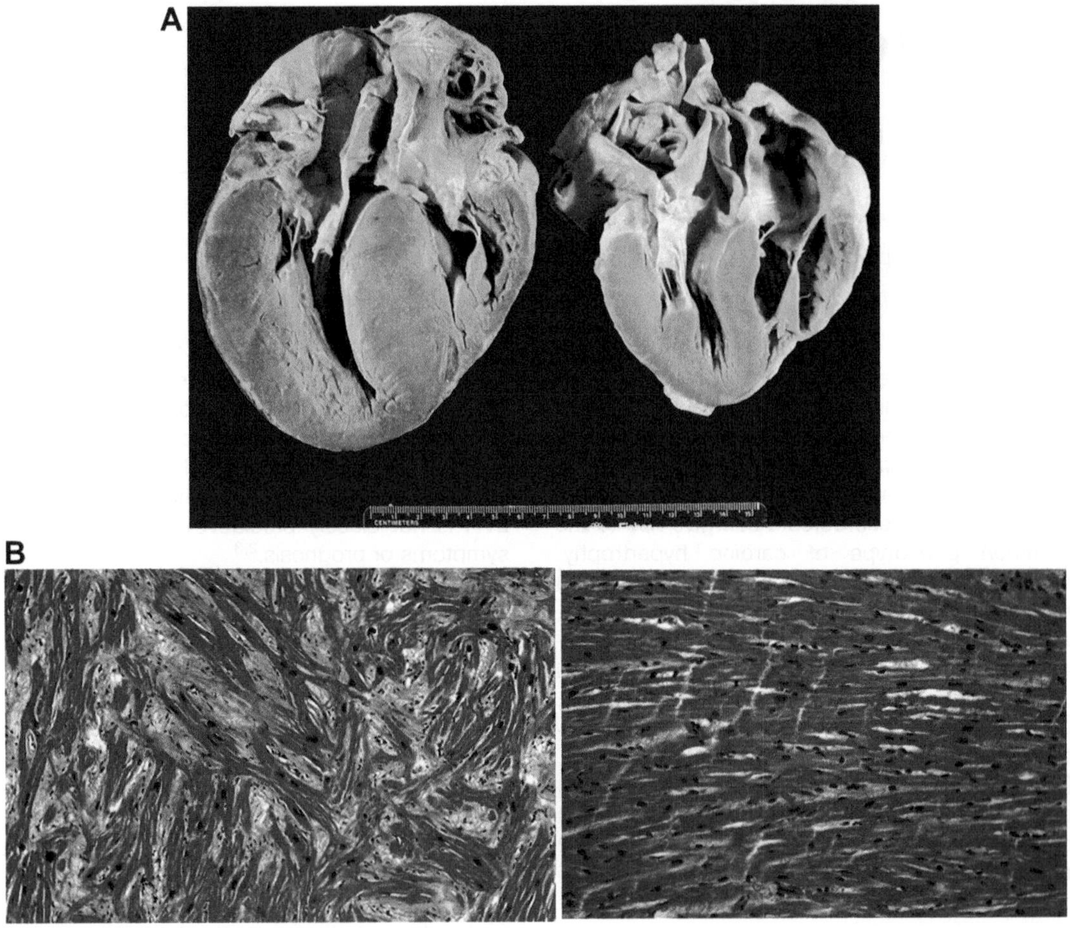

Fig. 1. Pathologic features of HCM. (*A*) Gross pathology showing markedly increased LV wall thickness associated with hypertrophic cardiomyopathy (*left*) as compared with normal cardiac morphology (*right*). (*B*) Histologic sections stained with hematoxylin and eosin demonstrate myocyte disarray, where myocytes are oriented at bizarre and variable angles to each other, and increased myocardial fibrosis (*left*), the pathognomonic features of HCM. In contrast, normal myocardium demonstrates a very orderly arrangement of myocytes (*right*). Images are at ×10 magnification. (*Courtesy of* Dr Robert Padera, Department of Pathology, Brigham and Women's Hospital, Boston, MA.)

The mechanism for outflow tract obstruction in most patients is systolic anterior motion of the mitral valve causing mechanical obstruction to the flow of blood out of the heart. Although older reports have not demonstrated a close relationship with outcomes, a recent large retrospective study indicated that the presence of outflow tract obstruction (>30 mm Hg) is associated with increased disease-related morbidity and mortality.[7] The magnitude of the gradient did not correlate with clinical outcomes; however, patients with obstruction were nearly five times more likely to progress to severe symptoms of heart failure and heart failure–related death.

Although left ventricular ejection fraction is typically preserved or even hyperdynamic in HCM, up to 5% to 10% of patients may progress to the "burnt-out" or end-stage phase of HCM. This is marked by left ventricular systolic dysfunction, worsening symptoms, and occasionally progressive left ventricular wall thinning, and chamber enlargement. The prognosis of patients who develop this end-stage phenotype is worse, with an increased risk of cardiovascular events and need for transplantation as compared with typical HCM.[8,9] Patients with end-stage development are more likely to have a family history of HCM, suggesting a genetic association; however, specific genetic factors that predict or correlate with this phenotypic variant have not been identified.

Estimates of annual mortality rates for HCM range from 4% to 6% in referral-based populations to 1% to 2% in community-based studies.[10] Overall, life expectancy is not dramatically

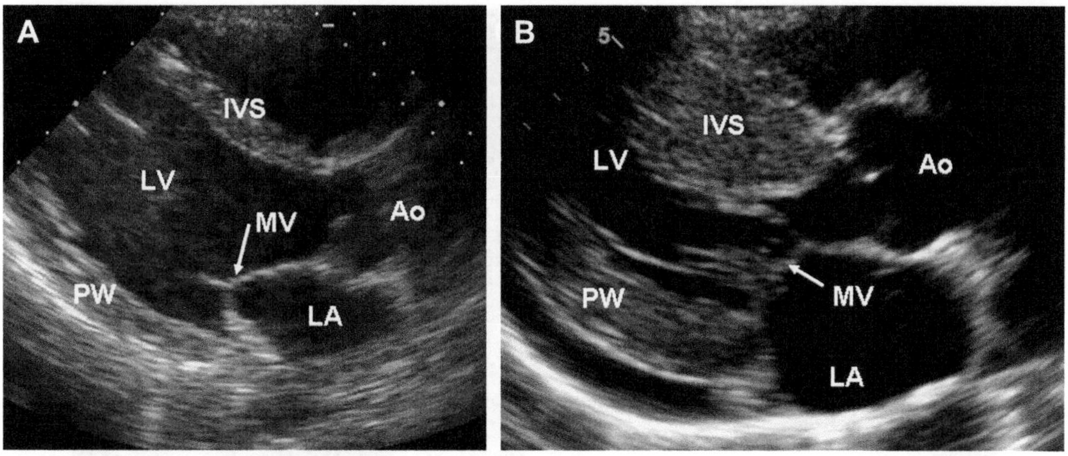

Fig. 2. Echocardiographic appearance of HCM. (*A*) Normal parasternal long axis view demonstrating normal LV wall thickness, with both interventricular septum and posterior wall measuring 8 mm. (*B*) Parasternal long axis view from a patient with HCM demonstrating severe asymmetric septal hypertrophy. The interventricular septum measures 24 mm, the posterior wall measures 11 mm. Ao, aorta; IVS, interventricular septum; LA, left atrium; LV, left ventricle; MV, mitral valve (marked by *arrow*); PW, posterior wall.

impacted in most patients with HCM. SCD (accounting for approximately half of HCM-related deaths), progressive heart failure, atrial fibrillation, and stroke are leading contributors to the morbidity and mortality associated with HCM.

Management

Strategies to prevent or modify disease progression in asymptomatic patients are not yet available. Therefore current treatment focuses on symptom management, assessment for risk of SCD, and family screening as summarized in **Box 1**. Medical therapy is the first-line approach for symptomatic disease, typically using β-blockers or L-type calcium channel blockers (verapamil or diltiazem) to lengthen diastolic filling period and diminish left ventricular gradients. If obstruction is present and symptoms persist, the addition of disopyramide may provide additional symptomatic benefit by reducing left ventricular pressure gradients by its negative inotropic effects. If symptoms from left ventricular outflow tract obstruction are refractory to medical management, invasive approaches, such as ethanol septal ablation or surgical myectomy, may be used to mechanically decrease outflow tract gradients.[2,3,11] Patients with nonobstructive disease and those with end-stage HCM should be managed with appropriate therapy for advanced heart failure and may ultimately require cardiac transplantation.

HCM is associated with an increased risk of SCD; rarely, such an event may be the presenting manifestation of disease.[2,3,5,11] HCM is the leading cause of sudden death among adolescents and young adults, and competitive athletes in the United States.[12] Assessment of SCD risk and determination of appropriate therapy are important, although challenging, components of clinical management. Clinical predictors associated with an increased risk of SCD include a family history of sudden death or known malignant genotype, unexplained syncope, hypotensive blood pressure response to exercise, significant spontaneous ventricular ectopy on Holter monitoring, and extreme LVH (>30 mm), as summarized in **Table 1**.[11,13] Implantable cardiovertor-defibrillator therapy has been shown to be effective and life saving in appropriate patients.[3,11,13,14] Because the positive predictive value of these predictors individually is relatively low, however, accurate risk assessment is difficult. Making the decision to implant an implantable cardiovertor-defibrillator for primary prevention is guided by the number and nature of predictors, and individualized clinical judgment and personal input from well-educated and informed patients.[15] Individuals who do not demonstrate any of these risk predictors are at low risk and do not require more aggressive management, although longitudinal reassessment of risk is appropriate. Patients who have survived cardiac arrest or sustained ventricular tachycardia are at high risk for recurrent events and should receive implantable cardiovertor-defibrillator for secondary prevention.

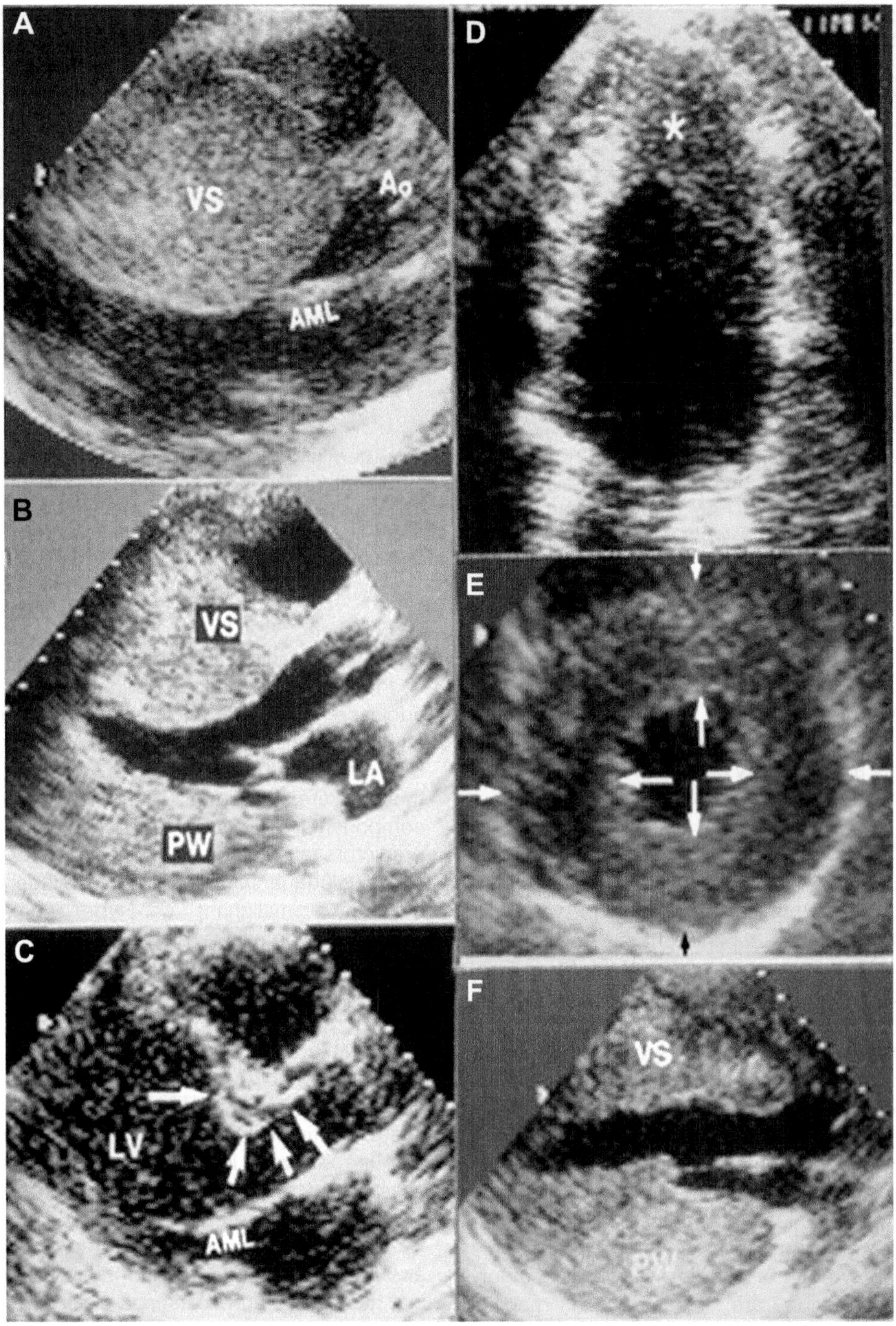

Fig. 3. Morphologic spectrum of HCM. Asymmetric septal hypertrophy is the most common morphologic pattern in HCM; however, a myriad of different locations and extent of LVH have been described, as demonstrated in these still-frame images. No direct correlation between the distribution of LVH and clinical outcomes has been demonstrated. (*A*) Massive asymmetric septal hypertrophy with septal wall thickness >50 mm. (*B*) Septal hypertrophy with more prominent mid and distal portion involvement. (*C*) Hypertrophy confined to the proximal septum, just below the aortic valve (*arrows*). (*D*) Apical HCM (asterisk). (*E*) Relatively mild hypertrophy in a concentric pattern showing similar thicknesses within each segment (*paired arrows*). (*F*) Inverted pattern with posterior free wall (PW) thicker (40 mm) than anterior ventricular septum. AML, anterior mitral valve leaflet; calibration marks, 1 cm; LV, left ventricle; PW, posterior wall; VS, ventricular septum. (*Courtesy of* Dr Barry J. Maron, Minneapolis Heart Institute Foundation, Minneapolis, MN.)

Box 1
Standard management strategies for HCM

All patients

Family screening

Genetic counseling

Periodic assessment for SCD risk

Education on recommended exercise restrictions

Mild to moderate symptoms (exercise intolerance, SOB, CP)

β -blockers

Calcium channel blockers (diltiazem or verapamil)

Symptomatic volume overload

Consider diuretics (caution; hypovolemia may worsen obstructive physiology)

Persistent or worsening symptoms plus obstructive physiology

Consider adding disopyramide

Medically refractory symptoms plus obstructive physiology

Septal myectomy

Alcohol septal ablation

Heart failure, end-stage HCM without obstructive physiology

Diuretics

Angiotensin-converting enzyme inhibitors, angiotensin receptor blockers (if left ventricular systolic dysfunction)

β -blockers

Consider cardiac transplantation

GENETICS OF HCM: A DISEASE OF THE SARCOMERE

The heritable nature and autosomal-dominant pattern of inheritance of HCM have long been appreciated. Family linkage studies in the 1980s led to the discovery of pathogenic mutations in genes encoding different components of the contractile apparatus[16–18] and established the paradigm that HCM is a disease of the sarcomere (**Fig. 4**). The prevalence of unexplained LVH in the general adult population is estimated to be 1 in 500, but not all have an underlying sarcomere mutation.[19,20] The proportion of disease caused by sarcomere mutations is estimated to range from 45% to 70%, with a higher prevalence if a family history of HCM is present.[21–23] As such, HCM is the most common monogenic cardiovascular disorder. As with the clinical heterogeneity seen with HCM, however, there is also substantial genetic heterogeneity, at both allelic and nonallelic levels. Over 1000 distinct mutations have been identified in 11 different contractile genes, with no specific racial or ethnic predilections. Genes that have been causally associated with HCM are summarized in **Table 2**. In addition to the genes listed in **Table 2**, mutations in other sarcomere-associated genes have been described in HCM, including cardiac troponin C (*TNNC1*), telethonin (*TCAP*), and muscle LIM protein (*CRP3*).[24–26] Mutations in these genes are rare and the strength of evidence that they are truly disease-causing is not yet definitive.

Currently, most mutations identified (approximately 30%–60% in *MYBPC3* and *MYH7*) are novel sequence variants, not previously identified as pathogenic mutations.[21,22,27,28] Furthermore, when novel sequence variants are identified, family analysis to confirm appropriate cosegregation is valuable. Demonstrating that the variant is present in other relatives with HCM and not present in clinically unaffected family members provides further support to allow a more confident conclusion that the variant is clinically significant and responsible for causing disease in the family. A relatively high 3% to 10% rate of compound heterozygosity (two sarcomere mutations present in a single individual with HCM) has also been observed.[22,29]

Mutations in the genes encoding cardiac β-myosin heavy chain (*MYH7*), cardiac myosin binding protein C (*MYBPC3*), cardiac troponin T (*TNNT2*), and cardiac troponin I (*TNNI3*) are the most prevalent and, in aggregate, account for over 80%–90% of HCM.

Cardiac β-MYOSIN HEAVY CHAIN (MYH7, β-MHC)

In 1989, linkage analysis of a large family led to the discovery of the first mutation associated with HCM, identified in *MYH7*.[16,30] Since then, over 200 different *MYH7* mutations have been reported in both familial and sporadic disease, accounting for approximately 30% to 40% of cases[21,27,28] (http://cardiogenomics.med.harvard.edu). Myosin heavy chain is an abundant protein that has two functional domains: an amino terminal globular head and a carboxyl terminal rod.[31] The head domain binds ATP, contains the ATPase activity to power the lever arm, and contains the actin-binding domain to form the actinomyosin complex crucial for force generation. The rod domain interacts with the myosin light chains. Mutations that cause HCM are almost exclusively missense (resulting in amino acid substitution) and clustered

Table 1
Risk predictors for sudden death in HCM

	Criteria	Comments
History	Exertional or recurrent syncope Family history of sudden death or known malignant genotype	Risk is greatest in children Risk is related to family size and number of family members with sudden cardiac death
Diagnostic evaluation	Severe left ventricular hypertrophy (maximal wall thickness ≥30 mm) Nonsustained ventricular tachycardia (ambulatory Holter monitoring) Abnormal hemodynamic response to exercise (failure to augment systolic blood pressure by at least 20 mm Hg)	Risk increases as wall thickness increases Higher predictive value in children and patients with history of syncope Less applicable to patients >40 y

within the globular head or head-rod junction, as illustrated in the molecular model shown in **Fig. 5**. In general, *MYH7* mutations have been associated with a gain of function, resulting in increased actin-dependent ATPase activity, in vitro sliding velocity, and force production (discussed later).[32,33] Gain of function effects have also been suggested in studies on thin filament mutations and MYBPC3.[34,35]

Cardiac Myosin Binding Protein C (MYPBC3, cMyBPC)

The function of cardiac myosin binding protein C is unknown, but it is thought to provide structural integrity to the sarcomere (binding MHC and titin), play a role in sarcomeric assembly,[35] and may modulate myosin ATPase activity and cardiac contractility in response to adrenergic stimulation.[36] Missense mutations occur; however, nonsense (leading to premature termination of translation), splice site, and small deletion- insertion mutations are common, leading to a truncated protein or null allele.[22] Over 200 mutations have been reported to date, accounting for approximately 30% to 40% of cases of HCM.[21,27,28] Mutations in *MYBPC3* have been associated with late-onset disease[37]; however, they are also a frequent cause of pediatric-onset HCM.[38]

Cardiac Troponin T (TNNT2, cTnT)

Troponin T links the troponin complex to α-tropoymyosin, playing a central role in the regulation of contraction. Alternative splicing results in multiple isoforms of troponin T, including a cardiac-specific

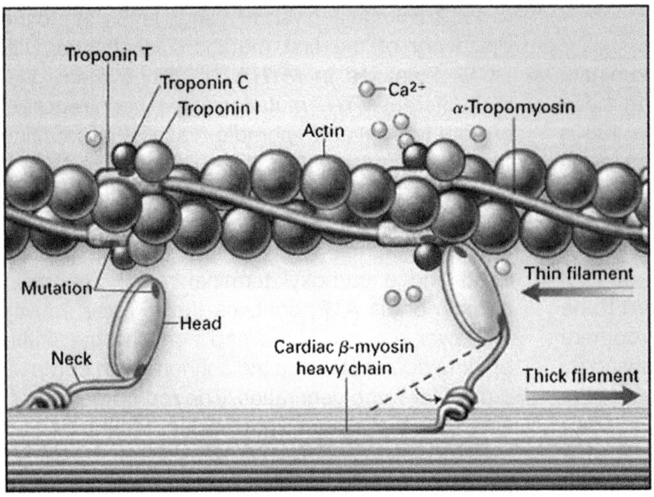

Fig. 4. HCM is caused by mutations in the sarcomere, the molecular motor of the heart. The sarcomere is the fundamental unit of contraction in the cardiac myocyte. It is composed of interdigitating thick and thin filaments that generate force by cyclical crossbridge formation between actin and myosin. Dominantly inherited mutations in β-myosin heavy chain, myosin binding protein C, and cardiac troponins T and I are most common. (*From* Kamisago M, Sharma SD, DePalma SR, et al. Mutations in sarcomere protein genes as a cause of dilated cardiomyopathy. N Engl J Med 2000;343:1688–96; with permission. Copyright © 2003, Massachusetts Medical Society.)

Table 2
Sarcomere mutations in hypertrophic cardiomyopathy

Protein	Gene	Chromosome	% Prevalence	Function	Comments
Cardiac β-myosin heavy chain[a]	*MYH7*	14q1	~40	Thick filament-force generation	Younger onset is typical
Cardiac myosin binding protein C[a]	*MYBPC3*	11q1	~40	Structural support	Association with later-onset left ventricular hypertrophy
Cardiac troponin T[a]	*TNNT2*	1q3	~5	Thin filament-regulation	Increased sudden cardiac death risk in some
Cardiac troponin I[a]	*TNNI3*	19p1	~5	Thin filament-regulation	
α-Tropomyosin[a]	*TPM1*	15q2	~2	Thin filament-regulation	
Myosin essential[a] and regulatory[a] light chains	*MYL2, MYL3*	3p, 12q	~1	Thick filament	
Actin[a]	*ACTC*	11q	~1	Thin filament-force generation	
Titin	*TTN*	2q3	Rare		
Myozenin	*MYOZ2*	4q26	Rare	Z-disk	
α-Myosin heavy chain	*MYH6*	14q1	Rare	Thick filament-force generation	

[a] Clinical genetic testing available.

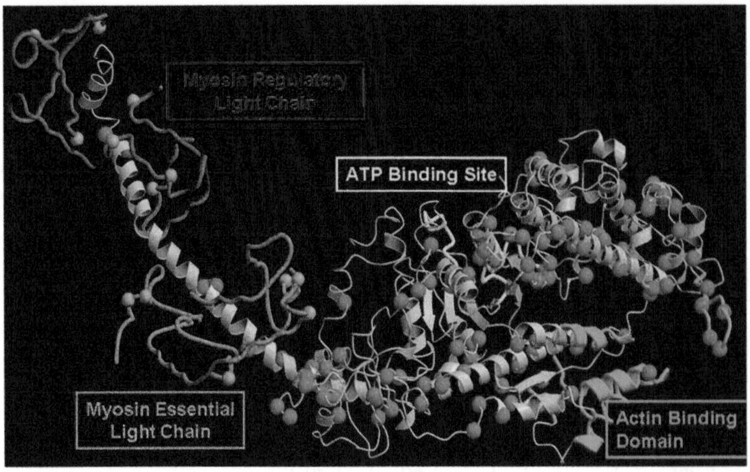

Fig. 5. Molecular structure of myosin heavy chain and location of mutations associated with HCM. This three-dimensional molecular model is based on the x-ray crystallographic structure of chicken skeletal myosin heavy chain.[31] The residues shown correspond to human residues Asp3 through Lys841. The actin binding domain is shown in green; the ATP binding site is in yellow. The myosin regulatory and essential light chains are overlaid in violet and orange, respectively. Mutations that cause HCM are shown in blue, superimposed onto the molecular structure. Light chain mutations are shown in light blue. (*Courtesy of* Steven DePalma, PhD, Department of Genetics, Harvard Medical School, Boston, MA.)

isoform. To date over 50 missense, splice site, and deletion mutations have been reported in *TNNT2*, accounting for approximately 5% of HCM.[22] Initial reports suggested that disease caused by *TNNT2* mutations was associated with an increased risk of sudden death despite only modest hypertrophy[18,39]; however, exceptions have been well documented.

SARCOMERE GENE MUTATIONS ARE A COMMON ETIOLOGY FOR CARDIAC HYPERTROPHY IN DIFFERENT PATIENT POPULATIONS

The clinical diagnosis of HCM is typically made in adolescence or young adulthood, but patients may present at any age. Whether childhood-onset HCM represents the same disease as HCM that presents in adulthood has recently been evaluated. Direct sequence analysis of sarcomere genes was performed in children with isolated, idiopathic LVH diagnosed before the age of 15 years (mean age, 7 ± 6.1 years).[38] The prevalence of sarcomere mutations was found to be essentially the same as that seen in adult-onset HCM. Mutations were identified in 49% of children with apparently sporadic disease and 64% of children with a family history of HCM. Also, as in adult-onset disease, approximately 75% of cases were attributable to mutations in *MYH7* or *MYBPC3*, although *MYBPC3* mutations in children were more likely to be missense (predicted to result in an amino acid substitution), rather than truncation mutations, which predominate in adults. Unrecognized familial disease was also well-documented, where direct family evaluation revealed that one of the parents of an affected child carried the causal sarcomere mutation, but were without symptoms or clinical features of HCM on echocardiography.

At the other end of the age spectrum, sarcomere mutations have been identified in adults with late-onset cardiac hypertrophy, presenting after age 40 years.[37] Approximately 20% had an underlying sarcomere mutation; however, a distinctive feature of this population was the relative underrepresentation of mutations in *MYH7*, *TNNT2*, and *TNNI3*, which together typically account for greater than 45% of HCM, accounted for only approximately 5% of late-onset disease. Mutations were most frequently identified in *MYBPC3*, *TPM1*, and *MYH6* (encoding α-myosin heavy chain).

Sarcomere mutations are also present in individuals in a community-based population with incidentally identified unexplained LVH, but without a formal clinical diagnosis of HCM. A cohort from the Framingham Heart Study (N = 1869; mean age, 59 ± 9 years) demonstrated an approximately 3% prevalence of unexplained increased LV wall thickness. Sarcomere gene mutations were identified in 15% of these subjects, but were notably absent in control subjects without LVH and in those with secondary cardiac hypertrophy from hypertension or aortic stenosis.[40] These studies indicate that sarcomere mutations are an important and shared contribution to HCM throughout different ages and demographic groups. Because a similar genetic contribution to disease is seen, the reasons underlying differences in natural history are unclear and speak to the importance of genetic and environmental modifiers that have not yet been characterized.

GENOTYPE-PHENOTYPE CORRELATIONS

The factors that drive the diverse phenotypic spectrum of HCM and the clinical significance of prominent features of disease are unclear. Genetic heterogeneity is equally marked and likely accounts for some of the clinical diversity; however, robust genotype-phenotype correlations have not emerged. Although genotype certainly influences phenotype, most mutations are individually rare, private to a particular family and infrequently recurring in unrelated individuals. Furthermore, clinical outcomes of individual mutations are not consistently benign or malignant. There is great diversity in the degree of symptoms, age of onset, extent and location of LVH, and sudden death risk, even among family members who have inherited the same causal mutation, indicating that variation in genotype alone does not account for all of the variation in clinical features. In most cases, determining the exact identity of the causal gene mutation confirms the clinical diagnosis, defines the exact genetic etiology, and may importantly inform family management, but typically does not alter specific management or provide prognostic insight.

A small number of specific point mutations have recurred more frequently and have demonstrated more consistent phenotypes in unrelated families. For example, the clinical course of *MYH7* mutations Arg403Gln, Arg719Trp, and Arg719Gln have tended to be severe, associated with an increased risk of sudden death or development of end-stage heart failure. Certain *TNNT2* mutations (Arg92Trp, Arg92Gln, Ile79Asn) have been associated with mild LVH but an increased risk of sudden death in certain families.[18,27,35,39] Caution must be used, however, in generalizing these specific observations to other patients and families, because exceptions are well documented.

Although the causal sarcomere mutation is inherited or introduced at the time of fertilization, the clinical expression or penetrance of LVH is highly variable and age-dependent. Left ventricular wall thickness is often normal in infancy and early childhood, despite the presence of a sarcomere mutation. LVH more commonly becomes evident in adolescence, in conjunction with the pubertal growth spurt. Genotype may influence the age of onset of LVH, as illustrated in **Fig. 6**. Most *MYH7* mutation carriers develop demonstrable LVH by the second decade of life. In contrast, mutations in *MYBPC3* may not result in clinically evident hypertrophy until the fourth

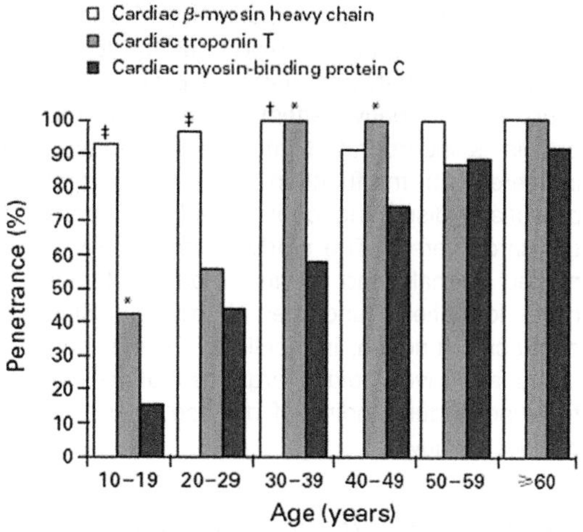

Fig. 6. The penetrance of left ventricular hypertrophy in HCM is dependent on age and influenced by the underlying sarcomere mutation. HCM caused by mutations in β-myosin heavy chain is typically associated with demonstrable LVH early in life, with near universal expression by the age 20 years. In contrast, HCM caused by mutations in the myosin binding protein C gene may not show clinically evident LVH until middle age or later. (*Adapted from* Niimura H, Bachinski LL, Sangwatanaroj S, et al. Mutations in the gene for cardiac myosin-binding protein C and late-onset familial hypertrophic cardiomyopathy [comments]. N Engl J Med 1998;338:1248. Copyright © 1998, Massachusetts Medical Society.)

or fifth decade of life, and mutations in this gene have been associated with elderly onset HCM.[37,41] The ultimate phenotype reflects a multitude of factors, including genetic background, comorbid illnesses, and lifestyle. Integrating genetic information, family history, and comprehensive clinical assessment leads to the best patient management. Longitudinal studies to follow genotyped patients, both apparently healthy mutation carriers who have not yet developed LVH and those with overt disease, will help address important unresolved issues, including more accurate determination of the true lifetime penetrance of sarcomere mutations, characterization of the full phenotypic spectrum, identification of more sensitive and early markers of disease, and description of disease evolution.

IMPLICATIONS OF GENETIC DISCOVERIES: REFINING THE PHENOTYPE OF HCM

Although unexplained LVH is the clinically defining feature of HCM, it is not an infallible marker for genetic status or future risk of developing disease or disease-related complications.[42,43] The steps leading from sarcomere gene mutation to clinical disease are largely unknown, but likely stem from a dominant negative effect in which the mutant protein is incorporated into the sarcomere and interferes with the function of the normal protein, potentially disrupting coordinated mechanics of the sarcomere.[34] The study of genetically engineered animals and in vitro models of disease have identified fundamental abnormalities of contractile function, intracellular calcium homeostasis, and myocardial energetics that are helping to refine understanding of disease phenotype at a molecular level.

Abnormalities of Diastolic Function

Abnormal diastolic function is a nearly universal feature of overt HCM and may largely account for common symptoms of pulmonary congestion and exercise intolerance. There are also compelling data from animal and human studies to indicate that diastolic dysfunction is an early manifestation of sarcomere mutations and an intrinsic feature of the HCM phenotype, present before the development of pathologic cardiac remodeling and LVH. A heterozygous knock-in mouse has been developed in which the Arg403Gln missense mutation in *MYH7* (αMHC$^{403/+}$) is introduced into the mouse genome and recapitulates many phenotypic features of human disease.[44] This mouse is a well-characterized model of disease and has demonstrated that diastolic abnormalities develop by 6 weeks of age, whereas gross or histopathologic LVH, fibrosis, and disarray are not consistently present until 20 to 25 weeks of age (**Fig. 7**A).[44,45] The mechanism of impaired relaxation in these animals may relate to alterations in intracellular calcium handling and slowed actin-myosin dissociation kinetics.[46–48] A *TNNT2* I79N transgenic mouse model also develops enhanced systolic function with increased diastolic stiffness in the absence of significant hypertrophy or fibrosis.[49]

More recently, tissue Doppler echocardiographic studies on genotyped human subjects have similarly demonstrated that individuals with sarcomere gene mutations have diastolic abnormalities early in life, before the development of LVH. Impaired relaxation is manifested by decreased early myocardial relaxation velocities, compared with normal controls without sarcomere mutations (**Fig. 7**B).[50,51] These studies provide further evidence that diastolic abnormalities are an early and direct manifestation of the underlying sarcomere mutation, rather than merely a secondary consequence of altered myocardial compliance characteristics caused by of the distinct changes in myocardial architecture that accompany development of clinically obvious disease.

Altered Intracellular Calcium Handling

Myocardial contraction and relaxation are coordinated by the orchestrated cycling of calcium from the cytoplasm, sarcoplasmic reticulum (SR), and sarcomere through excitation-contraction coupling (**Fig. 8**A). Altered calcium signaling has emerged as a potentially key link between sarcomere mutation, hypertrophic remodeling, contractile abnormalities, and arrhythmias. Biochemical studies using the αMHC$^{403/+}$ mouse model of HCM indicate that abnormalities in intracellular Ca^{2+} homeostasis (present at 4 weeks of age) are one of the earliest manifestations of sarcomere mutations, preceding the development of diastolic abnormalities (approximately age 6 weeks), and histologic changes (approximately age 20 weeks).[47,52] Evidence for altered intracellular calcium handling has been detected at multiple levels. Biophysical studies across a spectrum of sarcomere genes with HCM-associated mutations have demonstrated increased calcium sensitivity resulting in increased tension generation and ATPase activity.[32,46] Calcium cycling between the sarcomere and SR also seems to be altered in HCM. There is blunted release of calcium from the SR in response to caffeine stimulation in αMHC$^{403/+}$ mice.[47] Furthermore, myocardial extracts from these mice show reduced expression of the cardiac ryanodine receptor (*RyR2)*, and SR Ca^{2+} storage protein calsequestrin (*CSQ*) and associated proteins junction and triadin.[52] Taken together, these results suggest that a key early event in HCM is dysregulation of the release of Ca^{2+} from the SR, possibly caused by "trapping" in the mutated sarcomere (**Fig. 8**B), and ultimately leading to reduced SR Ca^{2+} stores.

The identification of these early biochemical changes suggests that intracellular Ca^{2+} pathways may be targeted as a means to modify the phenotype of HCM. Pharmacologic studies on young, prehypertrophic αMHC$^{403/+}$ HCM mice demonstrated that treatment with the calcium channel blocker, diltiazem, attenuated phenotypic development with decreased myocyte hypertrophy, disarray, and fibrosis as compared with placebo-treated animals.[52] There was no benefit if drug administration was initiated after the development of LVH. These data have intriguing implications for future clinical management of HCM, suggesting that early pharmacologic intervention

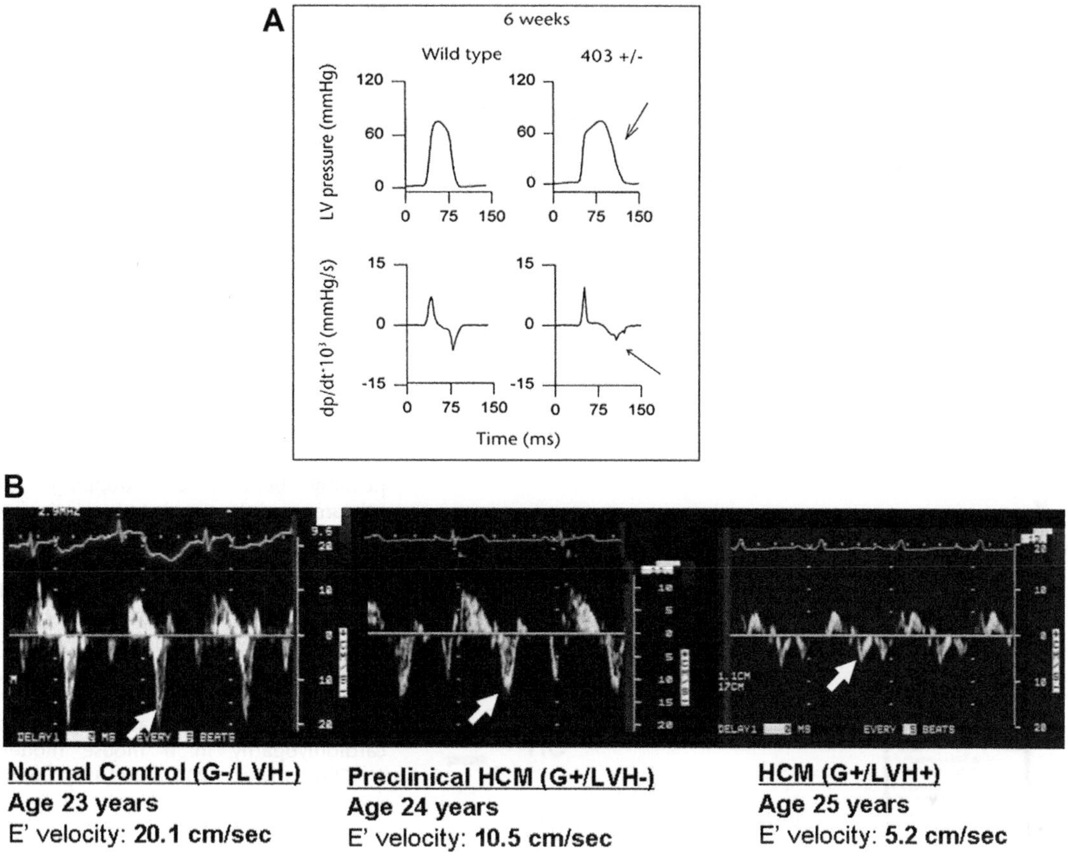

Fig. 7. Diastolic abnormalities are present before the development of LVH. (*A*) Invasive hemodynamic studies on isolated hearts and intact 6-week-old αMHC403/+ mice have shown decreased minimal peak –dP/dt (*arrow*), decreased rates of LV pressure decline (*arrow*), increased tau (the time constant of isovolumic relaxation), and increased time to peak filling. Gross and histologic LVH, myocyte disarray, and fibrosis are not consistently present until 20 to 25 weeks of age. (*B*) Echocardiographic studies on genotyped human populations with HCM also demonstrate impaired relaxation before the development of LVH in otherwise healthy family members who carry pathogenic sarcomere mutations. Reduced early myocardial relaxation velocity (E′ velocity; *white arrows*) on tissue Doppler interrogation indicates impaired relaxation. E′ velocity is normal and brisk in the genotype-negative control relative (*left panel*) but mildly reduced in a relative who carries a gene mutation but has not yet developed clinical disease (G+/LVH-; *center panel*). With development of overt disease, there is a marked reduction in E′ velocity (G+/LVH+, *right panel*). (Figure 7*A*—*Adapted from* Georgakopoulos D, Christe ME, Giewat M, et al. The pathogenesis of familial hypertrophic cardiomyopathy: early and evolving effects from an alphacardiac myosin heavy chain missense mutation. Nat Med 1999;5:327; with permission.)

to counteract biochemical abnormalities, started in advance of obvious disease expression, may diminish the expression of the underlying sarcomere gene mutation.

Arrhythmias

The determinants of SCD and ventricular arrhythmias in HCM remain incompletely defined and are likely complex and multifactorial. Focal ischemia, abnormalities of intramural arteries, abnormalities of calcium signaling, and changes in myocardial architecture have all been suggested as contributing factors to the atrial and ventricular arrhythmias that accompany HCM. Because myocardial fibrosis and disarray are prominent and characteristic features of HCM, and extrapolating from models of myocardial infarction, these histopathologic changes have been hypothesized to represent as the anatomic substrate for electrical instability in HCM, triggering ventricular tachycardia and SCD.[53] There is little direct evidence, however, linking fibrosis and disarray to arrhythmia. In *TNNT2* R92Q and I79N transgenic HCM mouse models, a strong association between hypertrophy or fibrosis and SCD was not demonstrated.[54,55] Studies on the $\alpha MHC^{403/+}$ knock-in HCM mouse model did not show a clear correlation between the location or extent of

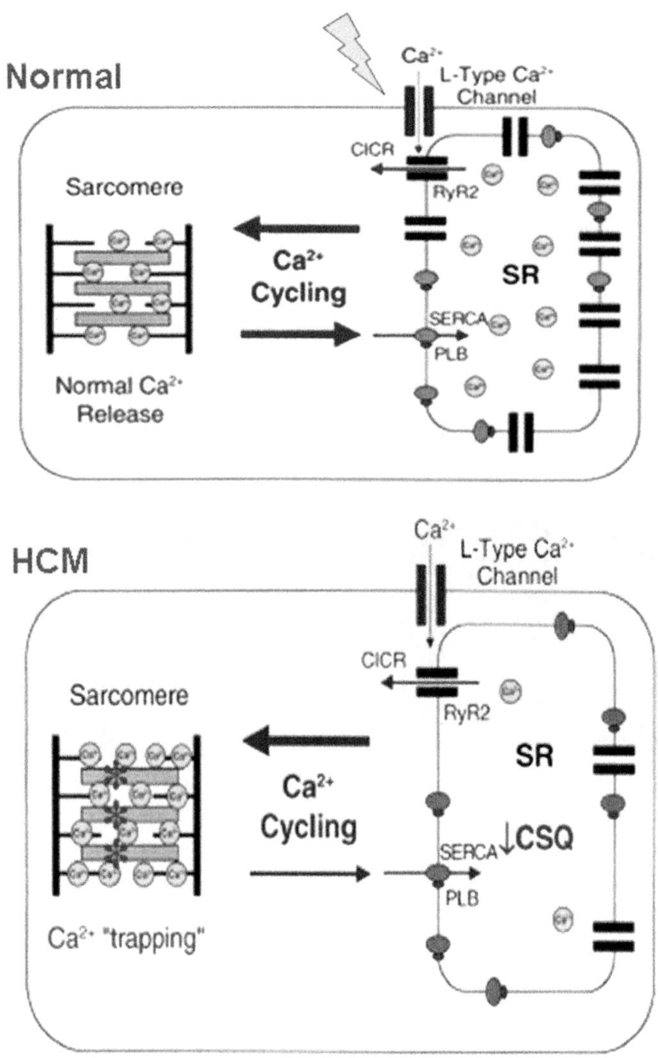

Fig. 8. Intracellular calcium homeostasis is altered in HCM. (*A*) Normal excitation-contraction coupling is initiated when membrane depolarization by the action potential opens voltage-gated L-type calcium channels on the cardiac myocyte membrane. The resultant influx of Ca2+ leads to calcium-induced calcium release (CICR) from stores in the sarcoplasmic reticulum (SR) and a more marked increase in intracellular Ca2+ concentration. Ca2+ binds to the sarcomere, allowing actin-myosin crossbridge formation and generation of the power stroke. Calcium is then taken back up into the SR by the SERCA pump (SR calcium ATPase). (*B*) In HCM, normal calcium cycling may be disrupted, possibly because of "trapping" of calcium in the mutated sarcomere (mutations indicated by asterisk). This may lead to altered intracellular calcium homeostasis with a relative excess of calcium in the sarcomere and relative depletion in the sarcoplasmic reticulum. (*Adapted from* Semsarian C, Ahmad I, Giewat M, et al. The L-type calcium channel inhibitor diltiazem prevents cardiomyopathy in a mouse model. J Clin Invest 2002;109:1013; with permission.)

fibrosis and arrhythmic inducibility on programmed stimulation. In contrast, increasing degrees of LVH and contractility correlated with inducibility.[56]

In humans, cardiac MRI studies have been performed to evaluate the association between delayed enhancement after administration of the extracellular contrast agent, gadolinium. Delayed enhancement is the presumptive imaging correlate of increased myocardial fibrosis or scar.[57–59] There has been only a modest correlation with presence, but not the degree, of delayed enhancement and the extent of hypertrophy,[60] left ventricular mass index, clinical risk factors for sudden death,[59] and ventricular ectopy on Holter monitoring[61] suggesting that there are additional factors beyond myocardial fibrosis that influence the expression of these important features of disease.

The alterations in intracellular Ca^{2+} homeostasis seen in HCM may be a common factor linking sarcomere mutations to both hypertrophy and increased risk for arrhythmias and SCD. Biophysical and genetic data from other inherited cardiac disease associated with an increased occurrence of sudden death has provided support for the role of calcium in arrhythmic risk. Calcium dysregulation and diastolic leak of Ca^{2+} from the SR have been implicated in catecholeminergic polymorphic ventricular tachycardia, a familial syndrome of exercise-induced sudden death, and arrhythmogenic right ventricular cardiomyopathy, a disease with fibrofatty infiltration of the right ventricular myocardium and increased ventricular arrhythmias.[62] Mutations in key calcium binding proteins have been implicated in both of these disorders; specifically, mutations in the cardiac ryanodine receptor (RyR2) have been identified in association with autosomal-dominant arrhythmogenic right ventricular cardiomyopathy and catecholeminergic polymorphic ventricular tachycardia[62,63]; mutations in calsequestrin have been associated with autosomal-recessive catecholeminergic polymorphic ventricular tachycardia.[64] Studies on patients and animal models suggest that the mechanism may involve delayed after-depolarizations, which may trigger membrane depolarization and arrhythmias.[65]

Abnormalities in Myocardial Energetics

Impaired myocardial energetics has been proposed as a unifying mechanism by which sarcomere mutations may result in both cardiac hypertrophy and heart failure.[48,66,67] ^{32}P magnetic resonance spectroscopy studies on the αMHC$^{403/+}$ mouse model have indicated that less force is generated per molecule of ATP hydrolyzed, which may result in reduced mechanical efficiency and compensatory hypertrophy.[48] ^{32}P magnetic resonance spectroscopy studies performed on a genotyped human population have also demonstrated impaired myocardial energetics, both in the early, prehypertrophic stage, and with clinically overt disease. Subjects with overt HCM and family members who carry sarcomere mutations but have not yet developed diagnostic clinical features had a significantly decreased ratio of phosphocreatine to ATP (P_{Cr}/ATP), indicating a compromised energetic state. These data lend further support to the primary role of energy deficiency and increased energy cost of force production in the pathogenesis of HCM.[67] Energy depletion may also be a common mechanism underlying the shared phenotype of cardiac hypertrophy, seen in HCM, mitochondrial disease, and in disease caused by mutations in genes involved in myocardial metabolism (reviewed later).

OTHER PARADIGMS OF GENETIC CARDIAC HYPERTROPHY

Sarcomere mutations are not identified in approximately 30% to 50% of individuals with a clinical diagnosis of HCM. This incomplete detection rate is partially explained by methodologic limitations. Although DNA sequencing technology is highly robust and reliable, in-frame deletions and promoter mutations that alter gene expression are not detected by current candidate gene sequencing strategies. Furthermore, clinical genetic testing is not available for certain sarcomere genes (titin, myozenin, α-myosin heavy chain) in which mutations have been rarely reported, but are known to cause HCM. The genetic basis of unexplained LVH in the absence of a sarcomere mutation has not yet been fully elucidated, either in familial or sporadic disease. Such subjects tend to be slightly older at presentation and lack a clear family history of HCM, but otherwise are difficult to differentiate from those with HCM from underlying sarcomere mutations.

Metabolic Cardiomyopathies

Phenocopies of HCM have been identified where cardiac hypertrophy is caused by mutations in genes distinct from those that encode sarcomere proteins (**Table 3**). By identifying these genes, different pathways leading to the common final disease phenotype can be discovered. Genetic studies in families and sporadic cases of unexplained LVH with conduction abnormalities (progressive atrioventricular block, atrial fibrillation, ventricular pre-excitation) have led to the discovery of a separate category of metabolic

Table 3
Mutations in genes that produce phenocopies of hypertrophic cardiomyopathy

Protein	Gene	Chromosome	Associated Disease	Comments
Metabolic cardiomyopathies				
γ-Subunit, AMP kinase	*PRKAG2*	7q3		Pre-excitation and conduction disease
Lysosome-associated membrane protein	*LAMP2*	Xq2	Danon disease	Cardiomyopathy, skeletal myopathy, and mental retardation; pre-excitation on EKG; rapid progression in adolescence, particularly males
α-Galactosidase	*GLA*	X	Fabry syndrome	Assess plasma or lymphocyte α-Gal activity (males); consider enzyme replacement

cardiomyopathies: genetic cardiac hypertrophy caused by mutations in *PRKAG2*, encoding the $\gamma 2$ regulatory subunit of adenosine monophosphate–activated protein kinase, and in the X-linked lysosome associated membrane protein (*LAMP2*) gene. Mutations in these genes may be present in roughly 2% to 12% of individuals who carry a clinical diagnosis of HCM in whom a sarcomere mutation is not identified, and 40% of individuals with combined features of LVH and pre-excitation.[68–71]

Histopathologically, cardiac hypertrophy caused by *PRKAG2* and *LAMP2* mutations does not display the prominent myocardial disarray or interstitial fibrosis pathognomonic for HCM. Instead, myocardial vacuolization with glycogen-filled myocytes (*PRKAG2*) or autophagic vacuoles (*LAMP2*) is seen (**Fig. 9**). Although incompletely defined, the molecular pathways triggered by *PRKAG2* and *LAMP2* mutations are almost certainly distinct from those triggered by sarcomere gene mutations. As such, practice guidelines developed for HCM may not be appropriate or applicable for treating these metabolic cardiomyopathies. Genetic testing for both *PRKAG2* and *LAMP2* is clinically available and may be considered when unexplained LVH is accompanied by pre-excitation, or if marked LVH is present in young men (*LAMP2*). In the case of *LAMP2* cardiomyopathy, genetic diagnosis provides important prognostic information by identifying individuals who may be destined for worse outcomes and warrant more aggressive management.

Fabry disease is an X-linked recessive disorder caused by mutations in the gene encoding the lysosomal hydrolase, α-galactosidase, and is etiologically similar to the less common *LAMP2* cardiomyopathy. Mutations cause enzyme deficiency and glycosphyngolipid accumulation in the heart, kidneys, nervous system, and skin. Classic Fabry disease occurs at a prevalence of approximately 1 per 40,000 and commonly presents in childhood or adolescence. A cardiac-predominant variant of Fabry disease has been described and may present later in life. Studies suggest that at least 2% to 3% of unexplained LVH in men may be caused by underlying Fabry disease.[72,73] Measuring plasma or leukocyte α-galactosidase activity can reliably diagnose males. α-Galactosidase mutation testing is also available and is particularly helpful to diagnose heterozygous females who may have normal α-galactosidase activity but nonetheless develop clinical disease caused by unfavorable X-inactivation. Identifying patients with Fabry disease is important because of the availability of potentially effective α-galactosidase enzyme replacement therapy.[74]

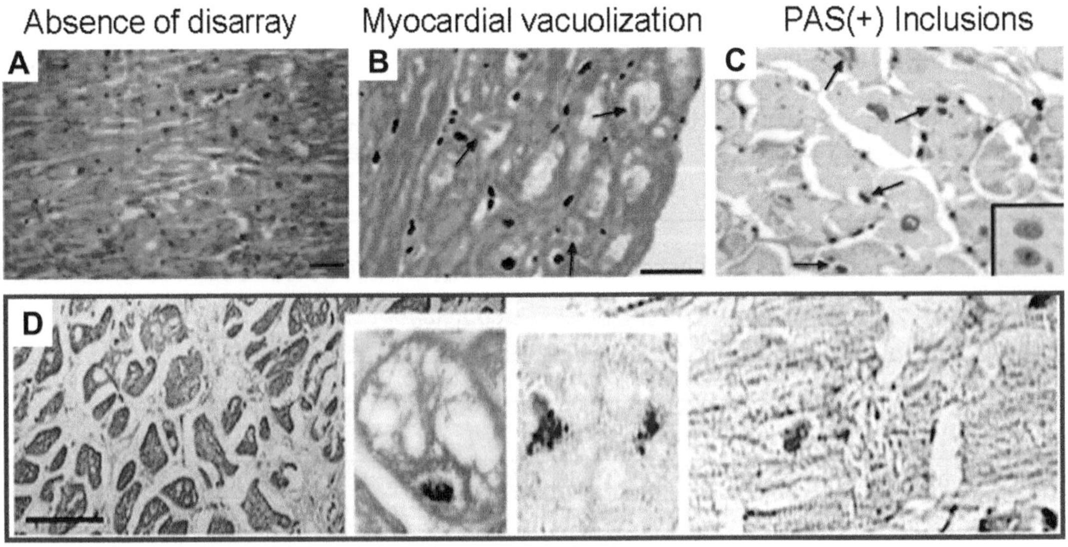

Fig. 9. The histopathology of metabolic cardiomyopthies caused by mutations in PRKAG2 (*A–C*) and LAMP2 (*D*) is distinct from HCM and characterized by glycogen-filled vacuoles without significant disarray, fibrosis, or myocyte hypertrophy. Panels *A* and *D* are stained with hematoxylin and eosin. With PRKAG2 mutations, note the presence of myocardial vacuolization (panel *B, arrows*) and inclusions which stain with periodic acid-Schiff (PAS, panel *C*), indicating the presence of glycogen. With LAMP2 mutations (*D*), vacuoles are also prominent. Immunohistochemical analysis demonstrate staining (*red*) with LAMP2-specific antibodies within the vacuoles. (Figure 9D—*From* Arad M, Maron BJ, Gorham JM, et al. Glycogen storage diseases presenting as hypertrophic cardiomyopathy. N Engl J Med 2005;352:362; with permission. Copyright © 2005, Massachusetts Medical Society.)

FROM BENCH TO BEDSIDE: INTEGRATING GENETIC INFORMATION INTO CLINICAL PRACTICE

Incorporating genetic information into clinical practice is increasingly important in the molecular era of medicine both to refine diagnosis and prognosis, and to provide optimal management for families with inherited disease.

Family Screening, Clinical Evaluation

HCM follows autosomal-dominant inheritance therefore clinical screening of first-degree relatives of affected individuals is recommended, consisting of history, physical examination, 12-lead EKG, and echocardiography. Because the penetrance of LVH is age-dependent, the absence of diagnostic clinical findings on initial assessment does not exclude the possibility of future disease development or the presence of an underlying sarcomere mutation, particularly in children, because left ventricular wall thickness is often normal early in life. Serial follow-up of apparently healthy members of families with HCM is required. The strategy outlined in **Fig. 10** has been proposed for following members of families with HCM for the development of clinical disease.[43]

Genetic Testing

The identification of a sarcomere gene mutation, in the appropriate clinical setting, can provide a definitive diagnosis of HCM, establish the exact genetic etiology of disease, and importantly guide the management of families. Testing can be fruitful in the context of familial disease, because a sarcomere mutation may be identified in approximately 60% of probands, and 50% of their first-degree relatives are predicted to carry the mutation. Mutation confirmation testing in relatives can definitively identify which currently unaffected family members are at risk for disease. Longitudinal clinical follow-up should be appropriately focused on these genotype-positive individuals, and this knowledge may relieve anxiety associated with the otherwise uncertain future risk of disease development. Family members who have not inherited the mutation can be reassured that they are not at risk for disease development or transmission to children, and do not require serial clinical evaluation. Family members who have inherited the causal mutation require serial clinical follow-up and counseling regarding the 50% risk of transmission to offspring.

Currently, genetic testing relies on DNA sequence analysis of candidate genes, and an

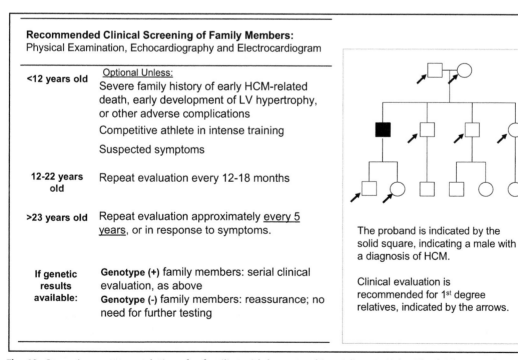

Recommended Clinical Screening of Family Members:
Physical Examination, Echocardiography and Electrocardiogram

<12 years old	Optional Unless: Severe family history of early HCM-related death, early development of LV hypertrophy, or other adverse complications Competitive athlete in intense training Suspected symptoms
12-22 years old	Repeat evaluation every 12-18 months
>23 years old	Repeat evaluation approximately every 5 years, or in response to symptoms.
If genetic results available:	**Genotype (+)** family members: serial clinical evaluation, as above **Genotype (-)** family members: reassurance; no need for further testing

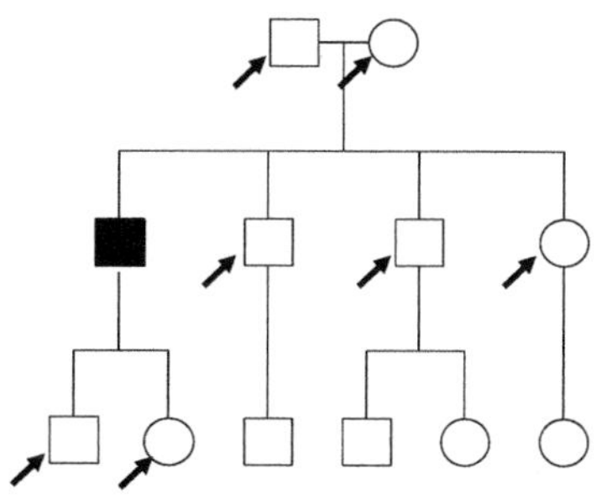

The proband is indicated by the solid square, indicating a male with a diagnosis of HCM.

Clinical evaluation is recommended for 1st degree relatives, indicated by the arrows.

Fig. 10. Screening recommendations for families with hypertrophic cardiomyopathy. The frequency of screening is based on the age of the patient, due to the age-dependent penetrance of LVH in HCM. (*Data from* Maron BJ, Seidman JG, Seidman CE. Proposal for contemporary screening strategies in families with hypertrophic cardiomyopathy. J Am Coll Cardiol 2004;44:2125–32.)

important caveat to this strategy is that the failure to identify a causal mutation by candidate gene sequencing is an inconclusive, noninformative result. It does not exclude the possibility of familial disease caused by rare genetic causes of HCM (not included in standard screening panels) or other types of inherited LVH.

Novel Treatment Strategies to Modify Disease

Greater understanding of the molecular pathogenesis of HCM fosters the development of new therapeutic approaches to disease designed to modify or prevent phenotypic development, rather than merely palliating symptoms or counteracting established hemodynamic abnormalities. For example, early treatment of mice carrying the Arg403Gln mutation in *MYH7* with the L-type calcium channel blocker, diltiazem, before overt disease development, appeared to mitigate development of hypertrophy and fibrosis.[52] Other strategies have been trialed in animal models to reverse the effects of established disease by decreasing myocardial fibrosis, a prototypic feature of HCM. Administration of angiotensin II receptor blockers (losartan),[75] HMG-CoA reductase inhibitors (simvastatin),[76] and aldosterone antagonists (spironolactone)[77] has shown encouraging results in decreasing myocardial fibrosis and collagen content, and identify other new targets for intervention in human studies.

SUMMARY

Elucidating the genetic basis of inherited cardiac hypertrophy provides important insights into the myriad of mechanisms involved in hypertrophic remodeling of the heart. Clinical translation of basic discoveries improves the practical management of patients by enabling precise diagnosis, identification of at-risk individuals, and determination of early markers of disease. These efforts will ultimately allow development of novel treatment paradigms designed to change the natural history of disease.

REFERENCES

1. Klues HG, Schiffers A, Maron BJ. Phenotypic spectrum and patterns of left ventricular hypertrophy in hypertrophic cardiomyopathy: morphologic observations and significance as assessed by two-dimensional echocardiography in 600 patients. J Am Coll Cardiol 1995;26:1699.
2. Elliott P, McKenna WJ. Hypertrophic cardiomyopathy. Lancet 2004;363:1881.
3. Maron BJ. Hypertrophic cardiomyopathy: a systematic review. JAMA 2002;287:1308.
4. Maron BJ, McKenna WJ, Danielson GK, et al. American College of Cardiology/European Society of Cardiology clinical expert consensus document on hypertrophic cardiomyopathy. A report of the American College of Cardiology Foundation Task Force on Clinical Expert Consensus Documents and the European Society of Cardiology Committee for Practice Guidelines. J Am Coll Cardiol 2003;42:1687.
5. Nishimura RA, Holmes DR Jr. Clinical practice: hypertrophic obstructive cardiomyopathy. N Engl J Med 2004;350:1320.
6. Maron MS, Olivotto I, Zenovich AG, et al. Hypertrophic cardiomyopathy is predominantly a disease of left ventricular outflow tract obstruction. Circulation 2006;114:2232.
7. Maron MS, Olivotto I, Betocchi S, et al. Effect of left ventricular outflow tract obstruction on clinical outcome in hypertrophic cardiomyopathy. N Engl J Med 2003;348:295.
8. Biagini E, Coccolo F, Ferlito M, et al. Dilated-hypokinetic evolution of hypertrophic cardiomyopathy: prevalence, incidence, risk factors, and prognostic implications in pediatric and adult patients. J Am Coll Cardiol 2005;46:1543.
9. Harris KM, Spirito P, Maron MS, et al. Prevalence, clinical profile, and significance of left ventricular remodeling in the end-stage phase of hypertrophic cardiomyopathy. Circulation 2006;114:216.
10. Maron BJ, Casey SA, Hauser RG, et al. Clinical course of hypertrophic cardiomyopathy with survival to advanced age. J Am Coll Cardiol 2003;42:882.
11. McKenna WJ, Behr ER. Hypertrophic cardiomyopathy: management, risk stratification, and prevention of sudden death. Heart 2002;87:169.
12. Maron BJ. Sudden death in young athletes. N Engl J Med 2003;349:1064.
13. Elliott PM, Poloniecki J, Dickie S, et al. Sudden death in hypertrophic cardiomyopathy: identification of high risk patients. J Am Coll Cardiol 2000;36:2212.
14. Elliott PM, Gimeno Blanes JR, Mahon NG, et al. Relation between severity of left-ventricular hypertrophy and prognosis in patients with hypertrophic cardiomyopathy. Lancet 2001;357:420.
15. Zipes DP, Camm AJ, Borggrefe M, et al. ACC/AHA/ESC 2006 Guidelines for Management of Patients With Ventricular Arrhythmias and the Prevention of Sudden Cardiac Death: a report of the American College of Cardiology/American Heart Association Task Force and the European Society of Cardiology Committee for Practice Guidelines (writing committee to develop Guidelines for Management of Patients With Ventricular Arrhythmias and the Prevention of Sudden Cardiac Death): developed in collaboration with the European Heart Rhythm

Association and the Heart Rhythm Society. Circulation 2006;114:e385.
16. Jarcho JA, McKenna W, Pare JA, et al. Mapping a gene for familial hypertrophic cardiomyopathy to chromosome 14q1. N Engl J Med 1989;321:1372.
17. Thierfelder L, Watkins H, MacRae C, et al. Alpha-tropomyosin and cardiac troponin T mutations cause familial hypertrophic cardiomyopathy: a disease of the sarcomere. Cell 1994;77:701.
18. Watkins H, McKenna WJ, Thierfelder L, et al. Mutations in the genes for cardiac troponin T and alpha-tropomyosin in hypertrophic cardiomyopathy. N Engl J Med 1995;332:1058.
19. Maron BJ, Gardin JM, Flack JM, et al. Prevalence of hypertrophic cardiomyopathy in a general population of young adults: echocardiographic analysis of 4111 subjects in the CARDIA study. Circulation 1995;92:785.
20. Zou Y, Song L, Wang Z, et al. Prevalence of idiopathic hypertrophic cardiomyopathy in China: a population-based echocardiographic analysis of 8080 adults. Am J Med 2004;116:14.
21. Richard P, Charron P, Carrier L, et al. Hypertrophic cardiomyopathy: distribution of disease genes, spectrum of mutations, and implications for a molecular diagnosis strategy. Circulation 2003;107:2227.
22. Richard P, Villard E, Charron P, et al. The genetic bases of cardiomyopathies. J Am Coll Cardiol 2006;48:A79.
23. Van Driest SL, Ellsworth EG, Ommen SR, et al. Prevalence and spectrum of thin filament mutations in an outpatient referral population with hypertrophic cardiomyopathy. Circulation 2003;108:445.
24. Bos JM, Poley RN, Ny M, et al. Genotype-phenotype relationships involving hypertrophic cardiomyopathy-associated mutations in titin, muscle LIM protein, and telethonin. Mol Genet Metab 2006;88:78.
25. Geier C, Perrot A, Ozcelik C, et al. Mutations in the human muscle LIM protein gene in families with hypertrophic cardiomyopathy. Circulation 2003;107:1390.
26. Osio A, Tan L, Chen SN, et al. Myozenin 2 is a novel gene for human hypertrophic cardiomyopathy. Circ Res 2007;100:766.
27. Marian AJ, Roberts R. The molecular genetic basis for hypertrophic cardiomyopathy. J Mol Cell Cardiol 2001;33:655.
28. Seidman JG, Seidman C. The genetic basis for cardiomyopathy: from mutation identification to mechanistic paradigms. Cell 2001;104:557.
29. Van Driest SL, Vasile VC, Ommen SR, et al. Myosin binding protein C mutations and compound heterozygosity in hypertrophic cardiomyopathy. J Am Coll Cardiol 2004;44:1903.
30. Geisterfer-Lowrance AA, Kass S, Tanigawa G, et al. A molecular basis for familial hypertrophic cardiomyopathy: a beta cardiac myosin heavy chain gene missense mutation. Cell 1990;62:999.
31. Rayment I, Holden HM, Whittaker M, et al. Structure of the actin-myosin complex and its implications for muscle contraction. Science 1993;261:58.
32. Palmiter KA, Tyska MJ, Haeberle JR, et al. R403Q and L908V mutant beta-cardiac myosin from patients with familial hypertrophic cardiomyopathy exhibit enhanced mechanical performance at the single molecule level. J Muscle Res Cell Motil 2000;21:609.
33. Tyska MJ, Hayes E, Giewat M, et al. Single-molecule mechanics of R403Q cardiac myosin isolated from the mouse model of familial hypertrophic cardiomyopathy. Circ Res 2000;86:737.
34. Ahmad F, Seidman JG, Seidman CE. The genetic basis for cardiac remodeling. Annu Rev Genomics Hum Genet 2005;6:185.
35. Tardiff JC. Sarcomeric proteins and familial hypertrophic cardiomyopathy: linking mutations in structural proteins to complex cardiovascular phenotypes. Heart Fail Rev 2005;10:237.
36. Freiburg A, Gautel M. A molecular map of the interactions between titin and myosin-binding protein C: implications for sarcomeric assembly in familial hypertrophic cardiomyopathy. Eur J Biochem 1996;235:317.
37. Niimura H, Patton KK, McKenna WJ, et al. Sarcomere protein gene mutations in hypertrophic cardiomyopathy of the elderly. Circulation 2002;105:446.
38. Morita H, Rehm HL, Menesses A, et al. Shared genetic causes of cardiac hypertrophy in children and adults. N Engl J Med 2008;358:1899.
39. Moolman JC, Corfield VA, Posen B, et al. Sudden death due to troponin T mutations. J Am Coll Cardiol 1997;29:549.
40. Morita H, Larson MG, Barr SC, et al. Single-gene mutations and increased left ventricular wall thickness in the community: the Framingham Heart Study. Circulation 2006;113:2697.
41. Niimura H, Bachinski LL, Sangwatanaroj S, et al. Mutations in the gene for cardiac myosin-binding protein C and late-onset familial hypertrophic cardiomyopathy [comments]. N Engl J Med 1998;338:1248.
42. Charron P, Heron D, Gargiulo M, et al. Genetic testing and genetic counselling in hypertrophic cardiomyopathy: the French experience. J Med Genet 2002;39:741.
43. Maron BJ, Seidman JG, Seidman CE. Proposal for contemporary screening strategies in families with hypertrophic cardiomyopathy. J Am Coll Cardiol 2004;44:2125.
44. Geisterfer-Lowrance AA, Christe M, Conner DA, et al. A mouse model of familial hypertrophic cardiomyopathy. Science 1996;272:731.

45. Georgakopoulos D, Christe ME, Giewat M, et al. The pathogenesis of familial hypertrophic cardiomyopathy: early and evolving effects from an alpha-cardiac myosin heavy chain missense mutation [comments]. Nat Med 1999;5:327.
46. Blanchard E, Seidman C, Seidman JG, et al. Altered crossbridge kinetics in the alphaMHC403/+ mouse model of familial hypertrophic cardiomyopathy. Circ Res 1999;84:475.
47. Fatkin D, McConnell BK, Mudd JO, et al. An abnormal Ca (2+) response in mutant sarcomere protein-mediated familial hypertrophic cardiomyopathy. J Clin Invest 2000;106:1351.
48. Spindler M, Saupe KW, Christe ME, et al. Diastolic dysfunction and altered energetics in the alphaMHC403/+ mouse model of familial hypertrophic cardiomyopathy. J Clin Invest 1998;101:1775.
49. Westermann D, Knollmann BC, Steendijk P, et al. Diltiazem treatment prevents diastolic heart failure in mice with familial hypertrophic cardiomyopathy. Eur J Heart Fail 2006;8:115.
50. Ho CY, Sweitzer NK, McDonough B, et al. Assessment of diastolic function with Doppler tissue imaging to predict genotype in preclinical hypertrophic cardiomyopathy. Circulation 2002;105:2992.
51. Nagueh SF, Bachinski LL, Meyer D, et al. Tissue Doppler imaging consistently detects myocardial abnormalities in patients with hypertrophic cardiomyopathy and provides a novel means for an early diagnosis before and independently of hypertrophy. Circulation 2001;104:128.
52. Semsarian C, Ahmad I, Giewat M, et al. The L-type calcium channel inhibitor diltiazem prevents cardiomyopathy in a mouse model. J Clin Invest 2002;109:1013.
53. Varnava AM, Elliott PM, Mahon N, et al. Relation between myocyte disarray and outcome in hypertrophic cardiomyopathy. Am J Cardiol 2001;88:275.
54. Knollmann BC, Blatt SA, Horton K, et al. Inotropic stimulation induces cardiac dysfunction in transgenic mice expressing a troponin T (I79N) mutation linked to familial hypertrophic cardiomyopathy. J Biol Chem 2001;276:10039.
55. Maass AH, Ikeda K, Oberdorf-Maass S, et al. Hypertrophy, fibrosis, and sudden cardiac death in response to pathological stimuli in mice with mutations in cardiac troponin T. Circulation 2004;110:2102.
56. Wolf CM, Moskowitz IP, Arno S, et al. Somatic events modify hypertrophic cardiomyopathy pathology and link hypertrophy to arrhythmia. Proc Natl Acad Sci U S A 2005;102:18123.
57. Kim RJ, Judd RM. Gadolinium-enhanced magnetic resonance imaging in hypertrophic cardiomyopathy: in vivo imaging of the pathologic substrate for premature cardiac death? J Am Coll Cardiol 2003;41:1568.
58. Kim RJ, Wu E, Rafael A, et al. The use of contrast-enhanced magnetic resonance imaging to identify reversible myocardial dysfunction. N Engl J Med 2000;343:1445.
59. Moon JC, McKenna WJ, McCrohon JA, et al. Toward clinical risk assessment in hypertrophic cardiomyopathy with gadolinium cardiovascular magnetic resonance. J Am Coll Cardiol 2003;41:1561.
60. Choudhury L, Mahrholdt H, Wagner A, et al. Myocardial scarring in asymptomatic or mildly symptomatic patients with hypertrophic cardiomyopathy. J Am Coll Cardiol 2002;40:2156.
61. Adabag AS, Maron BJ, Appelbaum E, et al. Occurrence and frequency of arrhythmias in hypertrophic cardiomyopathy in relation to delayed enhancement on cardiovascular magnetic resonance. J Am Coll Cardiol 2008;51:1369.
62. MacRae CA, Birchmeier W, Thierfelder L. Arrhythmogenic right ventricular cardiomyopathy: moving toward mechanism. J Clin Invest 2006;116:1825.
63. Priori SG, Napolitano C, Tiso N, et al. Mutations in the cardiac ryanodine receptor gene (hRyR2) underlie catecholaminergic polymorphic ventricular tachycardia. Circulation 2001;103:196.
64. Eldar M, Pras E, Lahat H. A missense mutation in the CASQ2 gene is associated with autosomal-recessive catecholamine-induced polymorphic ventricular tachycardia. Trends Cardiovasc Med 2003;13:148.
65. Bauce B, Rampazzo A, Basso C, et al. Screening for ryanodine receptor type 2 mutations in families with effort-induced polymorphic ventricular arrhythmias and sudden death: early diagnosis of asymptomatic carriers. J Am Coll Cardiol 2002;40:341.
66. Ashrafian H, Watkins H. Reviews of translational medicine and genomics in cardiovascular disease: new disease taxonomy and therapeutic implications cardiomyopathies: therapeutics based on molecular phenotype. J Am Coll Cardiol 2007;49:1251.
67. Crilley JG, Boehm EA, Blair E, et al. Hypertrophic cardiomyopathy due to sarcomeric gene mutations is characterized by impaired energy metabolism irrespective of the degree of hypertrophy. J Am Coll Cardiol 2003;41:1776.
68. Arad M, Benson DW, Perez-Atayde AR, et al. Constitutively active AMP kinase mutations cause glycogen storage disease mimicking hypertrophic cardiomyopathy. J Clin Invest 2002;109:357.
69. Arad M, Maron BJ, Gorham JM, et al. Glycogen storage diseases presenting as hypertrophic cardiomyopathy. N Engl J Med 2005;352:362.
70. Blair E, Redwood C, Ashrafian H, et al. Mutations in the gamma (2) subunit of AMP-activated protein kinase cause familial hypertrophic cardiomyopathy: evidence for the central role of energy compromise in disease pathogenesis. Hum Mol Genet 2001;10:1215.

71. Gollob MH, Green MS, Tang AS, et al. Identification of a gene responsible for familial Wolff-Parkinson-White syndrome. N Engl J Med 2001; 344:1823.
72. Nakao S, Takenaka T, Maeda M, et al. An atypical variant of Fabry's disease in men with left ventricular hypertrophy. N Engl J Med 1995;333:288.
73. Sachdev B, Takenaka T, Teraguchi H, et al. Prevalence of Anderson-Fabry disease in male patients with late onset hypertrophic cardiomyopathy. Circulation 2002;105:1407.
74. Banikazemi M, Bultas J, Waldek S, et al. Agalsidase-beta therapy for advanced Fabry disease: a randomized trial. Ann Intern Med 2007;146:77.
75. Lim DS, Lutucuta S, Bachireddy P, et al. Angiotensin II blockade reverses myocardial fibrosis in a transgenic mouse model of human hypertrophic cardiomyopathy. Circulation 2001;103:789.
76. Patel R, Nagueh SF, Tsybouleva N, et al. Simvastatin induces regression of cardiac hypertrophy and fibrosis and improves cardiac function in a transgenic rabbit model of human hypertrophic cardiomyopathy. Circulation 2001;104:317.
77. Tsybouleva N, Zhang L, Chen S, et al. Aldosterone, through novel signaling proteins, is a fundamental molecular bridge between the genetic defect and the cardiac phenotype of hypertrophic cardiomyopathy. Circulation 2004;109:1284.

Arrhythmogenic Right Ventricular Cardiomyopathy

Patrick T. Ellinor, MD, PhD[a],
Calum A. MacRae, MB, ChB, PhD[b,*],
Ludwig Thierfelder, MD[c,d]

KEYWORDS

- Arrhythmogenic right ventricular cardiomyopathy
- Sudden death • Desmosome • Genetic

Arrhythmogenic right ventricular cardiomyopathy (ARVC) is a syndrome characterized by myocardial disease, predominantly involving the right ventricle (RV) and associated with ventricular tachycardia arising from this chamber (left bundle branch block [LBBB] morphology), syncope, and sudden death. At autopsy, there is an unusual distribution of fatty and fibrotic tissue within the RV, preferentially affecting 3 areas, namely, the apex, the inflow tract, and the outflow tract.[1,2] In typical cases of ARVC there is evidence of a familial trait, but this may only be revealed when relatives are examined directly.[3] Clinical genetic studies performed to date have established that ARVC is not a single disorder but a syndrome consisting of multiple entities with discrete clinical features. There is significant variation in the natural history of the underlying diseases, but there is also substantial pleiotropy of clinical expression of the same single disease gene segregating within individual families.[3,4] The mutated genes identified so far strongly suggest that ARVC is the result of perturbation in specialized intercellular adhesion junctions known as desmosomes,[5–17] and thus is mechanistically distinct from either hypertrophic or dilated cardiomyopathy.[18]

Data-driven diagnosis and management are difficult in rare disorders. These problems are further compounded in ARVC, where the causal heterogeneity results in differential representation of specific forms of the disease in smaller studies. This representation is particularly problematic in inherited diseases whereby many individuals in smaller series are likely to be related. As the RV has become more accessible through improved imaging techniques, the number of individuals diagnosed with ARVC has increased substantially. However, it is clear that many subjects who carry the label of ARVC exhibit a natural history different from that seen in early reports.[19] It remains unclear whether this is the result of the inadvertent inclusion of discrete disorders and normal variants or the reflection of a reservoir of ARVC in which ventricular arrhythmias and sudden death are infrequent complications. The investigation and management of this expanding group of indeterminate patients is now a common clinical dilemma.

This work was supported by grants from the National Institutes of Health and the Ernst and Berta Grimmke Stiftung, Duesseldorf, Germany.

[a] Cardiovascular Research Center and Cardiology Division, Massachusetts General Hospital, Charlestown, Boston, MA, USA
[b] Cardiovascular Division, Brigham and Women's Hospital and Harvard Medical School, 75 Francis Street, Boston, MA 02115, USA
[c] Department of Cardiology, Max-Delbrueck Center for Molecular Medicine, Robert-Roessle Strabe 10, D-13092 Berlin, Germany
[d] Franz-Volhard Clinic, Charité, Campus Buch, Helios Clinic, Robert-Roessle Strabe 10, D-13092 Berlin, Germany
* Corresponding author. Cardiovascular Division, Brigham and Women's Hospital, 75 Francis Street, Boston, MA 02115.
E-mail address: camacrae@bics.bwh.harvard.edu

Heart Failure Clin 6 (2010) 161–177
doi:10.1016/j.hfc.2009.12.003
1551-7136/10/$ – see front matter

International registries have been established, but will take time to accumulate the numbers and outcomes data required to make rigorous conclusions.[20–22]

These problems led to the proposal of standardized diagnostic criteria by an international Task Force in 1994 (**Box 1**).[23] Multiple disease features were classified as major or minor by consensus, and an empiric scoring system was developed incorporating insights from autopsy studies, noninvasive investigation, and family studies. However, the original criteria and subsequent proposed modifications were defined retrospectively from aggregated series of referrals to tertiary care institutions and have never been prospectively validated as was originally intended.[3,23,24] The criteria are increasingly applied in situations where the prior probability of ARVC is different from the initial derivation set of patients, and thus the sensitivity and specificity of the scoring system are less robust than anticipated.[3,19] This difference is highlighted by recent genetic work whereby it

Box 1
Task Force criteria, qualifiers, and limitations

Family history

Major: familial disease confirmed at necropsy or surgery

Evaluation should be done by a cardiac pathologist.

Minor: family history of premature, sudden death or of clinical diagnosis based on present criteria

Clinical and autopsy data (if available) from premature, sudden deaths should be reevaluated by a specialist.

Electrocardiographic (ECG) depolarization or conduction abnormalities

ECG criteria are particularly dependent on prior probability of ARVC.

Major: epsilon waves or localized prolongation of QRS (>110 ms) in right precordial leads

Minor: late potentials on signal-averaged ECG

ECG repolarization abnormalities

ECG criteria are particularly dependent on prior probability of ARVC.

Minor: inverted T waves in right precordial leads in individuals older than 12 years in absence of right bundle branch block

Arrhythmias

Minor: sustained or nonsustained LBBB-type ventricular tachycardia documented on ECG, Holter or during exercise testing; frequent ventricular extrasystoles (>1000/24 hours on Holter)

Recent data suggest electrophysiology study (EPS) may be helpful in discriminating between ARVC and right ventricular outflow tract tachycardias.

Global or regional right ventricular dysfunction or structural abnormality

Reproducible quantitative indices of RV function (using magnetic resonance imaging [MRI], computed tomography [CT], cardiac catheterization, or echo) remain specialist tools.

Major: severe dilatation and reduction of RV ejection fraction with minimal or no left ventricle (LV) involvement; localized right ventricular aneurysms (akinetic or dyskinetic areas with diastolic bulging); severe segmental dilation of RV

Minor: mild global RV dilatation or reduction in ejection fraction with normal LV: mild segmental dilatation of RV; regional RV hypokinesis

Tissue characteristics of walls

Major: fibrofatty replacement of myocardium on endomyocardial biopsy

Biopsy is insensitive, but may help exclude other disorders restricted to RV. MRI tissue characterization was not included in original criteria.

Note that for at-risk relatives of definitively affected probands, virtually any cardiac abnormality may represent ARVC. This representation does not imply that the clinical course will be similar to the probands or other definitively affected individuals.

was demonstrated that Task Force criteria were poor predictors of carrier status in family members.[8] In the setting of familial disease, where the prior probability of ARVC may approach 0.50, the original Task Force criteria are greatly reduced in sensitivity, and modifications already have been proposed.[3] Conversely, in the context of incidental clinical abnormalities the criteria lack specificity, and the number of indeterminate individuals generated by their application suggests that a comprehensive reevaluation is necessary, particularly to determine thresholds for implantation of cardioverter defibrillators.[19]

In this article, focus is on diagnosis and management of ARVC, while highlighting central issues in the rigorous assessment of RV disease and emphasizing the practical management of indeterminate individuals. The investigators have concentrated on larger published series that are less likely to have been distorted by referral biases or local genetic founder effects, and have deliberately excluded current dogma based on small studies that are difficult to interpret. This approach is intended not to be nihilistic but to avoid overstatement of current knowledge while highlighting areas for future investigation.

CLINICAL PRESENTATION AND NATURAL HISTORY

The defining reports in ARVC were pathologic series based on premature sudden deaths.[1,2] Modern pathologic studies suggest that ARVC is the primary cause in as many as 10% to 15% of cases of sudden death in those younger than 65 years, but nonischemic causes are likely to be overrepresented in these data.[25] Unheralded cardiac arrest remains the typical mode of presentation for a substantial subset of those with ARVC. Not surprisingly, clinical series based on antemortem diagnosis offer a more varied picture (**Box 2**). The largest studies suggest that most living ARVC patients present with palpitations or presyncope, whereas as many as one-third would have had a documented syncopal episode.[26,27] Less common presentations include ventricular tachycardia originating in the RV, isolated and unexplained RV failure, or even biventricular heart failure. Clinical screening of the families of probands with definitive ARVC also identifies significant numbers of asymptomatic but affected relatives.[3,4,28] Perhaps more common than these groups is the increasing number of individuals with 1 or more incidentally discovered abnormalities suggestive of ARVC, but in whom no definitive diagnosis is possible.[19] The combined prevalence of each of these clinical entities is unknown, but in aggregate is likely to be considerably more common than suggested by autopsy series.

Box 2
Presentation in ARVC

- Cardiac arrest
- Palpitations
- Presyncope
- Syncope
- Sustained LBBB pattern ventricular tachycardia
- Unexplained heart failure
- Asymptomatic relative
- Incidental RV abnormality

Note the relative frequency of each of these presentations is unknown. It is possible that most of those with ARVC are undetected until they suffer a cardiac arrest.

As might be expected from the range of potential presentations, there are few long-term follow-up studies of definitively affected ARVC subjects, and those that do exist are confounded to variable degrees by selection bias, causal heterogeneity, and local genetic founder effects.[4,29–31] Only 3 follow-up studies include more than 45 subjects, and these serve to illustrate the fundamental problems intrinsic to the study of this rare, familial syndrome. Hulot and colleagues[26] followed 130 selected patients for a mean of 8 years and noted an annual mortality rate of 2.3%, largely from progressive heart failure. In contrast, a follow-up of 151 affected relatives revealed electrocardiographic and echocardiographic evidence of progression, but only 1 individual died over an 8-year period, indicating a annual mortality rate of only 0.08%.[4] In this series, there were no episodes of clinical heart failure. These 151 subjects represented only a few causal genotypes as multiple families mapped to the same loci, and there was clear evidence of local genetic founder effects. Most recently, the initial experience with 100 subjects from Johns Hopkins was reported confirming the substantial variation in presentation and natural history seen in other studies.[27]

These data strongly suggest that smaller studies are likely to be heavily weighted in favor of specific forms of ARVC or individual ARVC families, and thus are nonrepresentative of the syndrome as a whole. Many of the disparities seen in the ARVC literature are likely to reflect this underlying causal heterogeneity.[20,23,31] For example, there are varying reports of a marked gender bias in the risk of sudden death, but these are most notable in single families[29] and not seen in unselected populations.[25]

PATHOLOGY

Pathologic examination is the effective gold standard in ARVC, but correlation with antemortem clinical features has proven difficult. The original descriptions of ARVC focused on the fatty replacement seen in the RV.[1,2] The use of the term replacement infers that the muscle develops normally, and subsequently undergoes dysplastic degeneration with replacement of muscle by fibrous scarring and fatty tissue. Although this sequence of events has never been conclusively demonstrated, progressive deterioration of RV structure and function undoubtedly occur.[26,30] Focal RV wall thinning and RV aneurysms have been reported on gross pathologic examination, and are considered by some investigators to be pathognomonic of ARVC.[32]

Histologic examination reveals a range of myocardial injury and repair similar to that seen in other forms of cardiomyopathy.[1,2,25,33] Aside from the chronic stage at which isolated myocytes are seen within large tracts of fibrous tissue and adipocytes, there are no unique microscopic features. Some investigators have made distinctions between bland adipose replacement and fibrofatty disease with inflammatory infiltrates, but whether these represent distinct clinical or biologic entities remains unclear.[32,34] There are studies suggesting that inflammatory infiltrates are more common in the context of sudden death, and recent work has demonstrated evidence of RV apoptotic activity in individuals who have died.[35] There is important histologic evidence of fibrofatty involvement of the left ventricle (LV) in a significant proportion (30%–75%) of ARVC cases.[25,33] Similar histologic findings restricted to the LV also have been seen in so-called arrhythmogenic LV cardiomyopathy.[15,36]

Ultimately, large prospective studies may be able to address the relationship between the clinical and pathologic features of ARVC, but at present only retrospective data exist. Tabib and colleagues[25] defined the circumstances of death associated with gross and microscopic evidence of ARVC in 200 individuals. These cases represent approximately 10% of the unexpected sudden cardiac deaths in a large municipal autopsy series. Most individuals in this series died suddenly during daily activities, with a small number of subjects collapsing during exercise (3.5%). Most died in their forties, but only 6 individuals had any arrhythmia diagnosed before death, and none of those who died suddenly from ARVC had suffered any symptoms of heart failure. This study is the largest single series of definitive ARVC cases and offers several important insights. Fatty replacement in virtually all cases extended from the septum or anterior interventricular groove into the anterior RV wall to a variable extent (correlation with magnetic resonance imaging [MRI] is seen in **Fig. 1**A and B). Fibrofatty lesions were restricted to the external margin of the RV in only 2% of cases. Other notable findings were the unusually wide distribution of heart weights, which was not reflected in the normal mean values. Although rarely noted in other studies of ARVC, significant left ventricular hypertrophy was seen in 15% of subjects and was particularly prevalent in younger age groups. The predominant histologic lesions seen were fine interstitial fibrosis and adipose replacement. Fibrosis involved the His bundles in most of the hearts studied. Inflammatory infiltrates were rare and, when present, were sparse. LV involvement was present in around 30% of cases but was largely fibrotic rather than adipose in nature, correlating closely with heart weight. Smaller series have identified more frequent LV involvement and more impressive inflammatory infiltrates.[33]

Taken together, these data serve to highlight the problems correlating rigorous, pathologically confirmed ARVC with clinical features other than sudden death. Many of the current problems in diagnosis and management reflect the lack of a gold standard in most clinical studies of ARVC. Progress in the field depends on establishing a tight relationship between each of the constituent clinical entities within ARVC and the underlying gross, microscopic, or molecular pathology.[33]

GENETICS

Clinical Genetics

Early in the study of ARVC, it became evident that many of the relatives of probands also exhibited arrhythmias, syncope, or sudden death. Systematic studies of family members suggest that up to 50% of individuals with ARVC have evidence of a Mendelian disease.[3,37] Smaller kindred, with only 1 or 2 affected first-degree relatives, seem to be the rule. This evidence could reflect reduced penetrance or be a result of disease morbidity in utero and prior to reproductive years. Larger kindreds suitable for gene mapping and cloning do exist, but these may represent only specific causal forms of ARVC.

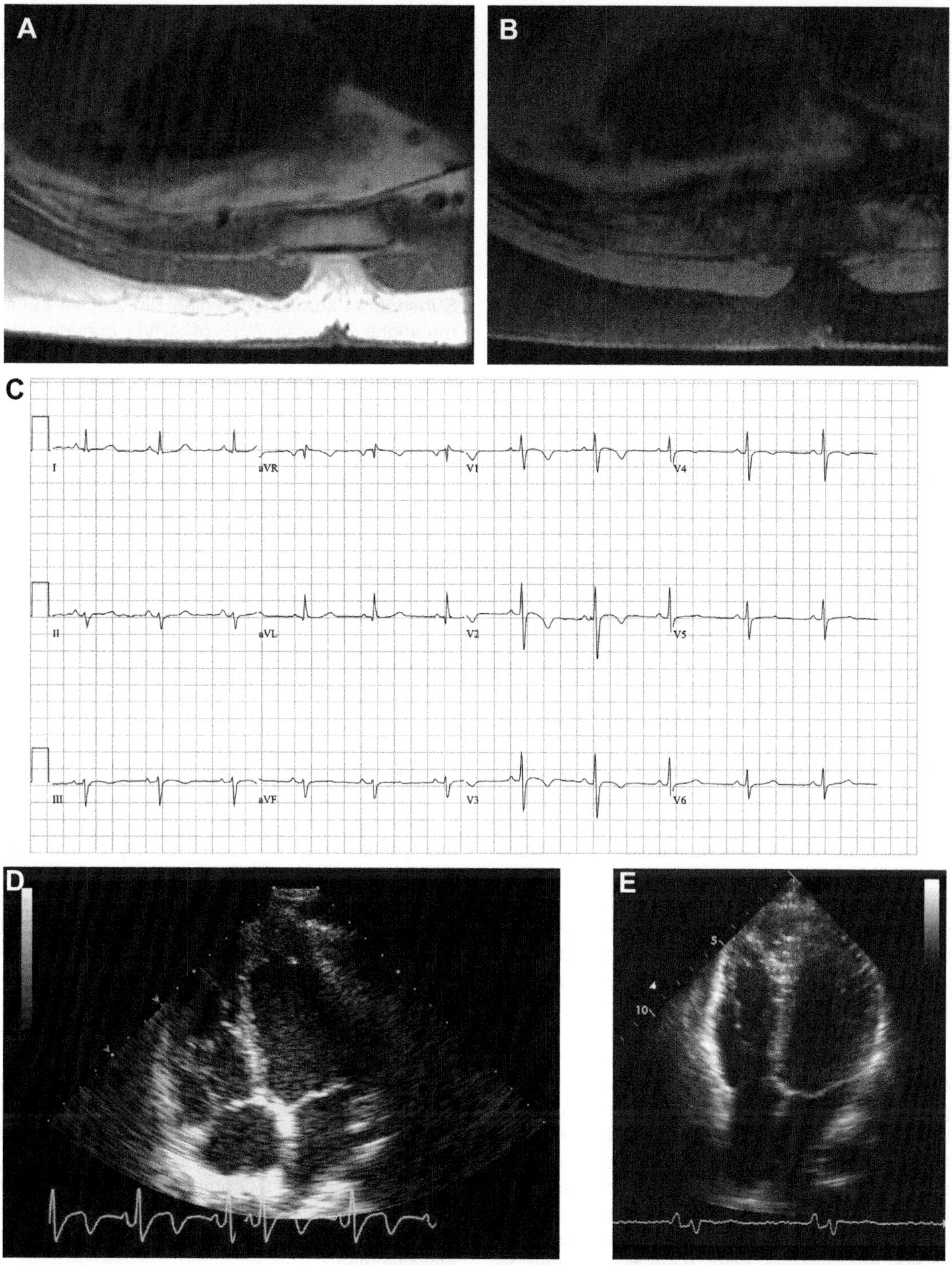

Fig. 1. Clinical findings in ARVC. (*A*) A T1-weighted spin-echo image of the RV. The myocardium is extensively infiltrated with areas of bright signal suggestive of fat. (*B*) Identical to A but now, in addition, a chemical fat saturation prepulse has been applied. The areas of signal hyperenhancement on the first image are clearly suppressed on the fat-saturated image, confirming that the RV free wall myocardium is infiltrated with fat extending into the anterior interventricular groove. (*C*) A typical 12-lead ECG with repolarization abnormalities in the right precordial leads (V_2–V_4). No specific features are present, and the diagnosis of ARVC is completely dependent on the prior probability of this disease or additional abnormalities on other testing. (*D*) Echocardiographic features of ARVC evident on the apical 4-chamber view demonstrating excessive trabeculations. (*E*) Echocardiographic features of ARVC evident on the apical 4-chamber view with evidence of an apical aneurysmal segment. (MRI images: *Courtesy of* Dr David E. Sosnovik and Dr Fred Holmvang, Massachusetts General Hospital; echocardiographic images: *Courtesy of* Dr Danita M. Yoerger, Massachusetts General Hospital.)

The high rates of familiality support the systematic clinical screening of at-risk relatives.[4,28,29] The identification by screening of presymptomatic individuals or subclinical disease raises many questions regarding their subsequent management.[31] Although these individuals carry the same mutated gene as their relatives with ARVC, the natural history of such formes frustes of the disorder remains to be determined by long-term studies and likely varies widely with the specific causal gene.[4,29] Family studies also may offer insights into the factors modifying progression to clinical disease.

Molecular Genetics

Like other highly morbid inherited diseases, ARVC is genetically heterogeneous. There are now 12 genetic loci described for various forms of the disorder, and several unmapped families also are known to exist (**Table 1**). It is likely that at each locus there will be a high de novo mutation rate and consequent allelic heterogeneity. For these reasons, genetic diagnosis will be subject to many of the technical and interpretive issues already seen with other inherited cardiac syndromes such as hypertrophic cardiomyopathy and long QT syndrome.[49]

The clinical study of extended families suggested a shared pathophysiology between some skin disorders and RV cardiomyopathy. Perhaps the best known of these is Naxos disease, in which palmoplantar keratoderma, woolly hair, and ARVC cosegregate as a recessive syndrome.[5] Similar recessive cardiocutaneous syndromes have been described in other consanguineous populations.[50] Distinct epithelial defects including anterior polar cataracts also have been described in association with ARVC.[48]

These clinical clues led to the identification of a recessive mutation in Naxos disease in the gene encoding plakoglobin, a desmosomal structural protein.[5,6] In turn, this insight led to the detection of homozygous mutations in the desmoplakin gene in an Ecuadorian family with recessive biventricular dilated cardiomyopathy, keratoderma, and woolly hair.[13,50] Subsequently, distinct mutations of the desmoplakin gene have been found to cause autosomal dominant forms of ARVC (such as ARVC8) and arrhythmogenic LV cardiomyopathy.[14,15] Recently, an autosomal dominant mutation of plakoglobin in a patient with ARVC has also been identified.[7]

Taken together, mutations in plakoglobin and desmoplakin represent only a small proportion of ARVC. However, the recent description of plakophilin 2 (PKP2) mutations in a large proportion (25%–70%) of probands with ARVC suggests that this is a major disease locus and underscores the unique role of desmosomal biology in this syndrome.[8–10] Screening of 120 human probands revealed a range of mutations (largely truncations) in 32 individuals.[8] Mutation-positive subjects exhibited similar clinical features as the remaining cohort. The genetic analysis of 2 larger families in the study revealed markedly reduced penetrance, supporting previous clinical reports in ARVC.[3] Subsequent studies screening PKP2 have found mutations in up to 70% of ARVC cohorts with a preponderance of familial cases.[9] These efforts have led investigators to begin systematic screenings of the genes for many desmosomal proteins, and mutations have been identified in desmoglein 2 and desmocollin 2.[11,12,16,17]

Potential mutations have also been reported in the regulatory region of the transforming growth factor β3 gene,[38] but the pathogenicity of such mutations is difficult to establish, and confirmatory evidence is awaited. Mutations in the cardiac ryanodine receptor gene (RYR2) have also been described in a single kindred.[40,41] Mutations in the calcium release pathway previously have been associated with catecholaminergic ventricular tachycardia (VT), and it is unclear whether the affected individuals in this family shared such clinical features or exhibited evidence of more typical ARVC.

Potential overlap between ARVC and other clinical entities may be addressed by clinical and molecular genetic studies. For example, because end-stage ARVC is often indistinguishable from dilated cardiomyopathy, only the clinical study of relatives may reveal classic isolated RV involvement. The existence of desmoplakin-related arrhythmogenic left ventricular cardiomyopathy serves to emphasize the limits of clinical classifications.[15] Furthermore, PKP2 mutations do not appear to cause right ventricular outflow tract (RVOT), strongly supporting clinical and electrophysiologic evidence that this entity is distinct from ARVC (L. Thierfelder, unpublished data, 2009). Ultimately, a comprehensive molecular nosology for myocardial disease will resolve many of the inconsistencies in the current classification.[51]

Disease Mechanisms

Desmosomes are protein-rich plaques that form mechanically robust connections between cells and serve to organize other key intercellular junctions, including adherens junctions and gap junctions (**Fig. 2**).[52,53] Although their role in the structural integrity of epithelia and other tissues

Table 1
Known ARVC loci/disease genes

Locus Name	OMIM #	Genetic Locus	Causative Gene	Mode of Inheritance	Comments	References
ARVD1	107970 19230	14q23–q24	Transforming growth factor β3	AD	? Distinct from ARVC3 Pathogenic role unclear	38,39
ARVD2	600996 180902	1q42–q43	Cardiac ryanodine receptor (RYR2)	AD	CPVT No pathologic data	40,41
ARVD3	602086	14q12–q22	Unknown	AD	? Distinct from ARVC1	42
ARVD4	602087	2q32	Unknown	AD	Mutations found in plakophilin 2 (PKP2)	43
ARVD5	604400 612048	3p25	Transmembrane protein 43	AD	Founder mutation in large Newfoundland population	44,45
ARVD6	604401	10p12–p14	Unknown	AD		46
ARVD7	609160	10q22	Unknown	AD	? Distinct from DCM	47
ARVD8	607450 125647	6p24	Desmoplakin (DSP)	AD	Highly pleiotropic Occasionally LV cardiomyopathy only	14,15
ARVD9	609040 602861	12p11	PKP2	AD	Present in 25% of cases	8–10
ARVD10	610193 125671	18q12	Desmoglein 2	AD	Rare	16,17
ARVD11	610476 125645	18q12	Desmocollin 2	AD	Rare	11,12
ARVD12	611528 173325	17q21	Plakoglobin (JUP)	AD	Single case with nonsyndromic ARVC	7
Naxos disease	601214 173325	17q21	Plakoglobin (JUP)	AR	Palmoplantar keratoderma and wooly hair	5,6
Carvajal syndrome	605676 125647	6p24	Desmoplakin (DSP)	AR	LV involvement, aneurysm, palmoplantar keratoderma, woolly hair	13
ARVC/Cataract	115650	14q23–24	Unknown	AR	Anterior polar cataract	48

Abbreviations: AD, autosomal dominant; AR, autosomal recessive; CPVT, catecholaminergic polymorphic ventricular tachycardia; DCM, dilated cardiomyopathy; OMIM, online Mendelian inheritance in man; ?, significant questions re statements.

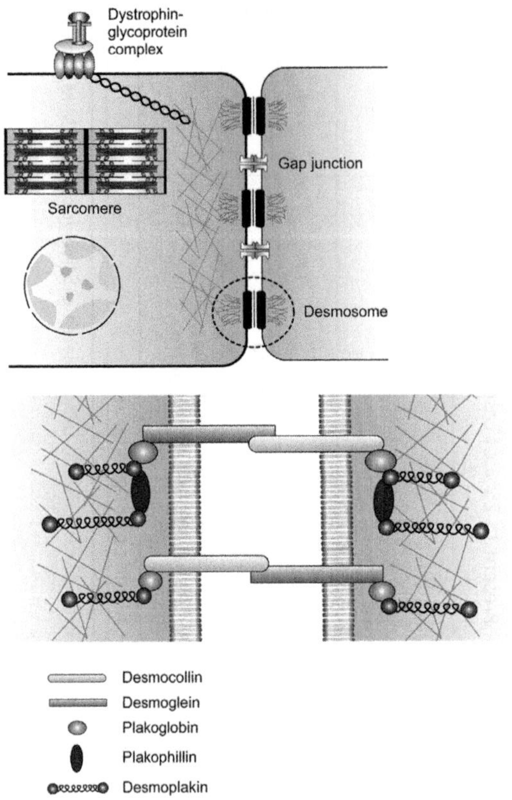

Fig. 2. Four known pathways for human cardiomyopathy. Desmosomal perturbations appear to uniquely affect the RV leading to ARVC. More typical dilated cardiomyopathy is a result of mutations, which affect the structural integrity of the cardiomyocyte through perturbations of the dystrophin-associated glycoprotein complex, the cytoskeleton, or more rarely the nuclear envelope. Mutations in sarcomeric contractile protein genes usually result in hypertrophic cardiomyopathy but can cause dilated ventricular phenotypes. It can be seen that these protein complexes are directly and indirectly linked to each other. This molecular overlap may at least partly explain the clinical overlap seen in these different disorders. Molecular composition of the desmosome is depicted (*inset*). The desmosomal cadherins desmocollin and desmoglein form classic homotypic and heterotypic interactions between cells. These membrane-bound proteins are linked through the armadillo family members, plakoglobin, and plakophilin to the intermediate filament binding protein desmoplakin. This complex anchors the desmosome to the cytoskeleton of the cell, and thus indirectly to the sarcomere, nuclear membrane, and the dystrophin-associated glycoproteins.

has been well defined, other aspects of desmosomal function, including putative roles in cell-cell signaling and intracellular calcium handling, are now being explored.[52,53] How disruption of these cell junctions by mutant proteins leads to cutaneous or myocardial disease remains unknown. Perturbed passive mechanical properties and remodeling of the intercalated disc have been documented,[54] but these alone are unlikely to be the sole explanations of the unique susceptibility of the RV in desmosomal disorders. Effects on myocyte differentiation and the development of the RV have been invoked, but experimental support is limited. Mice with a cardiac-specific deletion of desmoplakin recreate many of the pathologic features of ARVC. This work also demonstrated that the perturbation of the Wnt/β-catenin pathway in these hearts was sufficient to push the myocardial cells toward an adipocyte cell fate and away from a myocardial cell fate.[55] These data suggest that several steps in RV development and differentiation are likely to be disrupted in ARVC.[56] Spontaneous large animal models of ARVC may prove useful if molecular parallels with human disease are proven,[57] but understanding the entire pathophysiologic process may require the creation of genetically faithful knock-in mouse models.[58]

DIAGNOSIS

The intrinsic difficulties in making a definitive diagnosis in ARVC are evident from the existence of the Task Force criteria. Many of the management problems stem from overdiagnosis of isolated individuals with incidental findings or underdiagnosis of relatives of individuals with a clear history of ARVC or sudden death. The most helpful approach to diagnosis is prefaced by an initial estimate of the prior probability of ARVC in any given individual (**Fig. 3**). This estimate must be based on a careful consideration of the patient's history of syncope or palpitations, documented arrhythmias, and a rigorous family history. When weighting the family history, it is important to bear in mind the extent of the available information; for example, the absence of a history of sudden death is unhelpful in the face of a limited number of at-risk relatives. Difficult cases are best managed in centers with extensive expertise in the diagnosis and management of ARVC, ideally with systematic evaluation of the entire family.

Electrocardiography

Electrocardiography (ECG) may be useful in making the diagnosis of ARVC, but only in the appropriate clinical context (see **Fig. 1**C). The classic finding of an epsilon wave in the right-sided precordial leads occurred in 20% to 40% of subjects with definitive ARVC, but rarely in other disorders.[59] ECG findings such as T-wave inversion or prolonged S waves in precordial leads V_1 to V_3 may help discriminate between ARVC and RVOT but are not specific in the general

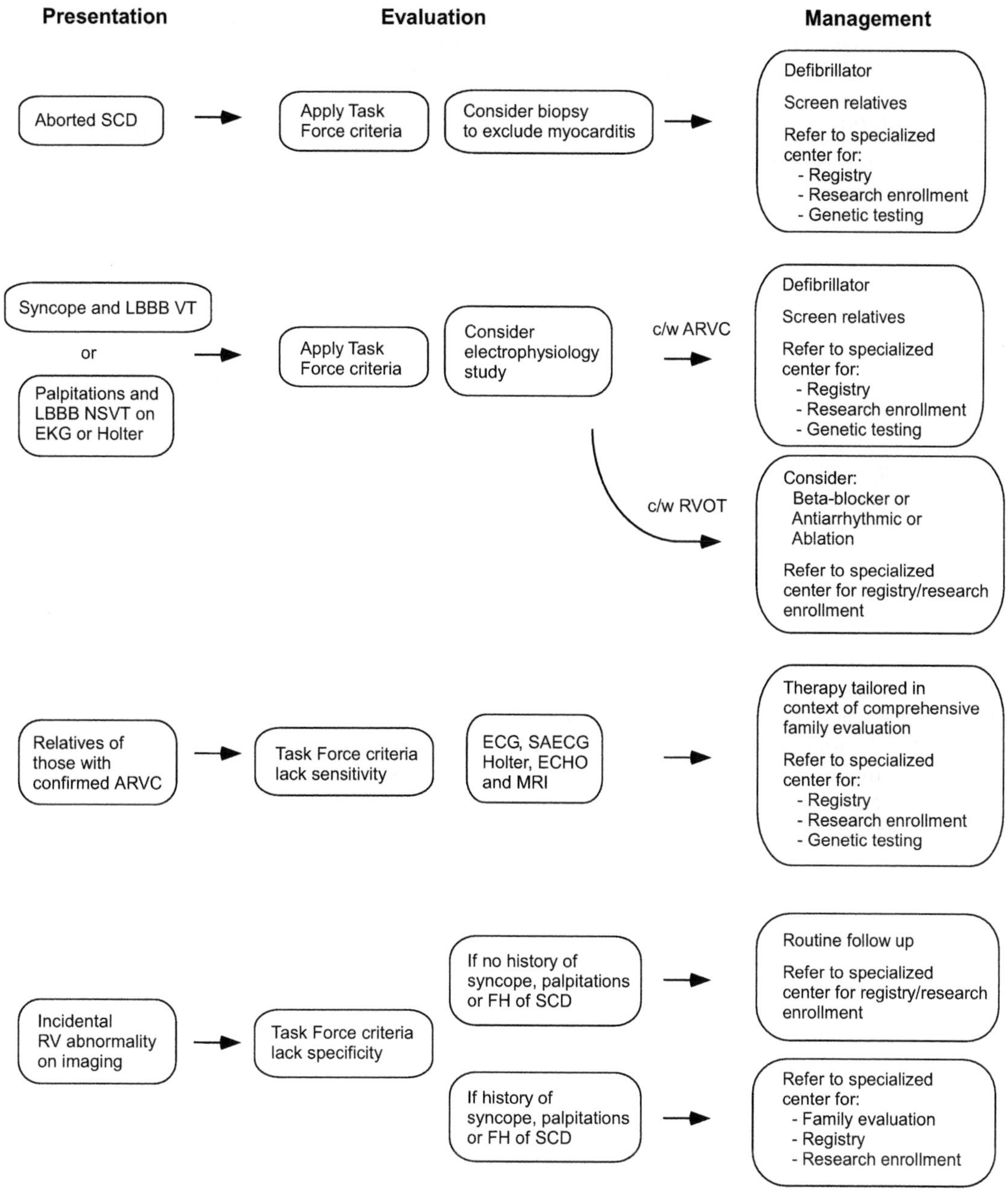

Fig. 3. A simplified management algorithm for commonly encountered presentations of ARVC.

population.[60] Some investigators have seen substantial progression in QRS duration in most of subjects over follow-up periods of 1 to 10 years, but others have seen no ECG progression over several years.[61,62]

Holter monitoring studies consistently identify high rates of ectopy arising from the RV, but here also, specificity is context dependent.[63] Sinoatrial disease and atrial fibrillation are not uncommon. The application of the signal-averaged ECG (SAECG) was expected to improve the sensitivity of noninvasive detection of RV disease, and this has been confirmed by several studies.[64,65] The use of total filtered QRS (fQRS) duration is sensitive in general as a marker of myocardial disease with several studies suggesting detection rates of more than 90%.[66] In ARVC cohorts, the fQRS duration is predictive of inducible VT at EPS. However, the specificity of SAECG for ARVC depends on the prior probability of disease, and the technique is most likely to be useful in the cases of family members of those already definitively diagnosed.[37] Other forms of ECG analysis such as measures of QT dispersion have failed to generate reproducible results.[67–70]

Echocardiography

Echocardiographic findings reported in definitive ARVC cases include RV dilation, reduced RV ejection fraction, and focal right ventricular aneurysms. Recent work paying particular attention to the acquisition of RV images revealed that most ARVC patients have some identifiable echocardiographic abnormality.[71] Only 35% of subjects had normal RV function, and most of these were found to have a focal-wall motion abnormality or morphologic abnormality (see **Fig. 1**D and E). The principal observation from this study was that RVOT enlargement (defined as a diastolic RVOT dimension of 30 mm or greater in the long-axis view) was a reproducible echocardiographic index of RV dilation. It remains to be seen whether such findings discriminate between ARVC and RVOT, and their specificity in unselected cohorts remains unknown.[72] Correlation with other techniques in validated ARVC patients and broader population studies are required to place these data in perspective. Echocardiographic assessment in ARVC requires considerable expertise given the complex 3-dimensional geometry of the RV, the lack of standard reference views, and the load dependence of RV function.

Magnetic Resonance Imaging

MRI enables tomographic imaging of the entire RV and combines functional data with tissue characterization capable of detecting fibrofatty replacement of the myocardium (see **Fig. 1**A and B). Although initial studies were encouraging, overdependence on this technique in the diagnosis of ARVC and the widespread application of cardiac MRI outside of specialized centers with consequent reduced specificity and sensitivity have led to its reappraisal.[19,73] MRI data from larger populations confirm that intramyocardial fat is seen in substantial numbers of normal individuals. In addition, there are cases of documented ARVC in which the fibrofatty infiltration was not detected by antemortem imaging. More recent work suggests that late enhancement with gadolinium may improve the detection of intramural fibrous regions. Several studies suggest that RV size and function may be more reproducible than the presence or absence of myocardial fibrofatty infiltration, but interobserver variability remains a major issue.[74,75] However, most of the current approaches have been tested only in small cohorts, and it requires considerable effort to derive rigorous quantitative end points that can reliably discriminate ARVC from other RV pathology or from normal cases.

Computed Tomographic Imaging

There is little experience with the use of computed tomographic (CT) scanning in ARVC, but more recent electron-beam multislice scanners may offer a reasonable alternative in cases where MRI is not feasible.[73] Current protocols are able to detect intramyocardial fat, define structural anomalies, and quantitate RV size and function. However, there are few data on the sensitivity or specificity of CT scanning for the diagnosis of ARVC.

Electrophysiology Study

The electrophysiologic evaluation of small series of individuals with an LBBB-morphology VT suggests that it may be possible to discriminate successfully between those with ARVC and benign RVOT. Subjects with ARVC were much more likely to have a reentrant tachycardia than those with RVOT who predominantly exhibited automatic tachycardias. In addition, subjects with ARVC were more likely to exhibit fragmented diastolic potentials, multiple inducible tachycardias, a lower success rate for ablation, and lower long-term success rates.[76,77] Electroanatomic mapping of affected regions in subjects with ARVC revealed lower unipolar amplitudes and a prolonged electrocardiographic duration compared with RVOT subjects or healthy controls.[78–80] The judicious use of invasive electrophysiologic studies may be helpful in the evaluation of intermediate phenotypes (see **Fig. 3**).

Cardiac Catheterization and RV Biopsy

The role of cardiac catheterization in the diagnosis or management of subjects with ARVC is limited. Individuals may undergo a cardiac catheterization to rule out occlusive coronary disease or to permit the evaluation of RV and LV function, but this is institution dependent. Investigators have identified subjective abnormalities of the RV in many individuals, including deep fissures in the anterior wall, moderator bands, apical aneurysms, and outflow tract dilation. Objective findings in support of the diagnosis of ARVC are uncommon.[81]

Endomyocardial biopsy has not been widely used in ARVC, largely because of concern about sampling errors in a regional disease and the risks of free-wall biopsy.[82,83] Several small studies have suggested that biopsy may be safe and a useful adjunct to noninvasive studies.[84] The greatest utility may be to identify other suspected causes of RV pathology.[83]

Genetic Testing

The identification of PKP2 mutations in up to 70% of selected cases suggests that defects in this gene may be a common cause of ARVC.[8–10] At present, there is no rationale for genetic testing outside of active research protocols, but as the causes of other forms of ARVC emerge and prognostic data accrue for these various entities, this may change. Deriving meaningful prognostic data from the small numbers of ARVC patients remains a challenge, and these difficulties are compounded by genetic and allelic heterogeneity.[49] These issues emphasize the need for the referral of probands and families to tertiary care centers with active genetic research programs, and the systematic collection of clinical data across the entire spectrum of idiopathic RV disease in large multicenter registries.[22]

DIFFERENTIAL DIAGNOSIS

Several other known conditions may exhibit some of the clinical features of ARVC and confound the diagnosis (**Table 2**). These disorders are associated with a spectrum of structural and functional involvement of the RV.

Idiopathic VT arising in the RV outflow tract is increasingly recognized as a benign form of arrhythmia occurring in the absence of any detectable structural heart disease. RVOT tachycardias are usually responsive to β-blockade, and at electrophysiology study (EPS), they are characteristically automatic in nature and amenable to ablation.[85,86] There is imaging, electrophysiologic and genetic evidence that ARVC and RVOT tachycardia are distinct processes.[76,85,87] Automatic RVOT tachycardia may be caused by somatic myocardial mutations in some cases,[88] but they do not appear to be associated with mutations in desmosomal genes.

Uhl anomaly classically presents as a completely atrophic RV, with little or no contractile tissue and functional tricuspid atresia in the neonatal period. Nevertheless, adult presentations have been described, occasionally with ventricular arrhythmias, but more often with intractable RV failure.[89] The distinction between Uhl and extreme forms of ARVC may not be possible even at autopsy. Multiple cases of Uhls have been reported on fetal echocardiography in single sibships, raising the possibility of a genetic basis.[90]

Perhaps the largest group of disorders within the differential diagnosis may be other right ventricular cardiomyopathies. Whether some of these represent distinct disease processes or simply milder variants of ARVC is unclear. Subtle forms of Ebstein anomaly, right ventricular noncompaction, or focal RV involvement with inflammatory disorders such as sarcoidosis, or even isolated RV infarction are among other reported confounders.[31,59,83] Disproportionate abnormalities of RV function are also seen in human immunodeficiency virus patients. Ultimately, the relationships between ARVC and other RV processes may be clarified by genetic techniques.

End-stage forms of ARVC are clinically indistinguishable from other forms of idiopathic biventricular failure. At present, the only convincing method of discriminating between ARVC and dilated cardiomyopathy is direct screening of the extended family to detect less advanced forms

Table 2
Differential diagnosis in ARVC

Diagnosis	Useful Discriminants
Right ventricular outflow tract tachycardia	Imaging Electrophysiology study
Uhl anomaly	Unknown
Idiopathic dilated cardiomyopathy	Evaluation of extended family
Focal RV myocarditis	RV biopsy
HIV-induced cardiomyopathy	Clinical context
Isolated RV infarction	Coronary angiography
Ebstein anomaly	Imaging Electrophysiology study
Sarcoidosis	RV biopsy
Carcinoid	Clinical context

of ARVC in relatives. Genetic testing eventually may be able to perform these diagnostic and screening functions.[49] Although left ventricular hypertrophy is seen in autopsy series of ARVC, it is not widely reported in clinical studies, and discrimination from hypertrophic cardiomyopathy is not a common problem.[25]

Clinical Management

The management of ARVC is focused largely on the prevention of sudden death. In those who experience syncopal events or have symptomatic VT or have survived a cardiac arrest, the appropriate interventions are obvious. However, an increasing number of individuals have some features of ARVC, but its correct diagnosis and management in them remain unclear. It is unlikely that rigorous, controlled data will become available for most interventions in ARVC; therefore, therapeutic decisions are driven by sensible extrapolation from related clinical settings. Until more rigorous data are available, the approach to ARVC is best viewed within the context of the Task Force criteria while highlighting necessary qualifiers and the overall limitations of this strategy (see **Fig. 3** and **Table 2**).

Antiarrhythmic Medications

Because most definitive ARVC cases are now treated with implantable cardioverter defibrillators (ICDs), pharmacologic antiarrhythmic therapy is typically adjunctive. In the absence of severe RV contractile dysfunction, β-blockers are well tolerated. The class III agent sotalol, which also exhibits some β antagonism, has emerged as a first-line therapy.[91,92] Amiodarone is a second line agent in patients with refractory ventricular arrhythmias.

Implantable Cardioverter Defibrillator

With the expanding indications for ICD use, prophylactic ICD implantation in definitive cases of ARVC has become the mainstay of therapy. Randomized controlled trials are not feasible in such a rare and heterogeneous syndrome, but observational studies confirm that defibrillators are effective in preventing sudden death in high-risk cohorts. The most extensive series consisted of 132 patients, and more than 70% of them presented with a ventricular fibrillation arrest or sustained VT.[93] During a mean follow-up of 39 months, nearly one-half of the patients had an appropriate therapy, 16% had an inappropriate therapy, and 14% had a device-related complication. ICD implantation in affected members of high-risk families confirms these findings.[29]

In cohorts with a lower incidence of aborted sudden cardiac death or unstable VT on presentation, the risk-benefit ratio may still favor an ICD.[94] The induction of LBBB morphology VT on a preimplantation EPS may predict appropriate ICD therapy. Similar outcomes were observed in several other smaller studies.[95,96] There may be a high rate of arrhythmia storm in this population, raising the possibility that sudden death is a result of an additional process, such as inflammation, superimposed on the basal ARVC substrate.[94] Increasingly, ICDs are implanted in individuals with little evidence of an elevated risk of sudden death.[19]

Catheter Ablation

The VTs observed in patients with ARVC are amenable to entrainment mapping similar to more common scar-mediated ventricular arrhythmias. Typical patients exhibit multiple inducible VTs, as expected in a diffuse cardiomyopathy. Nevertheless, ablation is successful in approximately 50% of the cases, suggesting that it may play a useful palliative role in the management of recurrent arrhythmias.[87,97]

Heart Failure Therapies

The precise incidence of heart failure in ARVC is unknown and probably varies widely with the specific underlying cause. The high frequency of RV hypokinesis, RV aneurysms, and regional wall motion abnormalities in ARVC suggests that formal anticoagulation might have a role to play.[33] There are reports of pulmonary or systemic embolism in ARVC; however, these are study specific. Angiotensin-converting enzyme inhibitors, or other vasodilators if these are contraindicated, seem reasonable if there is clinical evidence of heart failure, particularly in the presence of LV dysfunction. Cardiac transplantation is unusual in ARVC but has been performed for incessant VT and end-stage contractile failure.[98] It is possible that with the prevention of sudden death by ICD, ventricular dysfunction in later stages of ARVC will be uncovered.

Exercise Recommendations

Several smaller series have suggested a role for adrenergic drive or exercise in the precipitation of fatal arrhythmias.[31] However, the only large unselected series found that almost all sudden deaths occurred during normal daily activities.[25] Nevertheless, it may be reasonable to recommend the avoidance of strenuous activity.

Screening of Relatives

ARVC is frequently an inherited disease, exhibits reduced penetrance, and may present with sudden death. These observations, combined with the apparent success of the ICD therapy, predicate the directed screening of asymptomatic, at-risk (that is, at risk for having inherited the same genetic defect) family members. In the context of a probability of up to .50 that a given relative has inherited the gene defect causing ARVC in the proband, even minor cardiac abnormalities well below the threshold set by the Task Force guidelines take on great significance. In view of the reduced penetrance observed in most families, screening should be extended throughout the kindred to at least one generation beyond the last affected individual. In ARVC, as in other Mendelian forms of cardiomyopathy, the implications of subtle clinical findings often are only interpretable in the context of data from the entire extended family.[3] For this reason, such assessments are best undertaken at tertiary centers with a special interest in inherited forms of sudden death. Legislated investigation of unexplained sudden death by specialist teams is under evaluation in some countries.

Asymptomatic family members with a normal comprehensive evaluation are less likely to have inherited the gene defect, but should undergo follow-up at regular intervals (every 2–3 years) until definitive diagnostic tools are available. In the context of a proband with confirmed disease, family members with subtle signs of ARVC but no symptoms almost certainly are affected, but their risk of progressing to develop clinical problems is difficult to define. At present, decisions regarding ICD implantation in relatives are best undertaken in specialized centers with expertise in the management and counseling of families with ARVC. Until the different disease entities underlying ARVC are understood and robust clinical or molecular prognostic tools are available, decisions on prophylactic ICD placement should be circumspect.

FUTURE STUDIES AND SUMMARY

A central goal of future studies must be the systematic collection of unbiased cohorts not only of individuals who meet Task Force criteria, but also the relatives of probands with definitive ARVC and other individuals in whom the diagnosis is being considered. When combined with proband-based clinical and molecular genetic studies, such systematic data collection allows the prospective testing and weighting of any proposed diagnostic criteria. Wherever possible, the development of reproducible quantitative indexes of RV structure and function facilitates comparisons between cohorts and the normal population. Efforts to develop novel diagnostic modalities, including biomarkers, molecular imaging, and genetic testing are under way, and innovative approaches exploiting the pathophysiologic links with other tissues such as skin could be productive.

The identification of the causal mutations in different forms of ARVC may enable the discrimination of gene-specific features. Because the causal genes are so mechanistically faithful, animal models will become feasible. It is important to explore the pathways by which desmosomal dysfunction results in the perturbation of normal myocardial differentiation and ultimately leads to RV cardiomyopathy and arrhythmias. Understanding the basis of RV development and the unique features of RV structure and function assists the dissection of disease mechanisms and sheds light on potential therapies and prevention.

REFERENCES

1. Thiene G, Nava A, Corrado D, et al. Right ventricular cardiomyopathy and sudden death in young people. N Engl J Med 1988;318(3):129–33.
2. Marcus FI, Fontaine GH, Guiraudon G, et al. Right ventricular dysplasia: a report of 24 adult cases. Circulation 1982;65(2):384–98.
3. Hamid MS, Norman M, Quraishi A, et al. Prospective evaluation of relatives for familial arrhythmogenic right ventricular cardiomyopathy/dysplasia reveals a need to broaden diagnostic criteria. J Am Coll Cardiol 2002;40(8):1445–50.
4. Nava A, Bauce B, Basso C, et al. Clinical profile and long-term follow-up of 37 families with arrhythmogenic right ventricular cardiomyopathy. J Am Coll Cardiol 2000;36(7):2226–33.
5. Coonar AS, Protonotarios N, Tsatsopoulou A, et al. Gene for arrhythmogenic right ventricular cardiomyopathy with diffuse nonepidermolytic palmoplantar keratoderma and woolly hair (Naxos disease) maps to 17q21. Circulation 1998;97(20):2049–58.
6. McKoy G, Protonotarios N, Crosby A, et al. Identification of a deletion in plakoglobin in arrhythmogenic right ventricular cardiomyopathy with palmoplantar keratoderma and woolly hair (Naxos disease). Lancet 2000;355(9221):2119–24.
7. Asimaki A, Syrris P, Wichter T, et al. A novel dominant mutation in plakoglobin causes arrhythmogenic right ventricular cardiomyopathy. Am J Hum Genet 2007;81(5):964–73.
8. Gerull B, Heuser A, Wichter T, et al. Mutations in the desmosomal protein plakophilin-2 are common in

arrhythmogenic right ventricular cardiomyopathy. Nat Genet 2004;36(11):1162–4.
9. van Tintelen JP, Entius MM, Bhuiyan ZA, et al. Plakophilin-2 mutations are the major determinant of familial arrhythmogenic right ventricular dysplasia/cardiomyopathy. Circulation 2006;113(13):1650–8.
10. Dalal D, Molin LH, Piccini J, et al. Clinical features of arrhythmogenic right ventricular dysplasia/cardiomyopathy associated with mutations in plakophilin-2. Circulation 2006;113(13):1641–9.
11. Syrris P, Ward D, Evans A, et al. Arrhythmogenic right ventricular dysplasia/cardiomyopathy associated with mutations in the desmosomal gene desmocollin-2. Am J Hum Genet 2006;79(5):978–84.
12. Heuser A, Plovie ER, Ellinor PT, et al. Mutant desmocollin-2 causes arrhythmogenic right ventricular cardiomyopathy. Am J Hum Genet 2006;79(6):1081–8.
13. Norgett EE, Hatsell SJ, Carvajal-Huerta L, et al. Recessive mutation in desmoplakin disrupts desmoplakin-intermediate filament interactions and causes dilated cardiomyopathy, woolly hair and keratoderma. Hum Mol Genet 2000;9(18):2761–6.
14. Rampazzo A, Nava A, Malacrida S, et al. Mutation in human desmoplakin domain binding to plakoglobin causes a dominant form of arrhythmogenic right ventricular cardiomyopathy. Am J Hum Genet 2002;71(5):1200–6.
15. Norman M, Simpson M, Mogensen J, et al. Novel mutation in desmoplakin causes arrhythmogenic left ventricular cardiomyopathy. Circulation 2005;112(5):636–42.
16. Pilichou K, Nava A, Basso C, et al. Mutations in desmoglein-2 gene are associated with arrhythmogenic right ventricular cardiomyopathy. Circulation 2006;113(9):1171–9.
17. Awad MM, Dalal D, Cho E, et al. DSG2 mutations contribute to arrhythmogenic right ventricular dysplasia/cardiomyopathy. Am J Hum Genet 2006;79(1):136–42.
18. Seidman JG, Seidman C. The genetic basis for cardiomyopathy: from mutation identification to mechanistic paradigms. Cell 2001;104(4):557–67.
19. Bomma C, Rutberg J, Tandri H, et al. Misdiagnosis of arrhythmogenic right ventricular dysplasia/cardiomyopathy. J Cardiovasc Electrophysiol 2004;15(3):300–6.
20. Corrado D, Basso C, Thiene G. Arrhythmogenic right ventricular cardiomyopathy: diagnosis, prognosis, and treatment. Heart 2000;83(5):588–95.
21. Basso C, Wichter T, Danieli GA, et al. Arrhythmogenic right ventricular cardiomyopathy: clinical registry and database, evaluation of therapies, pathology registry, DNA banking. Eur Heart J 2004;25(6):531–4.
22. Marcus F, Towbin JA, Zareba W, et al. Arrhythmogenic right ventricular dysplasia/cardiomyopathy (ARVD/C): a multidisciplinary study: design and protocol. Circulation 2003;107(23):2975–8.
23. McKenna WJ, Thiene G, Nava A, et al. Diagnosis of arrhythmogenic right ventricular dysplasia/cardiomyopathy. Task Force of the Working Group Myocardial and Pericardial Disease of the European Society of Cardiology and of the Scientific Council on Cardiomyopathies of the International Society and Federation of Cardiology. Br Heart J 1994;71(3):215–8.
24. Priori SG, Aliot E, Blomstrom-Lundqvist C, et al. Task force on sudden cardiac death of the European Society of cardiology. Eur Heart J 2001;22(16):1374–450.
25. Tabib A, Loire R, Chalabreysse L, et al. Circumstances of death and gross and microscopic observations in a series of 200 cases of sudden death associated with arrhythmogenic right ventricular cardiomyopathy and/or dysplasia. Circulation 2003;108(24):3000–5.
26. Hulot JS, Jouven X, Empana JP, et al. Natural history and risk stratification of arrhythmogenic right ventricular dysplasia/cardiomyopathy. Circulation 2004;110(14):1879–84.
27. Dalal D, Nasir K, Bomma C, et al. Arrhythmogenic right ventricular dysplasia: a United States experience. Circulation 2005;112(25):3823–32.
28. Yoshioka N, Tsuchihashi K, Yuda S, et al. Electrocardiographic and echocardiographic abnormalities in patients with arrhythmogenic right ventricular cardiomyopathy and in their pedigrees. Am J Cardiol 2000;85(7):885–9, A889.
29. Hodgkinson KA, Parfrey PS, Bassett AS, et al. The impact of implantable cardioverter-defibrillator therapy on survival in autosomal-dominant arrhythmogenic right ventricular cardiomyopathy (ARVD5). J Am Coll Cardiol 2005;45(3):400–8.
30. Corrado D, Fontaine G, Marcus FI, et al. Arrhythmogenic right ventricular dysplasia/cardiomyopathy: need for an international registry. Study Group on Arrhythmogenic Right Ventricular Dysplasia/Cardiomyopathy of the Working Groups on Myocardial and Pericardial Disease and Arrhythmias of the European Society of Cardiology and of the Scientific Council on Cardiomyopathies of the World Heart Federation. Circulation 2000;101(11):E101–6.
31. Sen-Chowdhry S, Lowe MD, Sporton SC, et al. Arrhythmogenic right ventricular cardiomyopathy: clinical presentation, diagnosis, and management. Am J Med 2004;117(9):685–95.
32. Basso C, Thiene G, Corrado D, et al. Arrhythmogenic right ventricular cardiomyopathy. Dysplasia, dystrophy, or myocarditis? Circulation 1996;94(5):983–91.
33. Corrado D, Basso C, Thiene G, et al. Spectrum of clinicopathologic manifestations of arrhythmogenic right ventricular cardiomyopathy/dysplasia: a multicenter study. J Am Coll Cardiol 1997;30(6):1512–20.

34. Burke AP, Farb A, Tashko G, et al. Arrhythmogenic right ventricular cardiomyopathy and fatty replacement of the right ventricular myocardium: are they different diseases? Circulation 1998; 97(16):1571–80.
35. Mallat Z, Tedgui A, Fontaliran F, et al. Evidence of apoptosis in arrhythmogenic right ventricular dysplasia. N Engl J Med 1996;335(16):1190–6.
36. De Pasquale CG, Heddle WF. Left sided arrhythmogenic ventricular dysplasia in siblings. Heart 2001; 86(2):128–30.
37. Hermida JS, Minassian A, Jarry G, et al. Familial incidence of late ventricular potentials and electrocardiographic abnormalities in arrhythmogenic right ventricular dysplasia. Am J Cardiol 1997;79(10): 1375–80.
38. Beffagna G, Occhi G, Nava A, et al. Regulatory mutations in transforming growth factor-beta3 gene cause arrhythmogenic right ventricular cardiomyopathy type 1. Cardiovasc Res 2005;65(2):366–73.
39. Rampazzo A, Nava A, Danieli GA, et al. The gene for arrhythmogenic right ventricular cardiomyopathy maps to chromosome 14q23-q24. Hum Mol Genet 1994;3(6):959–62.
40. Rampazzo A, Nava A, Erne P, et al. A new locus for arrhythmogenic right ventricular cardiomyopathy (ARVD2) maps to chromosome 1q42-q43. Hum Mol Genet 1995;4(11):2151–4.
41. Tiso N, Stephan DA, Nava A, et al. Identification of mutations in the cardiac ryanodine receptor gene in families affected with arrhythmogenic right ventricular cardiomyopathy type 2 (ARVD2). Hum Mol Genet 2001;10(3):189–94.
42. Severini GM, Krajinovic M, Pinamonti B, et al. A new locus for arrhythmogenic right ventricular dysplasia on the long arm of chromosome 14. Genomics 1996;31(2):193–200.
43. Rampazzo A, Nava A, Miorin M, et al. ARVD4, a new locus for arrhythmogenic right ventricular cardiomyopathy, maps to chromosome 2 long arm. Genomics 1997;45(2):259–63.
44. Ahmad F, Li D, Karibe A, et al. Localization of a gene responsible for arrhythmogenic right ventricular dysplasia to chromosome 3p23. Circulation 1998; 98(25):2791–5.
45. Merner ND, Hodgkinson KA, Haywood AF, et al. Arrhythmogenic right ventricular cardiomyopathy type 5 is a fully penetrant, lethal arrhythmic disorder caused by a missense mutation in the TMEM43 gene. Am J Hum Genet 2008;82(4):809–21.
46. Li D, Ahmad F, Gardner MJ, et al. The locus of a novel gene responsible for arrhythmogenic right-ventricular dysplasia characterized by early onset and high penetrance maps to chromosome 10p12-p14. Am J Hum Genet 2000;66(1):148–56.
47. Melberg A, Oldfors A, Blomstrom-Lundqvist C, et al. Autosomal dominant myofibrillar myopathy with arrhythmogenic right ventricular cardiomyopathy linked to chromosome 10q. Ann Neurol 1999;46(5): 684–92.
48. Frances R, Rodriguez Benitez AM, Cohen DR. Arrhythmogenic right ventricular dysplasia and anterior polar cataract. Am J Med Genet 1997;73(2): 125–6.
49. MacRae CA, Ellinor PT. Genetic screening and risk assessment in hypertrophic cardiomyopathy. J Am Coll Cardiol 2004;44(12):2326–8.
50. Protonotarios N, Tsatsopoulou A. Naxos disease and Carvajal syndrome: cardiocutaneous disorders that highlight the pathogenesis and broaden the spectrum of arrhythmogenic right ventricular cardiomyopathy. Cardiovasc Pathol 2004;13(4):185–94.
51. Thiene G, Corrado D, Basso C. Cardiomyopathies: is it time for a molecular classification? Eur Heart J 2004;25(20):1772–5.
52. Jamora C, Fuchs E. Intercellular adhesion, signalling and the cytoskeleton. Nat Cell Biol 2002;4(4): E101–8.
53. Green KJ, Gaudry CA. Are desmosomes more than tethers for intermediate filaments? Nat Rev Mol Cell Biol 2000;1(3):208–16.
54. Basso C, Czarnowska E, Barbera MD, et al. Ultrastructural evidence of intercalated disc remodelling in arrhythmogenic right ventricular cardiomyopathy: an electron microscopy investigation on endomyocardial biopsies. Eur Heart J 2006;27(15):1847–54.
55. Garcia-Gras E, Lombardi R, Giocondo MJ, et al. Suppression of canonical Wnt/beta-catenin signaling by nuclear plakoglobin recapitulates phenotype of arrhythmogenic right ventricular cardiomyopathy. J Clin Invest 2006;116(7):2012–21.
56. Brembeck FH, Rosario M, Birchmeier W. Balancing cell adhesion and Wnt signaling, the key role of beta-catenin. Curr Opin Genet Dev 2006;16(1):51–9.
57. Basso C, Fox PR, Meurs KM, et al. Arrhythmogenic right ventricular cardiomyopathy causing sudden cardiac death in boxer dogs: a new animal model of human disease. Circulation 2004; 109(9):1180–5.
58. Milan DJ, MacRae CA. Animal models for arrhythmias. Cardiovasc Res 2005;67(3):426–37.
59. Santucci PA, Morton JB, Picken MM, et al. Electroanatomic mapping of the right ventricle in a patient with a giant epsilon wave, ventricular tachycardia, and cardiac sarcoidosis. J Cardiovasc Electrophysiol 2004;15(9):1091–4.
60. Piccini JP, Nasir K, Bomma C, et al. Electrocardiographic findings over time in arrhythmogenic right ventricular dysplasia/cardiomyopathy. Am J Cardiol 2005;96(1):122–6.
61. Jaoude SA, Leclercq JF, Coumel P. Progressive ECG changes in arrhythmogenic right ventricular disease. Evidence for an evolving disease. Eur Heart J 1996;17(11):1717–22.

62. Peters S, Trummel M. Diagnosis of arrhythmogenic right ventricular dysplasia-cardiomyopathy: value of standard ECG revisited. Ann Noninvasive Electrocardiol 2003;8(3):238–45.
63. Leclercq JF, Coumel P. Characteristics, prognosis and treatment of the ventricular arrhythmias of right ventricular dysplasia. Eur Heart J 1989;(10 Suppl D):61–7.
64. Turrini P, Angelini A, Thiene G, et al. Late potentials and ventricular arrhythmias in arrhythmogenic right ventricular cardiomyopathy. Am J Cardiol 1999; 83(8):1214–9.
65. Spier AW, Meurs KM. Use of signal-averaged electrocardiography in the evaluation of arrhythmogenic right ventricular cardiomyopathy in boxers. J Am Vet Med Assoc 2004;225(7):1050–5.
66. Nasir K, Tandri H, Rutberg J, et al. Filtered QRS duration on signal-averaged electrocardiography predicts inducibility of ventricular tachycardia in arrhythmogenic right ventricle dysplasia. Pacing Clin Electrophysiol 2003;26(10):1955–60.
67. Kazmierczak J, De Sutter J, Tavernier R, et al. Electrocardiographic and morphometric features in patients with ventricular tachycardia of right ventricular origin. Heart 1998;79(4):388–93.
68. Benn M, Hansen PS, Pedersen AK. QT dispersion in patients with arrhythmogenic right ventricular dysplasia. Eur Heart J 1999;20(10):764–70.
69. Wolk R. Is QT dispersion a reliable index of heterogeneity of ventricular repolarization and a proarrhythmic marker? Eur Heart J 2000;21(1):79–80.
70. Turrini P, Corrado D, Basso C, et al. Dispersion of ventricular depolarization-repolarization: a noninvasive marker for risk stratification in arrhythmogenic right ventricular cardiomyopathy. Circulation 2001; 103(25):3075–80.
71. Yoerger DM, Marcus F, Sherrill D, et al. Echocardiographic findings in patients meeting task force criteria for arrhythmogenic right ventricular dysplasia: new insights from the multidisciplinary study of right ventricular dysplasia. J Am Coll Cardiol 2005;45(6):860–5.
72. Scheinman MM, Crawford MH. Echocardiographic findings and the search for a gold standard in patients with arrhythmogenic right ventricular dysplasia. J Am Coll Cardiol 2005;45(6):866–7.
73. Tandri H, Bomma C, Calkins H, et al. Magnetic resonance and computed tomography imaging of arrhythmogenic right ventricular dysplasia. J Magn Reson Imaging 2004;19(6):848–58.
74. Bluemke DA, Krupinski EA, Ovitt T, et al. MR Imaging of arrhythmogenic right ventricular cardiomyopathy: morphologic findings and interobserver reliability. Cardiology 2003;99(3):153–62.
75. Tandri H, Calkins H, Marcus FI. Controversial role of magnetic resonance imaging in the diagnosis of arrhythmogenic right ventricular dysplasia. Am J Cardiol 2003;92(5):649.
76. O'Donnell D, Cox D, Bourke J, et al. Clinical and electrophysiological differences between patients with arrhythmogenic right ventricular dysplasia and right ventricular outflow tract tachycardia. Eur Heart J 2003;24(9):801–10.
77. Niroomand F, Carbucicchio C, Tondo C, et al. Electrophysiological characteristics and outcome in patients with idiopathic right ventricular arrhythmia compared with arrhythmogenic right ventricular dysplasia. Heart 2002;87(1):41–7.
78. Boulos M, Lashevsky I, Reisner S, et al. Electroanatomic mapping of arrhythmogenic right ventricular dysplasia. J Am Coll Cardiol 2001;38(7):2020–7.
79. Boulos M, Lashevsky I, Gepstein L. Usefulness of electroanatomical mapping to differentiate between right ventricular outflow tract tachycardia and arrhythmogenic right ventricular dysplasia. Am J Cardiol 2005;95(8):935–40.
80. Corrado D, Basso C, Leoni L, et al. Three-dimensional electroanatomic voltage mapping increases accuracy of diagnosing arrhythmogenic right ventricular cardiomyopathy/dysplasia. Circulation 2005;111(23):3042–50.
81. Hebert JL, Chemla D, Gerard O, et al. Angiographic right and left ventricular function in arrhythmogenic right ventricular dysplasia. Am J Cardiol 2004; 93(6):728–33.
82. Angelini A, Basso C, Nava A, et al. Endomyocardial biopsy in arrhythmogenic right ventricular cardiomyopathy. Am Heart J 1996;132(1 Pt 1):203–6.
83. Chimenti C, Pieroni M, Maseri A, et al. Histologic findings in patients with clinical and instrumental diagnosis of sporadic arrhythmogenic right ventricular dysplasia. J Am Coll Cardiol 2004;43(12):2305–13.
84. Wichter T, Hindricks G, Lerch H, et al. Regional myocardial sympathetic dysinnervation in arrhythmogenic right ventricular cardiomyopathy. An analysis using ^{123}I-meta-iodobenzylguanidine scintigraphy. Circulation 1994;89(2):667–83.
85. Lerman BB, Stein KM, Markowitz SM. Adenosine-sensitive ventricular tachycardia: a conceptual approach. J Cardiovasc Electrophysiol 1996;7(6): 559–69.
86. Joshi S, Wilber DJ. Ablation of idiopathic right ventricular outflow tract tachycardia: current perspectives. J Cardiovasc Electrophysiol 2005; 16(Suppl 1):S52–8.
87. Ellison KE, Friedman PL, Ganz LI, et al. Entrainment mapping and radiofrequency catheter ablation of ventricular tachycardia in right ventricular dysplasia. J Am Coll Cardiol 1998;32(3):724–8.
88. Lerman BB, Dong B, Stein KM, et al. Right ventricular outflow tract tachycardia due to a somatic cell mutation in G protein subunitalphai2. J Clin Invest 1998;101(12):2862–8.
89. Gerlis LM, Schmidt-Ott SC, Ho SY, et al. Dysplastic conditions of the right ventricular myocardium: Uhl's

anomaly vs arrhythmogenic right ventricular dysplasia. Br Heart J 1993;69(2):142–50.
90. Hornung TS, Heads A, Wright C, et al. Fetal diagnosis of lethal dysfunction of the right heart in three siblings. Cardiol Young 2000;10(6):621–4.
91. Wichter T, Borggrefe M, Haverkamp W, et al. Efficacy of antiarrhythmic drugs in patients with arrhythmogenic right ventricular disease. Results in patients with inducible and noninducible ventricular tachycardia. Circulation 1992;86(1):29–37.
92. Wichter T, Paul TM, Eckardt L, et al. Arrhythmogenic right ventricular cardiomyopathy. Antiarrhythmic drugs, catheter ablation, or ICD? Herz 2005;30(2):91–101.
93. Corrado D, Leoni L, Link MS, et al. Implantable cardioverter-defibrillator therapy for prevention of sudden death in patients with arrhythmogenic right ventricular cardiomyopathy/dysplasia. Circulation 2003;108(25):3084–91.
94. Roguin A, Bomma CS, Nasir K, et al. Implantable cardioverter-defibrillators in patients with arrhythmogenic right ventricular dysplasia/cardiomyopathy. J Am Coll Cardiol 2004;43(10):1843–52.
95. Tavernier R, Gevaert S, De Sutter J, et al. Long term results of cardioverter-defibrillator implantation in patients with right ventricular dysplasia and malignant ventricular tachyarrhythmias. Heart 2001;85(1):53–6.
96. Wichter T, Paul M, Wollmann C, et al. Implantable cardioverter/defibrillator therapy in arrhythmogenic right ventricular cardiomyopathy: single-center experience of long-term follow-up and complications in 60 patients. Circulation 2004;109(12):1503–8.
97. Fontaine G, Tonet J, Gallais Y, et al. Ventricular tachycardia catheter ablation in arrhythmogenic right ventricular dysplasia: a 16-year experience. Curr Cardiol Rep 2000;2(6):498–506.
98. Lemola K, Brunckhorst C, Helfenstein U, et al. Predictors of adverse outcome in patients with arrhythmogenic right ventricular dysplasia/cardiomyopathy: long term experience of a tertiary care centre. Heart 2005;91(9):1167–72.

Genetics of Restrictive Cardiomyopathy

Srijita Sen-Chowdhry, MBBS, MD (Cantab), MRCP[a],
Petros Syrris, PhD[b], William J. McKenna, MD, DSc, FRCP[b,*]

KEYWORDS

- Diastolic dysfunction • Constrictive pericarditis
- Myocardial restriction • Restrictive cardiomyopathy
- Sarcomeric disease

Restrictive physiology refers to a hemodynamic state characterized by rapid completion of ventricular filling in early diastole, with little or no further filling in late diastole, owing to compromised ventricular expansion. Ventricular contractility is often maintained. As the most severe form of isolated diastolic dysfunction, restrictive physiology is most usefully presented in the context of the full spectrum of diastolic abnormalities.

DIASTOLIC FUNCTION AND DYSFUNCTION

The diastolic phase of the cardiac cycle begins with active, isovolumic relaxation of the ventricles, which requires energy-dependent calcium uptake in the sarcoplasmic reticulum and uncoupling of actin-myosin cross-bridge bonds.[1] Elastic recoil of the ventricles ensues, with movement of the mitral annulus toward the base, represented on tissue Doppler imaging by the Ea wave.[2] This creates a suction effect that instigates early diastolic filling: the E wave of the mitral and tricuspid valve inflow. With the filling process underway, the ventricle distends to accommodate the influx of blood. This is a passive process that is again determined by the intrinsic elastic properties of the myocardium, collectively termed *compliance*. In late diastole, atrial contraction once again augments filling, generating the A wave of the mitral and tricuspid inflow.

In the young healthy heart, efficient relaxation causes a rapid early drop in intracavity pressure, resulting in high E velocity and an E/A ratio that typically exceeds 1.5. Left ventricular hypertrophy, ischemia, and the normal aging process may all contribute to a gradual reduction in ventricular compliance. The suction effect diminishes, and atrial systole plays a more prominent role in ventricular filling, resulting in E/A reversal, with a ratio of less than 1. The onset of atrial fibrillation may cause decompensation in patients with left ventricular hypertrophy of any etiology, or in the elderly, owing to increased reliance on the atrial kick. At this stage, however, filling pressures generally remain within the normal range.

As ventricular compliance decreases further, limited expansions in volume are associated with significant augmentations in intracavity pressure. The atrial kick becomes less effective and atrial pressure must inevitably increase to maintain an adequate gradient for filling. This, paradoxically, results in a reversion to the original E/A relationship (E/A>1). In the extreme scenario of restrictive physiology, small increments in diastolic volume lead to a precipitous rise in intraventricular pressure. Either or both ventricles may be affected, with elevation of pulmonary and/or systemic venous pressures, atrial dilation, and symptoms and signs of right- or left-sided heart failure.

MYOCARDIAL RESTRICTION VERSUS CONSTRICTIVE PERICARDITIS

Broadly, there are two possible etiologies for restrictive filling: either the myocardium itself has become stiff and noncompliant, or the pericardium has become rigid, constraining further expansion of the ventricles after rapid early filling. This latter

[a] Faculty of Medicine, Imperial College, St Mary's Campus, Norfolk Place, London W2 1NY, UK
[b] Inherited Cardiovascular Disease Group, University College London, The Heart Hospital, 16-18 Westmoreland Street, London W1G 8PH, UK
* Corresponding author.
E-mail address: william.mckenna@uclh.nhs.uk

Heart Failure Clin 6 (2010) 179–186
doi:10.1016/j.hfc.2009.11.005
1551-7136/10/$ – see front matter

phenomenon, termed *constrictive pericarditis*, is characterized pathologically by fibrotic and/or calcific thickening of the pericardium: a sequela of irradiation, hemorrhage, postoperative adhesions, or chronic inflammatory states, such as tuberculosis and uremia.[3] Recognition is critical since surgical pericardiectomy may be curative and undue delays may increase the risk of perioperative mortality.[3] Differentiating constrictive pericarditis from myocardial restriction is far from easy, however, because both the clinical manifestations and echocardiographic appearances may be similar. In the past, exploratory thoracotomy was not uncommonly required to clinch the diagnosis.[4]

One key distinction between the two entities is the presence of prominent respiratory variation in mitral inflow and pulmonary venous flow in patients with constrictive pericarditis. This variation is absent in myocardial restriction. The physiologic basis for this finding is the dissociation of respiratory influences on intrathoracic and intracardiac pressures, consequent to isolation of the heart from the lungs by the inelastic pericardium.[3] The reduction in pulmonary venous pressure during inspiration is therefore not transmitted to the left ventricle, causing a drop in the transmitral pressure gradient and flow velocity, discernible on the pulse wave Doppler signal.[5] At the same time, the right ventricle cannot expand sufficiently to accommodate the increased venous return during inspiration and the phenomenon of ventricular interdependence comes into play. Absent in myocardial restriction owing to septal involvement, ventricular interaction is exaggerated in constrictive pericarditis because of the relatively fixed cardiac volume. The combination of decreased left ventricular filling and rising right ventricular pressures results in leftward septal movement, augmenting tricuspid inflow. The reciprocal changes occur during expiration, with a significant decline in tricuspid flow and an increase in early mitral flow velocity.[3] Until recently, a combination of hemodynamic data from cardiac catheterization, imaging of pericardial thickness, and assessment of variations in pulse wave Doppler signal during respiration were the mainstay bases for evaluation. The reliability of these techniques has been questioned, however, particularly in the diagnosis of occult disease, where resting filling pressures may be normal. Variations in preload and coexisting pulmonary disease or systolic dysfunction may also act as confounders.[2]

The advent of tissue Doppler imaging has since provided an ancillary tool for discriminating constrictive pericarditis from myocardial restriction. The underlying premise is that ventricular wall motion velocities, which can be directly assessed by tissue Doppler imaging, will be deranged in myocardial disease but preserved in constrictive pericarditis.[2] Since isovolumic relaxation precedes the onset of filling, alterations in its rate are less likely to be influenced by preload. A peak early velocity of longitudinal expansion (peak Ea) of more than 8.0 cm/s has been shown to differentiate constriction from restriction with 89% sensitivity and 100% specificity.[5]

SECONDARY CAUSES OF CARDIAC RESTRICTION

In the presence of restrictive physiology, exclusion of constrictive pericarditis is strongly suggestive of myocardial dysfunction, the etiology of which may not be readily apparent. Secondary causes of restriction predominate and are conventionally classified into myocardial and endomyocardial pathologies (**Box 1**).[6] Myocardial causes of restriction may be further subdivided into infiltrative and storage disorders.

Most of the diseases listed in **Box 1** are systemic, although at any given time clinical manifestations may be confined to one organ system. Cardiac involvement is typically a major source of morbidity and mortality. External agents, including drugs and radiation, may be implicated in some cases, while parasitic infection, with its associated eosinophilia, is speculated to have a causative role in endomyocardial fibrosis. Metastatic cancer and carcinoid heart disease are rare causes of restrictive physiology.[6]

In most of the remaining causes of cardiac restriction, a genetic predisposition is either contributory or requisite (**Table 1**).[7] Hurler disease, Gaucher disease, and the glycogen storage disorders are inherited as Mendelian autosomal-recessive traits,[8,9] as are hemochromatosis types 1 through 3, while type 4 hemochromatosis demonstrates autosomal-dominant inheritance.[10] Fabry disease is transmitted in X-linked recessive fashion, although heterozygous women may show variable degrees of disease expression owing to random X-chromosome inactivation.[11,12] Sarcoidosis is a complex chronic inflammatory disorder that shows familial clustering. Hofmann and colleagues[13] conducted a genome-wide association study comparing around 500 cases of sarcoidosis with an equivalent number of controls. An association was found with a common nonsynonymous single nucleotide polymorphism in *ANXA11*, the annexin A11 gene, from the annexin family of calcium-dependent phospholipid-binding proteins. The annexin 11 protein

Box 1
Secondary causes of cardiac restriction

Myocardial
- Infiltrative
  - Amyloidosis
  - Sarcoidosis
- Storage disorders
  - Gaucher disease
  - Hurler disease
  - Glycogen storage disease
  - Fabry disease
  - Hemochromatosis
- Noninfiltrative
  - End-stage hypertrophic cardiomyopathy
  - End-stage dilated cardiomyopathy
  - Systemic sclerosis
  - Pseudoxanthoma elasticum
  - Diabetic cardiomyopathy

Endomyocardial
- Endomyocardial fibrosis
- Hypereosinophilic syndrome
- Carcinoid heart disease
- Metastatic cancer
- Radiation
- Cardiotoxicity from anthracycline derivatives
- Drugs causing fibrous endocarditis (serotonin, methysergide, ergotamine, mercurial agents, busulfan)

Data from Kushwaha SS, Fallon JT, Fuster V. Restrictive cardiomyopathy. N Engl J Med 1997;336:267–76.

product associates with mitotic spindles. Cells depleted of the protein product fail to complete cytokinesis and die by apoptosis, suggesting an essential role in proliferation.

Amyloidosis

One of the most well known causes of cardiac restriction is amyloidosis, a collective term for a group of disorders of protein folding. Soluble extracellular proteins are misfolded and deposited as insoluble fibrils in the tissues, leading to disruption of normal tissue structure and function. Both acquired and hereditary forms exist. Classification is based on the nature of the fibril precursor protein and associated clinical features.[14,15]

Of the acquired forms, *primary or AL amyloidosis* is a systemic disease frequently observed in conjunction with plasma cell dyscrasias, such as multiple myeloma or the monoclonal gammopathies. Around 50% have cardiac manifestations. The fibrillar protein is composed of kappa and lambda immunoglobulin light chains produced by a proliferating clone of plasma cells. In contrast, *secondary or AA amyloidosis* occurs in association with chronic inflammatory disorders, such rheumatoid arthritis, ankylosing spondylitis, and familial Mediterranean fever.[14] The amyloid fibrils are composed of serum amyloid A protein, an acute phase reactant. Nephrotic syndrome and renal failure are common at presentation. Cardiac involvement is rare, but a marker of adverse prognosis when present.[16] *β2-Microglobulin amyloidosis* is a complication of long-term hemodialysis that usually occurs in localized periarticular form but is occasionally systemic. Cardiac manifestations are prominent in *senile systemic amyloidosis*, which is typically seen in patients over the age of 80. The fibril precursor is normal, wild-type transthyretin. Recognized features include clinical heart failure, atrioventricular block, atrial fibrillation, and ventricular arrhythmia.[17] Progression, however, is often indolent. The median survival rate is almost 5 years, even in the presence of clinical heart failure, which may itself be more amenable to conventional therapy than that occurring in other types of amyloidosis.[17–19]

Hereditary amyloidosis is the result of a mutation in one of a number of fibril precursor proteins (see **Table 1**).[14] The most common pattern of inheritance is autosomal dominant with incomplete penetrance. The phenotype varies according to the specific protein affected. Under-recognition may contribute to the apparent rarity of familial forms. Lachmann and colleagues[20] performed systematic sequencing of the four main disease-causing genes in a series of 350 patients with systemic amyloidosis, the majority of whom had no relevant family history. The panel screened comprised coding regions of the transthyretin and apolipoprotein A-I genes, together with selected exons of fibrinogen Aα chain and lysozyme. Causative mutations were isolated in almost 10% (34 of 350) of the study patients, most frequently in the fibrinogen Aα and transthyretin genes. The implications are twofold. First, a negative family history appears insufficient per se to exclude genetically determined disease. Second, genetic screening has an important diagnostic role in patients with systemic amyloidosis in whom the AA form has been excluded (usually by immunohistochemistry) and the AL type cannot be confirmed. Distinguishing between inherited

Table 1
Genetic basis of diseases associated with secondary cardiac restriction

Disorder	Inheritance	Genes Implicated
Systemic sclerosis	Multifactorial	*PTPN22, MCP-1, IL-1α, IL-10, IL-13, FAS, AIF1, IL13RA2,* SPARC, *FBN1, TOPOI*
Pseudoxanthoma elasticum	Autosomal recessive	*ABCC6*
Sarcoidosis	Multifactorial	*BTNL2, ANXA11*
Gaucher disease	Autosomal recessive	*GBA*
Hurler disease	Autosomal recessive	*IDUA*
Glycogen storage disease[a]	Commonly autosomal recessive	*G6PC, SLC37A4, NPT4, GAA, AGL, GBE, PYGM, PYGL, PFKM, PBK, PBKPHKA2, PBKPHKB, PHKG2, PBK, PBKPHKA1, PHKA1, PHKG1, GYS2, GYS1*
Fabry disease	X-linked recessive	*GLA*
Hemochromatosis	Autosomal recessive Autosomal dominant	*HFE, HFE2, HAMP, TFR2* *SCL40A1*
Hereditary amyloidosis[a]	Autosomal dominant	*TTR, CST3, GSN, LYZ, APOA1, APOA2, FGA*

Abbreviation: SPARC, secreted protein, acidic, cystein-rich.
[a] Multiple different forms exist, with differing degrees of cardiac involvement.
Data from Refs.[6–20]

and AL amyloidosis has therapeutic consequences, since the latter often responds to chemotherapy aimed at suppressing the underlying clonal plasma cell disorder. In contrast, chemotherapy is of no benefit and potentially hazardous in hereditary amyloidosis.[20] Establishing that the disease has a genetic basis also paves the way for presymptomatic testing of relatives. Ultimately, elucidation of the molecular mechanisms underlying inherited amyloidosis may enable development of targeted therapies, as have already been tested in trials concerning familial periodic fevers.[21]

RESTRICTIVE CARDIOMYOPATHY

Although commonly applied to secondary forms of myocardial dysfunction, the term *cardiomyopathy*, in the strictest sense, refers to intrinsic disorders of the heart muscle. On this basis, restrictive cardiomyopathy (RCM) is best defined as a primary myocardial disorder in which restrictive ventricular physiology develops early in the disease course and is the dominant clinical feature. This designation excludes both the secondary causes of cardiac restriction discussed above, and the restrictive physiology that may be observed in the latter stages of hypertrophic cardiomyopathy, dilated cardiomyopathy, and valvular, hypertensive, and ischemic heart disease. Normal wall thickness and systolic function have traditionally been stipulated, but mild hypertrophy need not be exclusionary, and contractility is more often preserved than truly normal in RCM. Historically, this entity has been termed idiopathic RCM, but elucidation of its genetic basis in the past decade has rendered the "idiopathic" qualifier anachronistic.

RCM as such is the least common of the primary myocardial disorders, although its exact prevalence is not known. Ammash and colleagues[22] delineated its clinical profile in a series of 94 patients satisfying echocardiographic criteria for RCM (mainly biatrial enlargement and nondilated ventricles with normal wall thickness). None had known infiltrative disease or systemic diseases associated with restrictive filling. The average age of the patients in cohort was 64, range 10 to 90 years; the majority were over the age of 60, and the diagnosis appeared more common in older women than in men (male-to-female sex ratio of 1:1.5). Atrial fibrillation was observed in over 70%. Over a mean follow-up period of 68 months, cardiovascular mortality was 34%, with congestive heart failure accounting for the majority of deaths, although cerebrovascular accidents and arrhythmia also contributed. Outcomes are still less favorable in children, in whom RCM accounts for 2% to 5% of cases of primary myocardial disease.[23] Median survival without transplantation is reported at around 2 years.[23]

Endomyocardial histology was available in 37 patients from the cohort described by Ammash and colleagues,[22] commonly demonstrating interstitial fibrosis (81%) and myocyte hypertrophy (86%). Endocardial fibrosis was present in 45%, but without inflammatory changes.[22] The utility of endomyocardial biopsy is limited by the extent of sampling; in histology from postmortem or explanted hearts, a key finding is myocyte disarray akin to that observed in hypertrophic cardiomyopathy.

Before identification of disease-causing mutations, several lines of evidence supported a genetic etiology for RCM. Familial occurrence had long been established, although many early reports focused on variants associated with distal skeletal myopathy and atrioventricular block.[24,25] Autosomal-dominant RCM with variable penetrance was also recognized in conjunction with Noonan syndrome.[26] Nevertheless, it was the observation that RCM could coexist with hypertrophic cardiomyopathy in the same family that first shed light on its genetic basis.

Mogensen and colleagues[27] identified an index case with RCM involving a boy who had presented with clinical heart failure at the age of 11. Two-dimensional echocardiography demonstrated marked biatrial dilation and restrictive filling in the setting of normal left ventricular wall thickness and systolic function. Similar echocardiographic features were noted in his mother, who had developed symptoms of heart failure at the age of 29. The one additional finding of interest was localized apical thickening, to a maximum wall thickness of 14 mm.

The family history included 12 instances of sudden cardiac death, while several surviving relatives were known to have heart disease, including a cousin with a prior diagnosis of RCM. Subsequent investigation of around 30 surviving relatives revealed features consistent with hypertrophic cardiomyopathy in 9, sufficient to fulfill the extended diagnostic criteria for familial disease. Among affected individuals with left ventricular hypertrophy, the wall thickness varied from 13 to 20 mm. Diastolic filling patterns combined features of both impaired relaxation and restriction. Linkage analysis followed by direct sequencing identified a 87A-G nucleotide substitution in exon 8 of the cardiac troponin I gene (*TNNI3*), which cosegregated with disease status in the family.[27]

Based on the premise that RCM might be part of the clinical expression of troponin I disease, a further nine unrelated patients with RCM were subsequently investigated for mutations in the same gene, which were found in six. Two individuals among this latter subgroup had de novo mutations associated with early onset and clinically severe disease. Postmortem histology was available in two cases, which demonstrated myocyte hypertrophy, marked interstitial fibrosis, and myocyte disarray, thereby corroborating previous reports of typical hypertrophic cardiomyopathy histology in patients with a clinical diagnosis of RCM.[28]

The coexistence of the hypertrophic cardiomyopathy and RCM phenotypes in the same family, consequent to identical disease-causing mutations, highlights the importance of modifier genes and perhaps environmental influences in determining the ultimate phenotype. Demonstration of the causal involvement of cardiac troponin I in RCM, and the similarities in histology with hypertrophic cardiomyopathy, also paved the way for a more exhaustive enquiry into the overlap between the two phenotypes, and the genetic underpinning thereof. Kubo and colleagues[29] subsequently investigated the prevalence of the restrictive phenotype in 688 consecutive families with hypertrophic cardiomyopathy.

Of 1226 affected individuals, 19 (1.5%) fulfilled echocardiographic criteria for RCM. All had left atrial dilation, normal or reduced left ventricular end-diastolic diameter, maximum wall thickness of 15 mm or less, and preserved left ventricular systolic function. None developed the RCM phenotype de novo during the course of progressive left ventricular remodeling. Peak oxygen consumption on cardiopulmonary exercise testing was significantly lower in the subgroup with a restrictive phenotype than in other patients with hypertrophic cardiomyopathy (mean 49% vs 72% of predicted). During a mean follow-up period of 54 months, the majority (89%) of patients with the restrictive phenotype developed New York Heart Association (NYHA) class II to IV status, in contrast to only 24% of the other patients with hypertrophic cardiomyopathy. Paroxysmal or persistent atrial fibrillation was documented in 74% of the patients with RCM, but in only 12% of the remainder.[29]

Outcomes were significantly less favorable in the RCM subgroup, with five deaths occurring during follow-up, of which three were heart failure–related, one was sudden, and the remaining patient suffered a cerebrovascular accident. A sixth patient with RCM underwent cardiac transplantation. Whole-heart histology was available from five out of seven of these individuals and demonstrated abundant myocardial disarray, sufficient for a histopathological diagnosis of hypertrophic cardiomyopathy. Overall, the restrictive phenotype was associated with a fivefold higher risk for cardiac death, transplantation, or implantable cardioverter-defibrillator discharge.[29]

Fifteen of the index cases with RCM underwent mutation analysis. Direct sequencing was performed of the troponin I gene and four other genes previously implicated in hypertrophic cardiomyopathy (the myosin binding protein C gene [*MYBPC3*], the beta-myosin heavy chain gene [*MYH7*], the cardiac troponin T gene [*TNNT2*], and the alpha-tropomyosin gene [*TPM1*]). Four causative mutations were identified in both the troponin I gene and the beta-myosin gene.[29] A deletion in the troponin I gene (nt4762delG), resulting in frameshift and formation of a premature stop codon, has since been reported in a Swedish patient with RCM who died aged 28 from progressive heart failure.[30] In that case, the family history included the sudden death of her father and third-trimester fetal loss in two female relatives, although neither histopathology nor DNA were available to confirm familial cardiomyopathy as the etiology. Mutations in the β-myosin heavy chain gene and a de novo mutation in the troponin T gene have also been identified in infantile RCM.[31–33]

More recently, Menon and colleagues[34] reported on a family with autosomal-dominant heart disease encompassing three distinct phenotypes: RCM, hypertrophic cardiomyopathy, and dilated cardiomyopathy. Linkage analysis followed by sequencing identified a heterozygous missense mutation in the cardiac troponin T gene, resulting in substitution of isoleucine (I) with asparagine (N) at amino acid position 79. The I79N mutation has been previously reported in patients with hypertrophic cardiomyopathy and its functional consequences studied in a transgenic mouse model.[34] Mice with cardiac-targeted expression of human troponin T-I79N show enhanced calcium-activated force generation and adenosine triphosphatase activity, resulting in accelerated consumption of adenosine triphosphate stores. The rate of calcium dissociation from troponin C is reduced, slowing relaxation and augmenting baseline muscle tension, with elevation of end-diastolic pressure. The mice show no hypertrophy, but develop the RCM phenotype. Inhibition of the L-type calcium current with diltiazem prevents acute heart failure and sudden death from isoproterenol exposure, suggesting a possible role for calcium channel blockers in individuals carrying the mutation.[34–37]

Within the family described by Menon and colleagues,[34] all affected members demonstrated varying degrees of restrictive physiology. The individuals diagnosed with hypertrophic cardiomyopathy typically demonstrated asymmetric septal hypertrophy, with maximum wall thickness of 16 and 24 mm. Marked left atrial enlargement was a common finding, but none had systolic anterior motion of the mitral valve, left ventricular outflow tract obstruction, or significant mitral regurgitation. Echocardiographic data were available in one of the two relatives with dilated cardiomyopathy; the left ventricular end-diastolic dimension was 6.2 cm and the ejection fraction 21%; pulmonary artery systolic pressures were elevated.

The pivotal issue is whether the dilated cardiomyopathy phenotype identified in this family occurs de novo or as an end-stage complication of restrictive or hypertrophic cardiomyopathy. Menon and colleagues[34] point out that risk factors for progression to the "burnt out" phase include young age at diagnosis and increased left ventricular wall thickness, neither of which was observed in affected members of the family described. Nevertheless, the absence of serial echocardiograms precludes a definitive resolution to this question.

In an investigation into the clinical profile of the "burnt out" phase, Thaman and colleagues[38] evaluated a sample of 1080 patients with hypertrophic cardiomyopathy, comprising both probands and relatives. Systolic dysfunction, defined as a fractional shortening of 25% or less on two-dimensional echocardiography, had a prevalence of 2.4% and an annual incidence of 0.87% in the cohort. Among patients who had significant systolic dysfunction, the *mean* left ventricular end-diastolic dimension was about 5.2 cm (although the upper limit of the range was 8.2 cm). Serial echocardiography in patients who progressed to systolic dysfunction during follow-up showed a greater average increase in end-systolic than in end-diastolic dimension.[38] The characteristic pattern of "burnt out" hypertrophic cardiomyopathy is systolic dysfunction with relatively preserved end-diastolic dimension. In the individual described by Menon and colleagues,[34] the relatively prominent left ventricular dilation may indeed be more consistent with de novo dilated cardiomyopathy than with "burnt out" hypertrophic cardiomyopathy.

Conversely, transition from a classic hypertrophic cardiomyopathy picture to an apparently typical dilated cardiomyopathy phenotype has been reported, interestingly, in association with a troponin T gene mutation.[39] One mutation carrier showed gradual decline in interventricular septal thickness from 17 to 7 mm during a 12-year follow-up period. Over the same period, her left ventricular end-diastolic dimension increased from 50 to 67 mm, generating a phenotype that would be indistinguishable from de novo dilated cardiomyopathy without the benefit of access to previous imaging studies.[39] The evolution of the dilated cardiomyopathy phenotype in the family described by Menon and colleagues[34] therefore remains unresolved, although the genetic affiliation of restrictive and hypertrophic cardiomyopathy is underscored, and a novel association with troponin T is defined. Alpha-cardiac actin has since been implicated in familial RCM, in a small series that strengthened the premise that childhood RCM, like its adult counterpart, is predominantly sarcomeric in etiology.[40]

RCM is also part of the broad spectrum of desmin-related disease, which may encompass distal skeletal myopathy, dilated cardiomyopathy, and atrioventricular block.[41,42] One characteristic feature is the intracellular accumulation of electron-dense granulofilamentous aggregates containing, among other proteins, desmin and α-B-crystallin. Various causative mutations have been isolated in desmin, most of which show autosomal-dominant inheritance, although families with compound heterozygous and recessive defects are also described.[42,43] In general, however, defects in atrioventricular conduction are a prominent feature of the cardiac phenotype, distinguishing its clinical profile from that of sarcomeric RCM.

SUMMARY

Restrictive physiology, a severe form of diastolic dysfunction, is characteristically observed in the setting of constrictive pericarditis and myocardial restriction. The latter is commonly due to systemic diseases, some of which are inherited as Mendelian traits (eg, hereditary amyloidosis), while others are multifactorial (eg, sarcoidosis). When restrictive physiology occurs as an early and dominant feature of a primary myocardial disorder, it may be termed *restrictive cardiomyopathy*. In the past decade, clinical and genetic studies have demonstrated that restrictive cardiomyopathy as such is part of the spectrum of sarcomeric disease, and frequently coexists with hypertrophic cardiomyopathy in affected families.

REFERENCES

1. Kass DA, Bronzwaer JG, Paulus WJ. What mechanisms underlie diastolic dysfunction in heart failure? Circ Res 2004;94:1533–42.
2. Garcia MJ, Rodriguez L, Ares M, et al. Differentiation of constrictive pericarditis from restrictive cardiomyopathy: assessment of left ventricular diastolic velocities in longitudinal axis by Doppler tissue imaging. J Am Coll Cardiol 1996;27:108–14.
3. Goldstein JA. Cardiac tamponade, constrictive pericarditis, and restrictive cardiomyopathy. Curr Probl Cardiol 2004;29:503–67.
4. Hancock EW. Differential diagnosis of restrictive cardiomyopathy and constrictive pericarditis. Heart 2001;86:343–9.
5. Rajagopalan N, Garcia MJ, Rodriguez L, et al. Comparison of new Doppler echocardiographic methods to differentiate constrictive pericardial heart disease and restrictive cardiomyopathy. Am J Cardiol 2001;87:86–94.
6. Kushwaha SS, Fallon JT, Fuster V. Restrictive cardiomyopathy. N Engl J Med 1997;336:267–76.
7. Allanore Y, Wipff J, Kahan A, et al. Genetic basis for systemic sclerosis. Joint Bone Spine 2007;74:577–83.
8. Clarke LA. The mucopolysaccharidoses: a success of molecular medicine. Expert Rev Mol Med 2008; 10:e1.
9. Shin YS. Glycogen storage disease: clinical, biochemical, and molecular heterogeneity. Semin Pediatr Neurol 2006;13:115–20.
10. Adams PC, Barton JC. Haemochromatosis. Lancet 2007;370:1855–60.
11. Desnick RJ, Brady R, Barranger J, et al. Fabry disease, an under-recognized multisystemic disorder: expert recommendations for diagnosis, management, and enzyme replacement therapy. Ann Intern Med 2003;138:338–46.
12. MacDermot KD, Holmes A, Miners AH. Anderson-Fabry disease: clinical manifestations and impact of disease in a cohort of 60 obligate carrier females. J Med Genet 2001;38:769–75.
13. Hofmann S, Franke A, Fischer A, et al. Genome-wide association study identifies ANXA11 as a new susceptibility locus for sarcoidosis. Nat Genet 2008;40:1103–6.
14. Hirschfield GM. Amyloidosis: a clinico-pathophysiological synopsis. Semin Cell Dev Biol 2004;15:39–44.
15. Merlini G, Bellotti V. Molecular mechanisms of amyloidosis. N Engl J Med 2003;349:583–96.
16. Tanaka F, Migita K, Honda S, et al. Clinical outcome and survival of secondary (AA) amyloidosis. Clin Exp Rheumatol 2003;21:343–6.
17. Hassan W, Al-Sergani H, Mourad W, et al. Amyloid heart disease. New frontiers and insights in pathophysiology, diagnosis, and management. Tex Heart Inst J 2005;32:178–84.
18. Kyle RA, Spittell PC, Gertz MA, et al. The premortem recognition of systemic senile amyloidosis with cardiac involvement. Am J Med 1996;101:395–400.
19. Olson LJ, Gertz MA, Edwards WD, et al. Senile cardiac amyloidosis with myocardial dysfunction. Diagnosis by endomyocardial biopsy and immunohistochemistry. N Engl J Med 1987;317:738–42.
20. Lachmann HJ, Booth DR, Booth SE, et al. Misdiagnosis of hereditary amyloidosis as AL (primary) amyloidosis. N Engl J Med 2002;346:1786–91.

21. Hawkins PN, Lachmann HJ, McDermott MF. Interleukin-1-receptor antagonist in the Muckle-Wells syndrome. N Engl J Med 2003;348:2583–4.
22. Ammash NM, Seward JB, Bailey KR, et al. Clinical profile and outcome of idiopathic restrictive cardiomyopathy. Circulation 2000;101:2490–6.
23. Russo LM, Webber SA. Idiopathic restrictive cardiomyopathy in children. Heart 2005;91:1199–202.
24. Fitzpatrick AP, Shapiro LM, Rickards AF, et al. Familial restrictive cardiomyopathy with atrioventricular block and skeletal myopathy. Br Heart J 1990;63:114–8.
25. Ishiwata S, Nishiyama S, Seki A, et al. Restrictive cardiomyopathy with complete atrioventricular block and distal myopathy with rimmed vacuoles. Jpn Circ J 1993;57:928–33.
26. Cooke RA, Chambers JB, Curry PV. Noonan's cardiomyopathy: a non-hypertrophic variant. Br Heart J 1994;71:561–5.
27. Mogensen J, Kubo T, Duque M, et al. Idiopathic restrictive cardiomyopathy is part of the clinical expression of cardiac troponin I mutations. J Clin Invest 2003;111:209–16.
28. Angelini A, Calzolari V, Thiene G, et al. Morphologic spectrum of primary restrictive cardiomyopathy. Am J Cardiol 1997;80:1046–50.
29. Kubo T, Gimeno JR, Bahl A, et al. Prevalence, clinical significance, and genetic basis of hypertrophic cardiomyopathy with restrictive phenotype. J Am Coll Cardiol 2007;49:2419–26.
30. Kostareva A, Gudkova A, Sjöberg G, et al. Deletion in TNNI3 gene is associated with restrictive cardiomyopathy. Int J Cardiol 2009;131:410–2.
31. Ware SM, Quinn ME, Ballard ET, et al. Pediatric restrictive cardiomyopathy associated with a mutation in beta-myosin heavy chain. Clin Genet 2008;73:165–70.
32. Karam S, Raboisson MJ, Ducreux C, et al. A de novo mutation of the beta cardiac myosin heavy chain gene in an infantile restrictive cardiomyopathy. Congenit Heart Dis 2008;3:138–43.
33. Peddy SB, Vricella LA, Crosson JE, et al. Infantile restrictive cardiomyopathy resulting from a mutation in the cardiac troponin T gene. Pediatrics 2006;117:1830–3.
34. Menon S, Michels V, Pellikka P, et al. Cardiac troponin T mutation in familial cardiomyopathy with variable remodeling and restrictive physiology. Clin Genet 2008;74:445–54.
35. Miller T, Szczesna D, Housmans PR, et al. Abnormal contractile function in transgenic mice expressing a familial hypertrophic cardiomyopathy-linked troponin T (I79N) mutation. J Biol Chem 2001;276:3743–55.
36. Rust EM, Albayya FP, Metzger JM. Identification of a contractile deficit in adult cardiac myocytes expressing hypertrophic cardiomyopathy-associated mutant troponin T proteins. J Clin Invest 1999;103:1459–67.
37. Westermann D, Knollmann BC, Steendijk P, et al. Diltiazem treatment prevents diastolic heart failure in mice with familial hypertrophic cardiomyopathy. Eur J Heart Fail 2006;8:115–21.
38. Thaman R, Gimeno JR, Murphy RT, et al. Prevalence and clinical significance of systolic impairment in hypertrophic cardiomyopathy. Heart 2005;91:920–5.
39. Fujino N, Shimizu M, Ino H, et al. A novel mutation Lys273Glu in the cardiac troponin T gene shows high degree of penetrance and transition from hypertrophic to dilated cardiomyopathy. Am J Cardiol 2002;89:29–33.
40. Kaski JP, Syrris P, Burch M, et al. Idiopathic restrictive cardiomyopathy in children is caused by mutations in cardiac sarcomere protein genes. Heart 2008;94:1478–84.
41. Arbustini E, Morbini P, Grasso M, et al. Restrictive cardiomyopathy, atrioventricular block and mild to subclinical myopathy in patients with desmin-immunoreactive material deposits. J Am Coll Cardiol 1998;31:645–53.
42. Kostera-Pruszczyk A, Pruszczyk P, Kamińska A, et al. Diversity of cardiomyopathy phenotypes caused by mutations in desmin. Int J Cardiol 2007;117:244–53.
43. Goldfarb LG, Park KY, Cervenáková L, et al. Missense mutations in desmin associated with familial cardiac and skeletal myopathy. Nat Genet 1998;19:402–3.

Atrial Fibrillation in Congestive Heart Failure

Steven A. Lubitz, MD[a,b], Emelia J. Benjamin, MD, ScM[c,d,e], Patrick T. Ellinor, MD, PhD[f,*]

KEYWORDS

- Atrial fibrillation • Congestive heart failure
- Genetic mutations • Etiology
- Pathophysiology • Management

Atrial fibrillation (AF) and congestive heart failure (CHF) are among the most common medical conditions and are associated with significant morbidity. These two conditions share similar risk factors, frequently coexist, and have additive adverse effects when occurring in conjunction. Much evidence has amassed regarding the nature of the relations between AF and CHF. This review discusses AF in the context of CHF, with a particular emphasis on the underlying pathophysiologic mechanisms and genetic basis of AF. It also addresses the proper management, based on recent clinical trials and practice guidelines, of AF when it occurs in conjunction with CHF.

EPIDEMIOLOGY

AF is the most common arrhythmia seen in clinical practice and is responsible for significant morbidity.[1] More than 2.3 million individuals in the United States currently have AF,[2] and as many as 5.6 to 12.1 million individuals are projected to be affected by 2050.[2,3] The lifetime risk of developing AF after age 40 is 26% for men and 23% for women.[4] The presence of AF confers a fivefold increased risk of stroke,[5] a significantly increased risk of dementia,[6] and an almost twofold increased risk of death.[5] Moreover, the incidence of AF is rising,[7] presenting a significant health care burden as it accounts for an increasing proportion of hospitalizations.[8] Health care costs are approximately five times greater for individuals with AF than for those without AF.[9]

CHF has a similar prevalence, affecting more than 5 million individuals in the United States.[10] After age 40, the lifetime risk of developing CHF is more than 20%.[11] CHF portends a grave prognosis, with more than half of individuals dying within 5 years of diagnosis,[12] although some estimates indicate that survival may be improving.[12,13]

Dr Lubitz is supported by an NIH training grant (5T32HL007575). This work was supported by grants from the NIH: HL092577 to Drs Ellinor and Benjamin; AGO 28321 and RC1-HL01056 to Dr Benjamin; and DA027021 to Dr Ellinor. Dr Ellinor is a consultant to Sanofi-Aventis.

[a] Cardiovascular Research Center, Massachusetts General Hospital, 149 13th Street, Charlestown, MA 02129, USA
[b] Division of Preventive Medicine, Center for Cardiovascular Disease Prevention, Brigham and Women's Hospital, 900 Commonwealth Avenue, Boston, MA 02215, USA
[c] Section of Cardiology, Preventive Medicine, Whitaker Cardiovascular Institute, Boston University School of Medicine, Boston, MA, USA
[d] Department of Epidemiology, Boston University Schools of Medicine and Public Health, Framingham Heart Study, 73 Mount Wayte Avenue, Suite 2, Framingham, MA 01702-5827, USA
[e] National Heart, Lung and Blood Institute's Framingham Heart Study, Framingham, MA, USA
[f] Cardiac Arrhythmia Service & Cardiovascular Research Center, Massachusetts General Hospital, 149 13th Street, Charlestown, MA 02129, USA
* Corresponding author.
E-mail address: pellinor@partners.org

Heart Failure Clin 6 (2010) 187–200
doi:10.1016/j.hfc.2009.11.001
1551-7136/10/$ – see front matter

CHF accounts for a significant proportion of the health care budget, with an estimated cost of $34.8 billion in 2008.[10]

Prevalence of Comorbid Atrial Fibrillation and Congestive Heart Failure

As AF and CHF occur frequently, the simultaneous presence of these two conditions is common. The prevalence of AF in patients with systolic left ventricular dysfunction and CHF ranges from 6% for asymptomatic patients or for those with minimal symptoms[14] to between 15% and 35% for patients with New York Heart Association (NYHA) class II–IV symptoms.[15–23] In two large epidemiologic studies,[24,25] the prevalence of AF was greater in CHF patients with preserved ejection fractions than in those with left ventricular systolic dysfunction, although the rates of AF were similar in patients with systolic as compared to diastolic CHF in one clinical trial.[20]

The concomitant presence of AF and CHF in many patients may be explained by shared underlying risk factors and mechanisms or a causal relation between the entities. Many risk factors for AF have been recognized as leading risk factors for CHF (**Box 1**). The shared risk factors include hypertension, diabetes mellitus, ischemic heart disease, and valvular heart disease.[26] Additionally, evidence of myocarditis, one potential cause of dilated cardiomyopathy and CHF, has also been implicated in the genesis of AF.[27,28] In one series, AF was directly attributable to CHF in 5% of cases.[29]

Temporal Relations of Atrial Fibrillation and Congestive Heart Failure

The temporal relations of AF and CHF were examined in a study of 1470 patients from the Framingham Heart Study with new-onset AF or CHF.[30] The average follow-up was 5.6 years after the development of AF and 4.2 years after the development of CHF. Among patients who developed AF, 26% had a prior or concurrent diagnosis of CHF, and 16% of the remaining patients subsequently developed CHF during the follow-up period. Among patients who developed CHF, 24% had a prior or concurrent diagnosis of AF, and 17% developed AF during the subsequent follow-up period. For patients diagnosed with AF, the incidence of developing CHF was 33 per 1000 person-years. Conversely, among individuals diagnosed with CHF, the incidence of developing AF was 54 per 1000 person-years.

The association between AF and the development of CHF was also analyzed in a study of 3288 patients diagnosed with AF at the Mayo Clinic.[7] Twenty-four percent developed CHF during a mean follow-up of 6.1 years, with an incidence of 44 per 1000 patient-years. A spike in the incidence of CHF was seen early after the diagnosis of AF, with 7.8% of cases occurring within the first 12 months and approximately 3% per year thereafter. Patients with lone AF fared well, as only approximately 2% developed CHF within 5 years of being diagnosed with AF.[7]

Prognosis of Comorbid Atrial Fibrillation and Congestive Heart Failure

Whereas substantial morbidity and mortality are attributable to each of these individual conditions, the concomitant presence of AF and CHF identifies individuals with a higher risk for death than with either condition alone. The prognostic impact of incident AF or CHF among individuals diagnosed with the other comorbid condition was assessed by investigators from the Framingham Heart Study.[30] The development of AF in individuals with CHF was associated with a hazard ratio for death of 1.6 in men and 2.7 in women during follow-up of 4.2 years. Similarly, the development of CHF among individuals with AF was associated with a hazard ratio for death of 2.7 in men and 3.1 in women over a follow-up of 5.6 years.

The clinical consequences of AF are derived from the loss of organized atrial activity and absence of coordinated atrial mechanical function. Impaired contraction of the atria may cause blood stasis and the potential for thrombus formation, particularly in the left atrial appendage, with a resultant risk of stroke. This risk of stroke is increased in patients with CHF.[31] Hundreds of electrical impulses arrive at the atrioventricular node and are variably transmitted, resulting in fast or slow heart rates and irregular ventricular depolarization. Patients may experience symptoms, such as palpitations, dyspnea, or fatigue. The electrical and mechanical features of AF may also have hemodynamic consequences. A reduction in cardiac output is attributable to the irregularity of ventricular contractions and the loss of atrial mechanical activity, which impairs ventricular filling.[32,33] Restoration of sinus rhythm results in an approximately 30% increase in cardiac output,[34] although the significance of atrial contribution to cardiac output has been controversial in patients with pre-existing elevations in left atrial pressure.[35,36] Persistent tachycardia due to poor rate control has also been reported to result in a cardiomyopathy.[37]

Thus, AF and CHF commonly coexist, share a similar risk factor profile, and have adverse

Box 1
Shared risk factors for atrial fibrillation and congestive heart failure

Nonmodifiable risk factors
Aging
Male gender
Genetic predisposition

Modifiable risk factors
Hypertension
Diabetes mellitus
Obesity
Hyperthyroidism
Smoking
Excessive alcohol consumption

Heart disease
Ischemic heart disease
Valve disease
Infiltrative cardiomyopathies
Myocarditis
Left ventricular systolic dysfunction
Left ventricular diastolic dysfunction

Subclinical disease
Electrocardiographic left ventricular hypertrophy
Neurohormonal activation
Inflammation

hemodynamic effects. The simultaneous presence of both diseases identifies individuals at substantially increased risk of cardiovascular events and death.

PATHOPHYSIOLOGY OF ATRIAL FIBRILLATION IN CONGESTIVE HEART FAILURE

The pathophysiologic basis of AF is complex and incompletely understood.[38] Initial mechanistic explanations for AF cited reentry as a principal factor.[39–42] The multiple wavelet hypothesis, proposed by Moe and Abildskov,[41] stated that the development of AF depended on the perpetuation of a sufficient number of "randomly wandering wavelets" created as a normal occurrence due to heterogeneous repolarization. The hypothesis maintained that adequate atrial mass, short refractory periods, and conduction velocities slow enough to permit temporal disparities in depolarization and repolarization in the atria favored the development of these reentrant wavelets.

This argument is predicated on the concept that the wavelength of an electrical signal also represents the minimal pathway length that must be present to sustain a reentrant circuit. If a pathway is shorter, then a reentrant electrical stimulus will encounter refractory tissue on completing the circuit and terminate. In contrast, if the pathway is longer, then the electrical signal may encounter excitable tissue on completing the circuit, thereby perpetuating the previous cycle. The wavelength, and thus the pathway length, are proportional to the refractory period of the tissue and the conduction velocity. This model explains precipitants of AF that shorten the atrial effective refractory period or decrease conduction velocity.

The focal automaticity theory was an early competing hypothesis that explicitly challenged the role of reentrant rhythms in the genesis of AF, instead proposing that repetitively firing foci serve as the driving factor.[43] A contemporary paradigm acknowledges complexity in the development of AF, recognizing the role of susceptible atrial substrate, which may foster reentry, and focal electrophysiologic triggers (**Fig. 1**).[44]

Susceptible Atrial Substrate

Fibrosis

Atrial fibrosis is commonly observed in patients with AF, with and without underlying organic heart disease, and is considered a major factor contributing to the development and maintenance of AF.[27,28,45] Fibrosis results from increased interstitial collagen deposition, which may disrupt cell-to-cell coupling and thereby alter signal conduction. Areas with decreased conduction velocities and heterogeneous conduction have been observed in animal models of AF and fibrosis.[46,47]

Fibrosis accompanies aging and is observed with ischemia and with myocyte stretch.[48,49] Activation of the renin-angiotensin-aldosterone system provokes myocardial fibrosis, which appears to be mediated through up-regulation of the transforming growth factor ß1 pathway.[50] Indirect evidence of the contributory role of atrial fibrosis provoked by the renin-angiotensin-aldosterone neurohormonal axis is derived from clinical trials that have documented a significant reduction in the risk of new-onset or recurrent AF with angiotensin-converting enzyme (ACE) inhibitors or angiotensin receptor blockers.[51,52]

Myocyte stretch

Myocyte stretch is another important factor contributing to AF susceptibility. Several pathologic conditions associated with increased left atrial pressure are closely linked to the

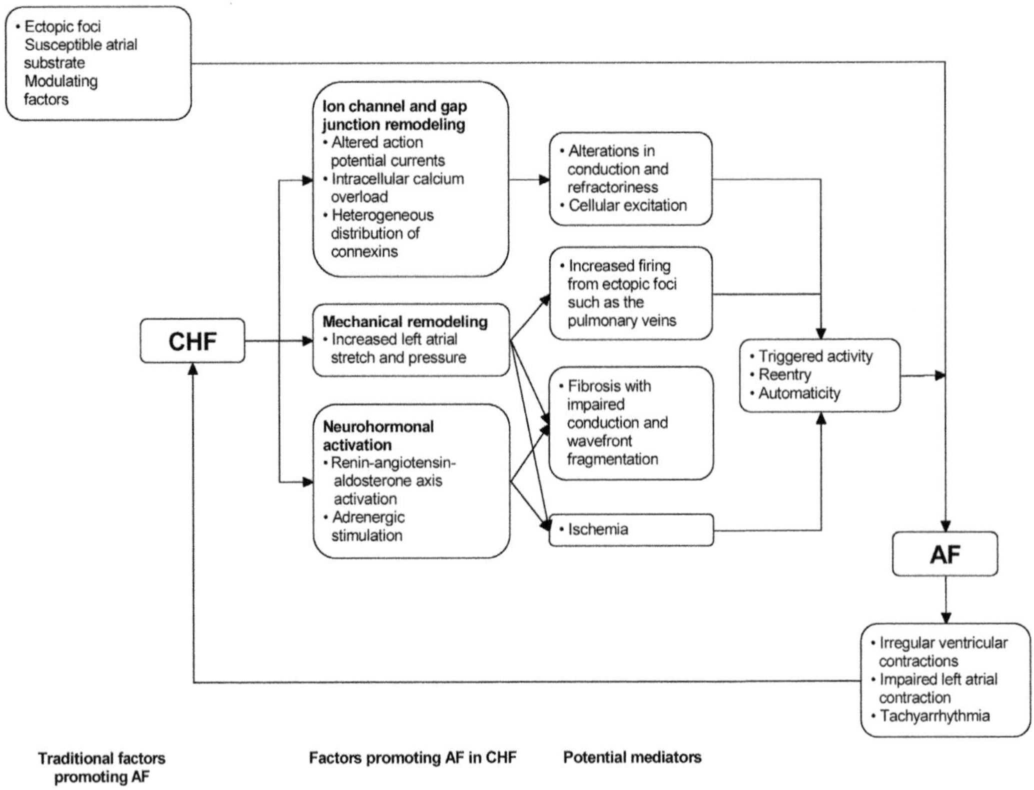

Fig. 1. Mechanisms promoting AF in CHF.

development of AF, including hypertension, mitral valve disease, and CHF. Myocyte stretch stimulates collagen deposition by fibroblasts, in part mediated via angiotensin II and transforming growth factor ß1 pathways.[48] Additionally, stretch causes acute alterations in electrophysiologic properties that are favorable to the development and maintenance of AF via mechanoelectric feedback mechanisms.[53]

Electromechanical remodeling

Experimental models in goats demonstrate that prior AF promotes an environment favorable to subsequent episodes of AF through electrophysiologic[54] and structural remodeling.[55] Intracellular calcium overload causing a reduction of L-type calcium currents may contribute to atrial remodeling.[56] Additional mechanisms of atrial remodeling may include intracellular glycogen accumulation accompanied by sarcomere loss[55] and diminished myocyte energy reserves.[53] Accompanying proarrhythmic electrophysiologic changes have been observed, such as decreases in myocyte resting potential, shortening of the atrial effective refractory period, and characteristic alterations in the morphology of the action potential.[54,56] Grossly, structural changes resulting from AF may manifest as left atrial enlargement,[57] which predisposes to recurrent AF.

Elements promoting susceptible atrial substrate are often interrelated, underscoring the difficulty of identifying discrete mechanisms that result in AF. For example, both myocyte stretch and prior AF have been linked to atrial fibrosis.[48]

Focal Triggers

In addition to the role of susceptible atrial substrate, recent evidence supports a critical role for focal triggers in the development of AF in many patients with this arrhythmia. These focal triggers most commonly arise from within the pulmonary veins[58,59] and conduct to the left atrium through sleeves of muscular tissue in the pulmonary veins.[60] The importance of these triggers has been underscored by the success of pulmonary vein isolation in preventing recurrences of AF in many patients.[61,62] The mechanisms resulting in these triggers remain unclear, although automaticity, triggered activity, and microreentry have all been implicated.[63] The observation that myocyte stretch increases pulmonary vein foci firing again illustrates the interdependence of mechanisms contributing to AF.[64] Ectopic foci have also been identified in other areas of the heart, such as the posterior left atrium, coronary sinus, superior vena cava, and ligament of Marshall.[65] Additionally, atrioventricular nodal reentrant tachycardias[66] and atrioventricular bypass tracts may trigger AF.[67]

Modulating Factors

In addition to susceptible atrial substrate and electrophysiologic triggers, modulating factors, such as autonomic tone, contribute to the development of AF.[68,69] Vagal denervation has been explored for the prevention of recurrent AF with promising initial results.[69] Inflammation may also be associated with the development of AF in patients with concomitant cardiovascular disease.[70] Treatment with corticosteroids in addition to β blockade during the postoperative period reduced the risk of developing postoperative AF by approximately 50% among patients undergoing cardiac surgery without any preexisting history of AF.[71]

Role of Genetics

An abundance of epidemiologic data implicate a heritable contribution to the development of AF. In a prospective cohort study encompassing patients from the original and offspring cohorts from the Framingham Heart Study, the odds ratio of developing AF over 4 years among participants with a parental history of AF was 1.85 and increased to 3.23 when limiting the analysis to parents and offspring who developed AF under age 75.[72] Other studies have confirmed that up to approximately one-third of individuals with AF have a positive family history of the condition.[73–76] In a study encompassing more than 5000 patients diagnosed with AF in Iceland, the relative risk of developing AF was 1.77 in those with an affected first-degree relative and declined with each successive degree of relation.[77]

Analyses of patients with familial AF have exposed mutations in genes encoding potassium[78–84] and sodium[75,76,85–87] channels (**Fig. 2**) as well as atrial natriuretic peptide,[88] and have identified several loci associated with AF.[89–93] Mutations in ion channels may contribute to AF by their effect on the atrial action potential, which is comprised of multiple tightly coordinated electrical currents. The majority of identified potassium channel mutations result in a gain of channel function. Such an increase in an outward potassium current would produce more rapid repolarization of atrial myocytes, shorten the atrial effective refractory period, and thus predispose to reentry.[78–81,83,84,94] A loss-of-function mutation in the ultrarapid delayed rectifier potassium current (I_{Kur}) has been identified, which prolongs the action potential and facilitates early afterdepolarizations, particularly under adrenergic stimulation.[82] As discussed later, prolongation of the action potential has been observed in patients with CHF, suggesting that triggered activity may play an important role in initiating AF in this setting.[95] Some loss-of-function mutations in sodium channels decrease ionic current, prolong the atrial action potential duration, and may predispose to AF in a similar manner. More recently, somatic mutations in gap junction proteins have been identified in patients with idiopathic AF,[96] but the prevalence of such mutations is unknown. Despite mechanistic insights gleaned from identification of these mutations, ion channel mutations are rare causes of AF.[97]

In some cases, identification of genes implicated in cardiomyopathies has shed light on possible shared biologic mechanisms between CHF and AF. In some patients with a familial cardiomyopathy and AF, mutations have been identified in *SCN5A* or the cardiac sodium channel gene also associated with the Brugada and long QT syndromes.[98,99] Similarly, mutations in the lamin A/C gene, a nuclear envelope protein, have been identified in patients with familial dilated cardiomyopathy that is preceded by the development of AF.[100,101] The mechanisms by which such mutations cause arrhythmias and a cardiomyopathy remain unclear.

Most mutations identified thus far have been discovered by linkage or candidate gene analysis. More recently, genome-wide association studies have been used to search for genetic variation that may underlie common diseases, such as AF.[102,103] Genome-wide association studies can identify genetic variants associated with a particular phenotype by scanning for hundreds of thousands of single nucleotide polymorphisms in patients with and without the condition of interest. The identified variants may have a direct pathogenic role in the development of the condition; however, in most cases, such variants are simply serving as a marker of a genetic region associated with a risk of the condition. Genome-wide association studies represent a major advance because they provide rapid assessment of thousands of markers throughout the genome and are not constrained by existing understanding of physiology.

A recent genome-wide association study in Iceland has identified two variants on chromosome 4q25 associated with AF.[102] Replication in two additional cohorts of European ancestry reproduced the associations, whereas replication

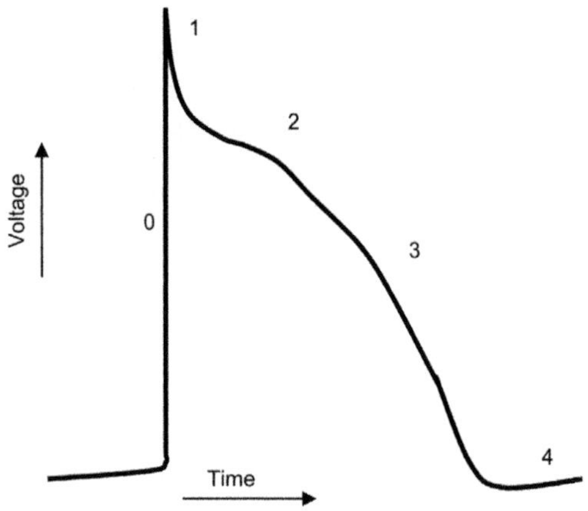

Ionic current	Predominant active phase	Gene	Gain or loss of function	Predicted effect on ARP	Reference
I_{Na}	0	*SCN5A*	Loss	↑	[85, 98]
I_{to}	1	*KCND3/KCNIP2*	-	-	-
I_{Kur}	2	*KCNA5*	Loss	↑	[82]
I_{CaL}	3	*CACNA1C*	-	-	-
I_{Kr}	3	*KCNH2/KCNE2*	Gain	↓	[80]
I_{Ks}	3	*KCNQ1/KCNE1*	Gain	↓	[78, 79, 83, 84, 94]
I_{NCX}	3		-	-	-
I_{K1}	4	*KCNJ2*	Gain	↓	[81]

Fig. 2. Genetic mutations affecting ionic currents that underlie the atrial action potential. ARP, atrial refractory period; GOF, gain-of-function mutation; LOF, loss-of-function mutation.

in a cohort of Chinese descent confirmed the association with one of the variants.[102] No known gene is present in the genomic block containing the two variants, although two potential candidate genes, *PITX2* and *ENPEP*, are located in close proximity. *PITX2* plays an important role in cardiac development by directing asymmetric morphogenesis of the heart.[104] Knockout of *PITX2* in a mouse model suppresses the default pathway for sinoatrial node formation in the left atrium.[105,106] *ENPEP* encodes an aminopeptidase responsible for breakdown of angiotensin II in the vascular endothelium. Knockout of *ENPEP* in a mouse model resulted in systemic hypertension but no arrhythmias.[107] Investigation of the causal mechanisms by which these variants are related to AF is ongoing. In two subsequent genome-wide association studies, a second common AF susceptibility locus was identified on chromosome 16q22 within the ZFHX3 gene.[108,109] This gene also encodes a transcription factor, though the mechanisms by which this gene promotes AF remain unclear.

Specific Implications in Congestive Heart Failure

Thus, electrical triggers, susceptible substrate, and modulating factors are important for the promotion of AF. Genetic factors may promote AF by increasing susceptibility to reentry, triggered activity, disrupting cell-to-cell communication, and other currently as yet undefined mechanisms. Several of the discussed pathophysiologic mechanisms are of particular importance in patients with CHF (see **Fig. 1**).

Increased atrial refractoriness has been observed in CHF patients who develop AF, suggesting that the origins of the arrhythmia in this patient population may differ from those classically described.[95] A variety of ion channel current abnormalities have been reported in experimental

CHF models, including a reduction in L-type Ca^{2+} current (I_{Ca}), transient outward K+ current (I_{to}), and slow delayed rectifier current (I_{Ks}).[110] CHF is accompanied by an increase in the Na^+/Ca^{2+} transmembrane exchange channel current, which exchanges three monovalent sodium ions for every one divalent calcium ion. This net positive intracellular imbalance can predispose to delayed afterdepolarizations, resulting in arrhythmias initiated by triggered activity. Data from a pacing-induced animal model of CHF demonstrate that abnormalities in calcium handling prolong the atrial action potential and foster AF through triggered activity.[111] Adrenergic stimulation occurs in CHF and is a well-known cause of triggered activity. The role of adrenergic stimulation in the genesis of AF is not clear.[112] In parallel to ion channel remodeling present in patients with CHF, heterogeneous distribution of connexins, which form gap junctions, has been observed in animal models of atrial hemodynamic overload and in humans with a history of CHF.[113]

Elevations in left atrial and pulmonary venous pressure present in CHF also promote AF. Myocyte stretch increases firing from ectopic foci, such as the pulmonary veins, through mechanoelectrical feedback.[64] Additionally, increased fibrosis results from myocyte stretch. Gross evidence of structural remodeling includes left atrial enlargement, which predisposes to AF.[114,115] Although increased atrial refractoriness has been observed clinically in patients with CHF, shortening of the atrial refractory period has been reported in experimental models of left atrial stretch, suggesting that many competing processes may be occurring simultaneously in these patients.[116]

Neurohormonal activation is another principal feature of CHF that promotes AF. Up-regulation of the renin-angiotensin-aldosterone and adrenergic systems causes myocardial fibrosis, which impairs impulse propagation.[46,117] Fibrosis is thought to play a prominent role in the development of AF in patients with CHF. In an experimental pacing model of CHF, fibrosis, rather than ion channel remodeling, produced lasting effects that correlated with the maintenance of induced AF.[118] Nonetheless, angiotensin II may have independent effects on ion currents that promote AF.[119]

TREATMENT

Thromboembolism Prophylaxis

Thromboembolism prophylaxis, ventricular rate control, and restoration of sinus rhythm, when indicated, are the goals of AF therapy.[1] The risk of cerebral thromboembolism in patients with AF is increased in those with CHF.[31] Annual stroke risk can be estimated using validated scoring schemes,[31,120] and guidelines provide a recommended approach to the prevention of thromboembolism in patients based on their underlying risk. Generally, warfarin is advisable for the prevention of ischemic cerebrovascular events in patients with CHF and an additional stroke risk factor.[1]

Rate and Rhythm Control

Recent controlled trials of patients with predominantly persistent and asymptomatic AF demonstrated no advantage of a rhythm control strategy comprised of antiarrhythmic drug therapy and electrical cardioversion over a rate control strategy in terms of survival or morbidity.[121–125] A meta-analysis of these trials demonstrated a reduction in the combined endpoint of all-cause death or thromboembolic stroke with a rate control strategy.[126]

Rhythm control strategies in these trials were only moderately successful, however, with the maintenance of sinus rhythm ranging from 23% to 64% over variable periods of follow-up. Post hoc analyses of these and other trials demonstrate that achievement of sinus rhythm is associated with improved survival[127] and quality of life.[128,129] The observation that noncardiovascular deaths were greater in the rhythm control arm than in the rate control arm of the Atrial Fibrillation Follow-up Investigation of Rhythm Management trial has provoked speculation that the benefits of maintaining sinus rhythm were offset by the harmful effects of antiarrhythmic drug therapy.[130]

These trials were not adequately powered to assess the optimal management strategy of AF in patients with CHF. More recently, the results of the Atrial Fibrillation and Congestive Heart Failure Trial were reported.[131] This randomized controlled trial assessed cardiovascular mortality among patients with concomitant AF and CHF treated with a rate or rhythm control strategy. More than 1300 patients were enrolled, with a mean left ventricular ejection fraction of 27%. One third of patients had NYHA class III or IV symptoms, and more than two-thirds had persistent AF. More than 80% of patients randomized to the rhythm control arm were treated with amiodarone, and 40% underwent electrical cardioversion. During a mean follow-up period of 37 months, sinus rhythm was documented in 75% to 80% of patients in the rhythm control arm by 12-lead electrocardiogram at each follow-up visit, whereas sinus rhythm was present in 30% to 40% of patients in the rate control arm at each visit. No difference was observed in cardiovascular mortality between strategies during the follow-up period. These data suggest that a rhythm control strategy consisting of pharmacologic and electrical cardioversion for stable patients with concomitant AF and CHF does not improve cardiovascular survival. These results may not pertain to patients who are hemodynamically unstable as a result of AF. Additionally, the impact of other rhythm or rate control strategies, such as catheter ablation for AF or atrioventricular node ablation with pacing, was not assessed adequately in this or other trials comparing rate and rhythm control strategies. In a smaller trial of 61 patients randomized to rhythm control with amiodarone and direct cardioversion or rate control and followed for one year, an improvement in left ventricular function and some quality of life parameters was observed among those in the rhythm control arm.[132]

Catheter Ablation

Catheter ablation for AF, specifically pulmonary vein isolation, has become an increasingly popular therapy for the treatment of AF. Recent controlled trials suggest that in carefully selected patients, catheter ablation is superior to a medical rhythm control strategy for the prevention of recurrent disease during short-term follow-up, with success rates ranging from 56% to 87%.[133] Yet subjects in these trials predominantly were healthy, had paroxysmal rather than persistent or permanent AF, and were typically without structural heart disease.

Catheter ablation for AF was assessed in 58 patients with CHF in one nonrandomized controlled trial.[134] Sinus rhythm was present in 78% of patients after ablation after approximately 1 year, although repeat ablations were required in half of the patients. Improvements in functional status, symptoms, and ejection fraction were noted with ablation.

Similarly, in a prospective cohort study, sinus rhythm was achieved in 73% of patients with left ventricular systolic dysfunction who underwent pulmonary vein isolation at approximately 14 months of follow-up as compared to 87% of patients with preserved left ventricular function.[135] Sixty-eight percent of the patients with left ventricular systolic dysfunction had NYHA class III symptoms.

Despite promising initial results, there are currently no data that demonstrate that catheter ablation improves survival in patients with CHF. Moreover, results from studies of catheter ablation for AF in the setting of CHF must be interpreted in the context of the study designs, which were not randomized, involved few patients, and provided only short-term follow-up.

Atrioventricular Nodal Ablation and Pacemaker Placement

Ablation of the atrioventricular node with implantation of a single right ventricular lead for permanent pacing, also referred to as the ablate and pace approach, is effective for the achievement of rate control in patients with AF and rapid ventricular response and results in greater symptom control than pharmacologic therapy aimed at controlling the ventricular rate in patients with left ventricular systolic dysfunction and CHF.[136] Yet right ventricular pacing can be associated with progressive left ventricular dysfunction, whereas biventricular pacing results in reduced morbidity and mortality in systolic CHF patients with NYHA class III or IV symptoms in sinus rhythm and with a prolonged QRS.[137] In a prospective cohort study of patients with conventional indications for biventricular pacemaker implantation, the benefits of biventricular pacing in a subgroup of patients with AF were maximized when biventricular pacing was induced nearly 100% of the time by atrioventricular node ablation.[138] Improvements in the ejection fraction and functional capacity were seen when compared to patients who received biventricular pacing less than 85% of the time. Other data demonstrate improvements in a variety of functional and symptomatic parameters in patients with AF and systolic CHF with a wide QRS who are treated with biventricular pacemakers.[139] The Atrioventricular Junction Ablation Followed by Resynchronization Therapy in Patients with CHF and AF trial[140] will compare pharmacologic rate control therapy to atrioventricular node ablation with biventricular pacemaker implantation in patients with symptomatic permanent AF and CHF, irrespective of underlying QRS duration.

Although the ablate and pace approach achieves rate control, it does not restore sinus rhythm and necessitates permanent implantation of a mechanical pacemaker. AV nodal ablation with biventricular pacing was compared to AF ablation in a pilot study of 35 subjects with CHF and systolic left ventricular dysfunction.[141] In the Comparison of Pulmonary Vein Isolation Versus AV Nodal Ablation With Biventricular Pacing for Patients With Atrial Fibrillation With Congestive Heart Failure study, pulmonary vein isolation was associated with greater improvement in symptoms and ejection fraction as compared with the ablate and biventricular pacing group.

Definitive trials assessing the effectiveness of AF ablation as compared with an ablate and ventricular pacing strategy are warranted. In the meantime, atrioventricular node ablation and ventricular pacing remains a reasonable option for the management of patients in whom the achievement of adequate rate control with pharmacologic therapy is inadequate.[1]

Renin-angiotensin-aldosterone Axis Inhibitors and β-Blockers

Pharmacologic agents commonly used in the management of patients with systolic CHF prevent incident AF and reduce recurrences in patients with concomitant AF and CHF, reinforcing the shared mechanisms of these diseases. ACE inhibitors and angiotensin receptor blockers are effective in preventing the onset of AF. In one meta-analysis of randomized trials assessing the use of an ACE inhibitor or angiotensin receptor blocker, the relative risk of developing AF among patients treated with either medication was reduced by 28%.[51] Patients with CHF enjoyed a relative risk reduction of 44%, with a greater benefit seen among those with more severe left ventricular systolic dysfunction. In another meta-analysis, the overall risk reduction for the development of new-onset AF in patients treated with an ACE inhibitor or angiotensin receptor blocker was 18%, and patients with a history of CHF had a particular benefit with a risk reduction of 43%.[52]

Furthermore, a systematic review of randomized placebo-controlled trials in patients with CHF demonstrated that the addition of β-blockers in addition to ACE-I therapy was associated with a relative risk reduction of 27% in the incidence of AF over an average follow-up of 1.35 years.[142] No preventative effect of β-blockade was observed in the Study of the Effects of Nebivolol Intervention on Outcomes and Rehospitalization in Seniors with Heart Failure trial, however, which studied the use of nebivolol in elderly patients (≥70 years old) with diastolic or systolic CHF.

SUMMARY

AF and CHF share many risk factors, frequently coexist, and identify individuals at high risk of cardiovascular morbidity. The pathophysiologic mechanisms of AF in patients with CHF are complex and potentially involve elements of reentry, triggered activity, and enhanced automaticity. Therefore, it is unlikely that a treatment strategy aimed at any one of these mechanisms alone will restore sinus rhythm. A rhythm control strategy consisting of antiarrhythmic drugs and electrical cardioversion in stable patients with AF and CHF adds no benefit to a rate control strategy. Newer therapies aimed at restoring sinus rhythm, such as catheter ablation for AF, and rate control therapies such as atrioventricular nodal ablation with biventricular pacing, have emerged as potential alternatives to conventional rhythm and rate control strategies. Future trials will be necessary to delineate the role for such techniques in the multitude of patients with these morbid conditions.

REFERENCES

1. Fuster V, Ryden LE, Cannom DS, et al. ACC/AHA/ESC 2006 guidelines for the management of patients with atrial fibrillation: a report of the American College of Cardiology/American Heart Association Task Force on practice guidelines and the European Society of Cardiology Committee for Practice Guidelines (Writing Committee to Revise the 2001 guidelines for the management of patients with atrial fibrillation): developed in collaboration with the European Heart Rhythm Association and the Heart Rhythm Society. Circulation 2006;114(7):e257–354.
2. Go AS, Hylek EM, Phillips KA, et al. Prevalence of diagnosed atrial fibrillation in adults: national implications for rhythm management and stroke prevention: the An Ticoagulation and Risk Factors in Atrial Fibrillation (ATRIA) study. JAMA 2001;285(18):2370–5.
3. Miyasaka Y, Barnes ME, Gersh BJ, et al. Secular trends in incidence of atrial fibrillation in olmsted county, minnesota, 1980 to 2000, and implications on the projections for future prevalence. Circulation 2006;114(2):119–25.
4. Lloyd-Jones DM, Wang TJ, Leip EP, et al. Lifetime risk for development of atrial fibrillation: the Framingham heart study. Circulation 2004;110(9):1042–6.
5. Kannel WB, Wolf PA, Benjamin EJ, et al. Prevalence, incidence, prognosis, and predisposing conditions for atrial fibrillation: population-based estimates. Am J Cardiol 1998;82(8A):2N–9N.
6. Ott A, Breteler MM, de Bruyne MC, et al. Atrial fibrillation and dementia in a population-based study. The Rotterdam study. Stroke 1997;28(2):316–21.
7. Miyasaka Y, Barnes ME, Gersh BJ, et al. Incidence and mortality risk of congestive heart failure in atrial fibrillation patients: a community-based study over two decades. Eur Heart J 2006;27(8):936–41.
8. Wattigney WA, Mensah GA, Croft JB. Increasing trends in hospitalization for atrial fibrillation in the united states, 1985 through 1999: implications for primary prevention. Circulation 2003;108(6):711–6.
9. Wu EQ, Birnbaum HG, Mareva M, et al. Economic burden and co-morbidities of atrial fibrillation in

a privately insured population. Curr Med Res Opin 2005;21(10):1693–9.
10. American heart association. Heart disease and stroke statistics—2008 update. Dallas (TX): American Heart Association; 2008.
11. Lloyd-Jones DM, Larson MG, Leip EP, et al. Lifetime risk for developing congestive heart failure: the Framingham heart study. Circulation 2002; 106(24):3068–72.
12. Levy D, Kenchaiah S, Larson MG, et al. Long-term trends in the incidence of and survival with heart failure. N Engl J Med 2002;347(18):1397–402.
13. Roger VL, Weston SA, Redfield MM, et al. Trends in heart failure incidence and survival in a community-based population. JAMA 2004;292(3):344–50.
14. Dries DL, Exner DV, Gersh BJ, et al. Atrial fibrillation is associated with an increased risk for mortality and heart failure progression in patients with asymptomatic and symptomatic left ventricular systolic dysfunction: a retrospective analysis of the solved trials. Studies of left ventricular dysfunction. J Am Coll Cardiol 1998;32(3):695–703.
15. van Veldhuisen DJ, Aass H, El Allaf D, et al. Presence and development of atrial fibrillation in chronic heart failure. Experiences from the merit-hf study. Eur J Heart Fail 2006;8(5):539–46.
16. De Ferrari GM, Klersy C, Ferrero P, et al. Atrial fibrillation in heart failure patients: prevalence in daily practice and effect on the severity of symptoms. Data from the alpha study registry. Eur J Heart Fail 2007;9(5):502–9.
17. Flather MD, Shibata MC, Coats AJ, et al. Randomized trial to determine the effect of nebivolol on mortality and cardiovascular hospital admission in elderly patients with heart failure (seniors). Eur Heart J 2005;26(3):215–25.
18. Poole-Wilson PA, Swedberg K, Cleland JG, et al. Comparison of carvedilol and metoprolol on clinical outcomes in patients with chronic heart failure in the carvedilol or metoprolol european trial (comet): randomised controlled trial. Lancet 2003; 362(9377):7–13.
19. Corell P, Gustafsson F, Schou M, et al. Prevalence and prognostic significance of atrial fibrillation in outpatients with heart failure due to left ventricular systolic dysfunction. Eur J Heart Fail 2007;9(3): 258–65.
20. Olsson LG, Swedberg K, Ducharme A, et al. Atrial fibrillation and risk of clinical events in chronic heart failure with and without left ventricular systolic dysfunction: results from the candesartan in heart failure-assessment of reduction in mortality and morbidity (charm) program. J Am Coll Cardiol 2006;47(10):1997–2004.
21. Deedwania PC, Singh BN, Ellenbogen K, et al. Spontaneous conversion and maintenance of sinus rhythm by amiodarone in patients with heart failure and atrial fibrillation: observations from the veterans affairs congestive heart failure survival trial of antiarrhythmic therapy (chf-stat). The department of veterans affairs chf-stat investigators. Circulation 1998;98(23):2574–9.
22. Maggioni AP, Latini R, Carson PE, et al. Valsartan reduces the incidence of atrial fibrillation in patients with heart failure: results from the valsartan heart failure trial (val-heft). Am Heart J 2005;149(3):548–57.
23. Swedberg K, Olsson LG, Charlesworth A, et al. Prognostic relevance of atrial fibrillation in patients with chronic heart failure on long-term treatment with beta-blockers: results from comet. Eur Heart J 2005;26(13):1303–8.
24. Bhatia RS, Tu JV, Lee DS, et al. Outcome of heart failure with preserved ejection fraction in a population-based study. N Engl J Med 2006;355(3): 260–9.
25. Owan TE, Hodge DO, Herges RM, et al. Trends in prevalence and outcome of heart failure with preserved ejection fraction. N Engl J Med 2006; 355(3):251–9.
26. Ho KK, Pinsky JL, Kannel WB, et al. The epidemiology of heart failure: the Framingham study. J Am Coll Cardiol 1993;22(4 Suppl A):6A–13A.
27. Frustaci A, Caldarulo M, Buffon A, et al. Cardiac biopsy in patients with "primary" atrial fibrillation. Histologic evidence of occult myocardial diseases. Chest 1991;100(2):303–6.
28. Frustaci A, Chimenti C, Bellocci F, et al. Histological substrate of atrial biopsies in patients with lone atrial fibrillation. Circulation 1997;96(4):1180–4.
29. Cowie MR, Wood DA, Coats AJ, et al. Incidence and aetiology of heart failure; a population-based study. Eur Heart J 1999;20(6):421–8.
30. Wang TJ, Larson MG, Levy D, et al. Temporal relations of atrial fibrillation and congestive heart failure and their joint influence on mortality: the Framingham heart study. Circulation 2003; 107(23):2920–5.
31. Gage BF, Waterman AD, Shannon W, et al. Validation of clinical classification schemes for predicting stroke: results from the national registry of atrial fibrillation. JAMA 2001;285(22):2864–70.
32. Naito M, David D, Michelson EL, et al. The hemodynamic consequences of cardiac arrhythmias: evaluation of the relative roles of abnormal atrioventricular sequencing, irregularity of ventricular rhythm and atrial fibrillation in a canine model. Am Heart J 1983;106(2):284–91.
33. Clark DM, Plumb VJ, Epstein AE, et al. Hemodynamic effects of an irregular sequence of ventricular cycle lengths during atrial fibrillation. J Am Coll Cardiol 1997;30(4):1039–45.
34. Scott ME, Patterson GC. Cardiac output after direct current conversion of atrial fibrillation. Br Heart J 1969;31(1):87–90.

35. Greenberg B, Chatterjee K, Parmley WW, et al. The influence of left ventricular filling pressure on atrial contribution to cardiac output. Am Heart J 1979; 98(6):742–51.
36. Mukharji J, Rehr RB, Hastillo A, et al. Comparison of atrial contribution to cardiac hemodynamics in patients with normal and severely compromised cardiac function. Clin Cardiol 1990;13(9):639–43.
37. Packer DL, Bardy GH, Worley SJ, et al. Tachycardia-induced cardiomyopathy: a reversible form of left ventricular dysfunction. Am J Cardiol 1986; 57(8):563–70.
38. Nattel S. New ideas about atrial fibrillation 50 years on. Nature 2002;415(6868):219–26.
39. Mines GR. On dynamic equilibrium in the heart. J Physiol 1913;46(4–5):349–83.
40. Garrey WE. The nature of fibrillary contraction of the heart; its relation to tissue mass and form. Am J Phys 1914;33(3):397–414.
41. Moe GK, Abildskov JA. Atrial fibrillation as a self-sustaining arrhythmia independent of focal discharge. Am Heart J 1959;58(1):59–70.
42. Lewis T. Observations upon flutter and fibrillation. Part IX. The nature of auricular fibrillation as it occurs in patients. Heart 1921;8:193–227.
43. Scherf D, Terranova R. Mechanism of auricular flutter and fibrillation. Am J Phys 1949;159(1): 137–42.
44. Natale A, Raviele A, Arentz T, et al. Venice chart international consensus document on atrial fibrillation ablation. J Cardiovasc Electrophysiol 2007; 18(5):560–80.
45. Kostin S, Klein G, Szalay Z, et al. Structural correlate of atrial fibrillation in human patients. Cardiovasc Res 2002;54(2):361–79.
46. Li D, Fareh S, Leung TK, et al. Promotion of atrial fibrillation by heart failure in dogs: atrial remodeling of a different sort. Circulation 1999;100(1):87–95.
47. Verheule S, Sato T, Everett TT, et al. Increased vulnerability to atrial fibrillation in transgenic mice with selective atrial fibrosis caused by overexpression of tgf-beta1. Circ Res 2004;94(11):1458–65.
48. Burstein B, Nattel S. Atrial fibrosis: mechanisms and clinical relevance in atrial fibrillation. J Am Coll Cardiol 2008;51(8):802–9.
49. Everett TH 4th, Olgin JE. Atrial fibrosis and the mechanisms of atrial fibrillation. Heart Rhythm 2007;4(Suppl 3):S24–7.
50. Chen K, Mehta JL, Li D, et al. Transforming growth factor beta receptor endoglin is expressed in cardiac fibroblasts and modulates profibrogenic actions of angiotensin ii. Circ Res 2004;95(12): 1167–73.
51. Healey JS, Baranchuk A, Crystal E, et al. Prevention of atrial fibrillation with angiotensin-converting enzyme inhibitors and angiotensin receptor blockers: a meta-analysis. J Am Coll Cardiol 2005;45(11):1832–9.
52. Anand K, Mooss AN, Hee TT, et al. Meta-analysis: inhibition of renin-angiotensin system prevents new-onset atrial fibrillation. Am Heart J 2006; 152(2):217–22.
53. Allessie MA, Boyden PA, Camm AJ, et al. Pathophysiology and prevention of atrial fibrillation. Circulation 2001;103(5):769–77.
54. Wijffels MC, Kirchhof CJ, Dorland R, et al. Atrial fibrillation begets atrial fibrillation. A study in awake chronically instrumented goats. Circulation 1995; 92(7):1954–68.
55. Ausma J, Wijffels M, Thone F, et al. Structural changes of atrial myocardium due to sustained atrial fibrillation in the goat. Circulation 1997; 96(9):3157–63.
56. Van Wagoner DR, Pond AL, Lamorgese M, et al. Atrial l-type Ca2+ currents and human atrial fibrillation. Circ Res 1999;85(5):428–36.
57. Petersen P, Kastrup J, Brinch K, et al. Relation between left atrial dimension and duration of atrial fibrillation. Am J Cardiol 1987;60(4):382–4.
58. Haissaguerre M, Jais P, Shah DC, et al. Spontaneous initiation of atrial fibrillation by ectopic beats originating in the pulmonary veins. N Engl J Med 1998;339(10):659–66.
59. Chen SA, Hsieh MH, Tai CT, et al. Initiation of atrial fibrillation by ectopic beats originating from the pulmonary veins: electrophysiological characteristics, pharmacological responses, and effects of radiofrequency ablation. Circulation 1999;100(18): 1879–86.
60. Nathan H, Eliakim M. The junction between the left atrium and the pulmonary veins. An anatomic study of human hearts. Circulation 1966;34(3):412–22.
61. Oral H, Pappone C, Chugh A, et al. Circumferential pulmonary-vein ablation for chronic atrial fibrillation. N Engl J Med 2006;354(9):934–41.
62. Wazni OM, Marrouche NF, Martin DO, et al. Radiofrequency ablation vs antiarrhythmic drugs as first-line treatment of symptomatic atrial fibrillation: a randomized trial. JAMA 2005;293(21):2634–40.
63. Nattel S. Basic electrophysiology of the pulmonary veins and their role in atrial fibrillation: precipitators, perpetuators, and perplexers. J Cardiovasc Electrophysiol 2003;14(12):1372–5.
64. Chang SL, Chen YC, Chen YJ, et al. Mechanoelectrical feedback regulates the arrhythmogenic activity of pulmonary veins. Heart 2007;93(1):82–8.
65. Lin WS, Tai CT, Hsieh MH, et al. Catheter ablation of paroxysmal atrial fibrillation initiated by non-pulmonary vein ectopy. Circulation 2003;107(25): 3176–83.
66. Sauer WH, Alonso C, Zado E, et al. Atrioventricular nodal reentrant tachycardia in patients referred for atrial fibrillation ablation: response to ablation that

incorporates slow-pathway modification. Circulation 2006;114(3):191–5.
67. Pappone C, Santinelli V, Manguso F, et al. A randomized study of prophylactic catheter ablation in asymptomatic patients with the Wolff-Parkinson-White syndrome. N Engl J Med 2003;349(19): 1803–11.
68. Chen YJ, Chen SA, Tai CT, et al. Role of atrial electrophysiology and autonomic nervous system in patients with supraventricular tachycardia and paroxysmal atrial fibrillation. J Am Coll Cardiol 1998;32(3):732–8.
69. Pappone C, Santinelli V, Manguso F, et al. Pulmonary vein denervation enhances long-term benefit after circumferential ablation for paroxysmal atrial fibrillation. Circulation 2004;109(3):327–34.
70. Aviles RJ, Martin DO, Apperson-Hansen C, et al. Inflammation as a risk factor for atrial fibrillation. Circulation 2003;108(24):3006–10.
71. Halonen J, Halonen P, Jarvinen O, et al. Corticosteroids for the prevention of atrial fibrillation after cardiac surgery: a randomized controlled trial. JAMA 2007;297(14):1562–7.
72. Fox CS, Parise H, D'Agostino RB Sr, et al. Parental atrial fibrillation as a risk factor for atrial fibrillation in offspring. JAMA 2004;291(23):2851–5.
73. Darbar D, Herron KJ, Ballew JD, et al. Familial atrial fibrillation is a genetically heterogeneous disorder. J Am Coll Cardiol 2003;41(12):2185–92.
74. Ellinor PT, Yoerger DM, Ruskin JN, et al. Familial aggregation in lone atrial fibrillation. Hum Genet 2005;118(2):179–84.
75. Chen LY, Ballew JD, Herron KJ, et al. A common polymorphism in scn5a is associated with lone atrial fibrillation. Clin Pharmacol Ther 2007;81(1): 35–41.
76. Darbar D, Kannankeril PJ, Donahue BS, et al. Cardiac sodium channel (scn5a) variants associated with atrial fibrillation. Circulation 2008; 117(15):1927–35.
77. Arnar DO, Thorvaldsson S, Manolio TA, et al. Familial aggregation of atrial fibrillation in iceland. Eur Heart J 2006;27(6):708–12.
78. Chen YH, Xu SJ, Bendahhou S, et al. Kcnq1 gain-of-function mutation in familial atrial fibrillation. Science 2003;299(5604):251–4.
79. Yang Y, Xia M, Jin Q, et al. Identification of a kcne2 gain-of-function mutation in patients with familial atrial fibrillation. Am J Hum Genet 2004;75(5): 899–905.
80. Hong K, Bjerregaard P, Gussak I, et al. Short qt syndrome and atrial fibrillation caused by mutation in kcnh2. J Cardiovasc Electrophysiol 2005;16(4):394–6.
81. Xia M, Jin Q, Bendahhou S, et al. A kir2.1 gain-of-function mutation underlies familial atrial fibrillation. Biochem Biophys Res Commun 2005;332(4): 1012–9.
82. Olson TM, Alekseev AE, Liu XK, et al. Kv1.5 channelopathy due to kcna5 loss-of-function mutation causes human atrial fibrillation. Hum Mol Genet 2006;15(14):2185–91.
83. Otway R, Vandenberg JI, Guo G, et al. Stretch-sensitive kcnq1 mutation a link between genetic and environmental factors in the pathogenesis of atrial fibrillation? J Am Coll Cardiol 2007;49(5): 578–86.
84. Das S, Makino S, Melman YF, et al. Mutation in the S3 segment of KCNQ1 results in familial lone atrial fibrillation. Heart Rhythm 2009;6(8):1146–53.
85. Ellinor PT, Nam EG, Shea MA, et al. Cardiac sodium channel mutation in atrial fibrillation. Heart Rhythm 2008;5(1):99–105.
86. Benito B, Brugada R, Perich RM, et al. A mutation in the sodium channel is responsible for the association of long QT syndrome and familial atrial fibrillation. Heart Rhythm 2008;5(10):1434–40.
87. Makiyama T, Akao M, Shizuta S, et al. A novel SCN5A gain-of-function mutation M1875T associated with familial atrial fibrillation. J Am Coll Cardiol 2008;52(16):1326–34.
88. Hodgson-Zingman DM, Karst ML, Zingman LV, et al. Atrial natriuretie peptide frameshift mutation in familial atrial fibrillation. N Engl J Med 2008; 359(2):158–65.
89. Brugada R, Tapscott T, Czernuszewicz GZ, et al. Identification of a genetic locus for familial atrial fibrillation. N Engl J Med 1997;336(13):905–11.
90. Ellinor PT, Shin JT, Moore RK, et al. Locus for atrial fibrillation maps to chromosome 6q14–16. Circulation 2003;107(23):2880–3.
91. Oberti C, Wang L, Li L, et al. Genome-wide linkage scan identifies a novel genetic locus on chromosome 5p13 for neonatal atrial fibrillation associated with sudden death and variable cardiomyopathy. Circulation 2004;110(25):3753–9.
92. Volders PG, Zhu Q, Timmermans C, et al. Mapping a novel locus for familial atrial fibrillation on chromosome 10p11–q21. Heart Rhythm 2007;4(4): 469–75.
93. Schott JJ, Charpentier F, Peltier S, et al. Mapping of a gene for long QT syndrome to chromosome 4q25-27. Am J Hum Genet 1995;57(5):1114–22.
94. Hong K, Piper DR, Diaz-Valdecantos A, et al. De novo kcnq1 mutation responsible for atrial fibrillation and short qt syndrome in utero. Cardiovasc Res 2005;68(3):433–40.
95. Sanders P, Morton JB, Davidson NC, et al. Electrical remodeling of the atria in congestive heart failure: Electrophysiological and electroanatomic mapping in humans. Circulation 2003;108(12): 1461–8.
96. Gollob MH, Jones DL, Krahn AD, et al. Somatic mutations in the connexin 40 gene (gja5) in atrial fibrillation. N Engl J Med 2006;354(25):2677–88.

97. Ellinor PT, MacRae CA. Ion channel mutations in AF: signal or noise? Heart Rhythm 2008;5(3):436–7.
98. Olson TM, Michels VV, Ballew JD, et al. Sodium channel mutations and susceptibility to heart failure and atrial fibrillation. JAMA 2005;293(4):447–54.
99. McNair WP, Ku L, Taylor MR, et al. Scn5a mutation associated with dilated cardiomyopathy, conduction disorder, and arrhythmia. Circulation 2004;110(15):2163–7.
100. Fatkin D, MacRae C, Sasaki T, et al. Missense mutations in the rod domain of the lamin a/c gene as causes of dilated cardiomyopathy and conduction-system disease. N Engl J Med 1999;341(23):1715–24.
101. Sebillon P, Bouchier C, Bidot LD, et al. Expanding the phenotype of lmna mutations in dilated cardiomyopathy and functional consequences of these mutations. J Med Genet 2003;40(8):560–7.
102. Gudbjartsson DF, Arnar DO, Helgadottir A, et al. Variants conferring risk of atrial fibrillation on chromosome 4q25. Nature 2007;448(7151):353–7.
103. Larson MG, Atwood LD, Benjamin EJ, et al. Framingham heart study 100k project: gGenome-wide associations for cardiovascular disease outcomes. BMC Med Genet 2007;8(Suppl 1):S5.
104. Franco D, Campione M. The role of pitx2 during cardiac development. Linking left-right signaling and congenital heart diseases. Trends Cardiovasc Med 2003;13(4):157–63.
105. Faucourt M, Houliston E, Besnardeau L, et al. The pitx2 homeobox protein is required early for endoderm formation and nodal signaling. Dev Biol 2001;229(2):287–306.
106. Mommersteeg MT, Hoogaars WM, Prall OW, et al. Molecular pathway for the localized formation of the sinoatrial node. Circ Res 2007;100(3):354–62.
107. Mitsui T, Nomura S, Okada M, et al. Hypertension and angiotensin ii hypersensitivity in aminopeptidase a-deficient mice. Mol Med 2003;9(1–2):57–62.
108. Gudbjartsson DF, Holm H, Gretarsdottir S, et al. A sequence variant in ZFHX3 on 16q22 associates with atrial fibrillation and ischemic stroke. Nat Genet 2009;41(8):876–8.
109. Benjamin EJ, Rice KM, Arking DE, et al. Variants in ZFHX3 are associated with atrial fibrillation in individuals of European ancestry. Nat Genet 2009;41(8):879–81.
110. Li D, Melnyk P, Feng J, et al. Effects of experimental heart failure on atrial cellular and ionic electrophysiology. Circulation 2000;101(22):2631–8.
111. Yeh YH, Wakili R, Qi X, et al. Calcium handling abnormalities underlying atrial arrhythmogenesis and contractile dysfunction in dogs with congestive heart failure. Circ Arrhythmia Electrophysiol 2008;1(2):93–102.
112. Tisdale JE, Borzak S, Sabbah HN, et al. Hemodynamic and neurohormonal predictors and consequences of the development of atrial fibrillation in dogs with chronic heart failure. J Card Fail 2006;12(9):747–51.
113. Rucker-Martin C, Milliez P, Tan S, et al. Chronic hemodynamic overload of the atria is an important factor for gap junction remodeling in human and rat hearts. Cardiovasc Res 2006;72(1):69–79.
114. Vaziri SM, Larson MG, Benjamin EJ, et al. Echocardiographic predictors of nonrheumatic atrial fibrillation. The Framingham heart study. Circulation 1994;89(2):724–30.
115. Psaty BM, Manolio TA, Kuller LH, et al. Incidence of and risk factors for atrial fibrillation in older adults. Circulation 1997;96(7):2455–61.
116. Bode F, Katchman A, Woosley RL, et al. Gadolinium decreases stretch-induced vulnerability to atrial fibrillation. Circulation 2000;101(18):2200–5.
117. Tanaka K, Zlochiver S, Vikstrom KL, et al. Spatial distribution of fibrosis governs fibrillation wave dynamics in the posterior left atrium during heart failure. Circ Res 2007;101(8):839–47.
118. Cha TJ, Ehrlich JR, Zhang L, et al. Dissociation between ionic remodeling and ability to sustain atrial fibrillation during recovery from experimental congestive heart failure. Circulation 2004;109(3):412–8.
119. Zankov DP, Omatsu-Kanbe M, Isono T, et al. Angiotensin ii potentiates the slow component of delayed rectifier k+ current via the at1 receptor in guinea pig atrial myocytes. Circulation 2006;113(10):1278–86.
120. Wang TJ, Massaro JM, Levy D, et al. A risk score for predicting stroke or death in individuals with new-onset atrial fibrillation in the community: the Framingham heart study. JAMA 2003;290(8):1049–56.
121. Carlsson J, Miketic S, Windeler J, et al. Randomized trial of rate-control versus rhythm-control in persistent atrial fibrillation: the strategies of treatment of atrial fibrillation (staf) study. J Am Coll Cardiol 2003;41(10):1690–6.
122. Hohnloser SH, Kuck KH, Lilienthal J. Rhythm or rate control in atrial fibrillation–pharmacological intervention in atrial fibrillation (PIAF): a randomised trial. Lancet 2000;356(9244):1789–94.
123. Opolski G, Torbicki A, Kosior DA, et al. Rate control vs rhythm control in patients with nonvalvular persistent atrial fibrillation: the results of the polish how to treat chronic atrial fibrillation (hot cafe) study. Chest 2004;126(2):476–86.
124. Van Gelder IC, Hagens VE, Bosker HA, et al. A comparison of rate control and rhythm control in patients with recurrent persistent atrial fibrillation. N Engl J Med 2002;347(23):1834–40.
125. Wyse DG, Waldo AL, DiMarco JP, et al. A comparison of rate control and rhythm control in patients

with atrial fibrillation. N Engl J Med 2002;347(23): 1825–33.
126. Testa L, Biondi-Zoccai GG, Dello Russo A, et al. Rate-control vs. Rhythm-control in patients with atrial fibrillation: a meta-analysis. Eur Heart J 2005;26(19):2000–6.
127. Corley SD, Epstein AE, DiMarco JP, et al. Relationships between sinus rhythm, treatment, and survival in the atrial fibrillation follow-up investigation of rhythm management (AFFIRM) study. Circulation 2004;109(12):1509–13.
128. Hagens VE, Ranchor AV, Van Sonderen E, et al. Effect of rate or rhythm control on quality of life in persistent atrial fibrillation. Results from the rate control versus electrical cardioversion (race) study. J Am Coll Cardiol 2004;43(2):241–7.
129. Singh BN, Singh SN, Reda DJ, et al. Amiodarone versus sotalol for atrial fibrillation. N Engl J Med 2005;352(18):1861–72.
130. Steinberg JS, Sadaniantz A, Kron J, et al. Analysis of cause-specific mortality in the atrial fibrillation follow-up investigation of rhythm management (AFFIRM) study. Circulation 2004; 109(16):1973–80.
131. Roy D, Talajic M, Nattel S, et al. Rhythm control versus rate control for atrial fibrillation and heart failure. N Engl J Med 2008;358(25):2667–77.
132. Shelton RJ, Clark AL, Goode K, et al. A randomised, controlled study of rate versus rhythm control in patients with chronic atrial fibrillation and heart failure: (CAFE-II Study). Heart 2009; 95(11):924–30.
133. Lubitz SA, Fischer A, Fuster V. Catheter ablation for atrial fibrillation. BMJ 2008;336(7648):819–26.
134. Hsu LF, Jais P, Sanders P, et al. Catheter ablation for atrial fibrillation in congestive heart failure. N Engl J Med 2004;351(23):2373–83.
135. Chen MS, Marrouche NF, Khaykin Y, et al. Pulmonary vein isolation for the treatment of atrial fibrillation in patients with impaired systolic function. J Am Coll Cardiol 2004;43(6):1004–9.
136. Brignole M, Menozzi C, Gianfranchi L, et al. Assessment of atrioventricular junction ablation and vvir pacemaker versus pharmacological treatment in patients with heart failure and chronic atrial fibrillation: a randomized, controlled study. Circulation 1998;98(10):953–60.
137. McAlister FA, Ezekowitz J, Hooton N, et al. Cardiac resynchronization therapy for patients with left ventricular systolic dysfunction: a systematic review. JAMA 2007;297(22):2502–14.
138. Gasparini M, Auricchio A, Regoli F, et al. Four-year efficacy of cardiac resynchronization therapy on exercise tolerance and disease progression: the importance of performing atrioventricular junction ablation in patients with atrial fibrillation. J Am Coll Cardiol 2006;48(4):734–43.
139. Linde C, Leclercq C, Rex S, et al. Long-term benefits of biventricular pacing in congestive heart failure: results from the multisite stimulation in cardiomyopathy (mustic) study. J Am Coll Cardiol 2002;40(1):111–8.
140. Hamdan MH, Freedman RA, Gilbert EM, et al. Atrioventricular junction ablation followed by resynchronization therapy in patients with congestive heart failure and atrial fibrillation (AVERT-AF) study design. Pacing Clin Electrophysiol 2006;29(10):1081–8.
141. Khan M, Jais P, Cummings JE, et al. American heart association 2006 scientific session. Pulmonary vein antrum isolation versus av node ablation with biventricular pacing for the treatment of atrial fibrillation in patients with congestive heart failure (PABA-CHF) [abstract]. Circulation 2006;114(22): 2426.
142. Nasr IA, Bouzamondo A, Hulot JS, et al. Prevention of atrial fibrillation onset by beta-blocker treatment in heart failure: a meta-analysis. Eur Heart J 2007; 28(4):457–62.

The Genetics of Conduction Disease

Roy Beinart, MD, Jeremy Ruskin, MD, David Milan, MD*

KEYWORDS

• Atrioventricular • Conduction diseases • Genetics

Conduction diseases (CD) include defects in impulse generation and conduction. Patients with CD may manifest in a wide range of clinical presentations, from asymptomatic to potentially life-threatening arrhythmias. Conduction disorders can occur at any point in the conduction system, but most are recognized between the sinus node and atrium (sinoatrial diseases); between the atria and ventricles (atrioventricular [AV] block); within the atria (intra-atrial block); or within the ventricles (intraventricular block).

The pathophysiologic mechanisms underlying CD are diverse and may have implications for diagnosis, treatment, and prognosis. In general, they are divided into acquired or inherited causes. The latter form may have implications for other family members of the affected individuals and for potential future genetic treatments.

In the past, CD was perceived as structural diseases per se, in which abnormalities in the conduction system structure caused disruption of impulse propagation. Conduction disturbances can be found even in the absence of anatomic abnormalities, a fact that suggests functional abnormalities and probably gene involvement. Several other observations support the role of genetics: first, there is overlap between classic CD and other cardiac disorders and this might suggest shared pathophysiologic mechanisms related to a common gene mutation; second, the underlying mechanism of so-called "degenerative conduction disorders" is attributed to fibrosis or atrophy of the specialized conduction tissues. The progression rates and extent of disease, however, could imply that additional factors play a role in determining the final outcomes. Individual susceptibility to the degenerative process might be predefined by genetic factors. Finally, the terminal events in many patients with CD are sudden death or heart failure rather than bradycardia, suggesting that there is more to the pathophysiology than simple failure of conduction.

Known causes of functional CD include cardiac ion channelopathies or defects in modifying proteins, such as cytoskeletal proteins. Although functional CD cannot be distinguished clinically from the classic structural CD, progress in molecular biology and genetics along with development of animal models has increased the understanding of the molecular mechanisms of these disorders. This article discusses the genetic basis for CD and its clinical implications.

CONDUCTION SYSTEM ANATOMY

The cardiac conduction system is composed of specialized cardiac structures that are responsible for impulse formation and propagation. The sinus node tissue is located in the right atrium and is normally responsible for impulse generation, which is conducted to the left atrium by the Bachmann bundle. From the atria, the impulse is conducted to the ventricular myocardium through the AV node, the bundle of His, the right and left bundle branches, and the Purkinje fibers.

Mechanisms of pacemaking in the sinus node are the subject of ongoing investigation, but there is evidence for involvement of a number of ion channels including the L- and T-type calcium channels and the delayed rectifier potassium channels.[1,2] In the myocardium, impulse propagation occurs predominantly by voltage-gated sodium channels and gap junctions.[3]

Massachusetts General Hospital, 55 Fruit Street, Boston, MA 02114, USA
* Corresponding author.
E-mail address: dmilan@partners.org

Heart Failure Clin 6 (2010) 201–214
doi:10.1016/j.hfc.2009.11.006

SEPTATION DEFECTS

Several mutations in genes encoding proteins that regulate septation of the heart have been documented. The phenotype includes atrial septal defects or ventricular septal defects.[4–10]

TBX5

Mutations in the T-box transcription factor TBX5 have been shown to cause Holt-Oram syndrome.[11,12] This autosomal-dominant inherited syndrome is typically characterized by cardiac septation defects and skeletal abnormalities that affect the upper limbs exclusively. These skeletal abnormalities are always bilateral and often asymmetric and predominantly involve the radial ray. The thumb is the most commonly affected structure and can be triphalangeal, hypoplastic, or completely absent.[8,11,13,14] Some mutation carriers have CD and atrial fibrillation in the absence of septation defects. A role for TBX5 in the specification and maintenance of the proximal conduction system is emerging from elegant studies in the mouse.[15–17]

NKX2.5

At least 12 distinctly different mutations of the NKX2.5 gene, mostly outside the homeodomain, have been reported. These mutations lead to a clinical picture ranging from atrial septal defects with AV block to ventricular septal defects and tetralogy of Fallot, without extracardiac abnormalities.[4,5,7,9,10] Recently, Bjornstad and Leren[18] reported a family with an autosomal-dominant inheritance of atrial septal defect with increasingly prolonged AV conduction time eventually producing AV block that segregates completely with mutation Q149X in the NKX2.5 gene. In addition, studies in Nkx2.5-deficient mice have shown that Nkx2.5 insufficiency may cause hypoplasia of the AV node, His bundle, and Purkinje system.[19,20] The precise genotype-phenotype correlations with respect to associated CD, however, have not emerged.

Currently, several familial cases of cardiac septation defects with AV block have been diagnosed in which the involved proteins and genes still await identification.

THE CYTOSKELETON

Mutations in genes encoding cytoskeletal proteins and nuclear membrane proteins have been found to be involved in inherited cardiomyopathies and muscular dystrophies.[21–28] Occasionally, the primary manifestation of inherited cardiomyopathy or muscular dystrophy is conduction disorder without detectable structural cardiac abnormalities. In view of that, mutations in cytoskeletal proteins might impair ion channel functions. For example, the intracellular protein syntrophin affects the pore-forming α subunit of the cardiac sodium channel and regulates its membrane expression.[29] Syntrophin additionally associates with dystrophin and ankyrin.[29–32] Disruption of cytoskeletal proteins may cause defects in ion channel function and lead to conduction abnormalities.[33–37]

Myotonic Dystrophy Protein Kinase

Myotonic dystrophy is the most common form of muscular dystrophy and is caused by an expansion of cytosine-thymine-guanine repeat on chromosome 19.[38–40] Cardiac manifestations include varying degrees of AV block and sudden death.[41–43] Occasional patients display atrial arrhythmias, which may dominate the clinical picture. Recently, Groh and his colleagues[44] found that "severe" ECG abnormalities (rhythm other than sinus, QRS >120 millisecond, PR interval >240 millisecond, or second- or third-degree AV block) and clinical diagnosis of atrial tachyarrhythmia are independent predictors, with moderate sensitivity, of sudden death in these patients. In addition, a mouse knockout model of the myotonic dystrophy protein kinase displays first-, second-, and third-degree AV block, and the haplo insufficient mice show first-degree AV block.[45] The mechanism of AV nodal pathology is thought to be caused by alterations in the activation kinetics or amplitude of the $I_{Ca,L}$ current.

Emerin, Lamin A/C, Nesprin

Mutations in these genes cause muscular dystrophy known as Emery-Dreifuss muscular dystrophy (EDMD) with manifestation as high-grade AV block.[46–50] It is classically X-linked, but also has autosomal-dominant variants. Clinical presentation is characterized by onset in the first to third decade with tendon contractures. Progressive CD is present in virtually all cases and leads to permanent pacing. The extent of the associated cardiomyopathy is variable as is the skeletal involvement.

Clinical genetics suggested that EDMD is a disorder of a distinct pathway and molecular studies confirmed this when a novel gene, emerin, encoding a nuclear membrane protein was identified as the cause of the X-linked form. The major autosomal form of EDMD is caused by mutations in the lamin A/C gene, encoding another nuclear envelope protein. Lamin mutations are also associated with a variety of other diseases, such as the Hutchinson-Gilford syndrome,[51] mandibuloacral dysplasia,[52] Charcot-Marie-Tooth disease type 2,[53] atypical Werner syndrome,[54] and the Dunnigan-type familial partial lipodystrophy,[55] most of which are also associated with CD.[56] Finally, it has been shown recently that mutations in nesprins 1 and 2 can also cause EDMD. The latter genes encode multi-isomeric, spectrin-repeat proteins that bind both emerin and lamins A/C and form a network in muscle linking the nucleoskeleton to the inner nuclear membrane, the outer nuclear membrane, membraneous organelles, the sarcomere, and the actin cytoskeleton. Hence, disruptions in nesprin-lamin-emerin interactions might play a role in the muscle-specific pathogenesis of EDMD.[49]

To date no unifying biologic mechanism has been discovered to explain the effects of these mutations on the cardiac conduction system, myocardial contractility, and skeletal muscle groups. Some animal models recapitulate the clinical features of these syndromes, but whereas effects on both transcription and nuclear integrity have been observed, the tissue-specific effects remain unexplained. The picture is further complicated by the marked clinical pleiotropy observed with lamin A/C mutations. Mutations in this single gene have been implicated in a remarkable array of clinical syndromes. Understanding how mutations in a single gene can result in such a diverse set of clinical syndromes is necessary if the fundamental biology of the disease is to be understood.

Interestingly, there may be a subtle gender difference in the severity of the cardiac phenotypes seen in lamin A/C disease. Males often have significant cardiac disease, with moderate or severe left ventricular (LV) dysfunction developing in the first two to three decades of life, whereas females bearing the same mutations are more likely to have progressive CD, with less severe LV dysfunction. It remains to be seen if a mechanistic interaction between lamin and emerin is the explanation for the similar clinical manifestations.

Dystrophin

Dystrophinopathies comprise Duchenne muscular dystrophy, Becker muscular dystrophy, and X-linked dilated cardiomyopathy. They are X-linked conditions and affect males. The primary defect is the deficiency of the sarcolemmal protein, dystrophin, which is part of a membrane-spanning dystrophin-associated protein complex. This protein complex can be divided into three major components: (1) the dystroglycan complex, which binds laminin in the extracellular matrix and dystrophin at the cytoplasmic face of the sarcolemma; (2) the sarcoglycan complex, which consists of four transmembrane glycoproteins and sarcospan; and (3) the cytoplasmic components, comprising the syntrophins, dystrobrevin, and neuronal nitric oxide synthase. In addition to providing a structural link between the subcortical actin and the extracellular matrix, the dystrophin-associated protein complex also seems to be involved in signaling with components, such as neuronal nitric oxide synthase, dystrobrevin, and syntrophin. Some proteins might play multiple roles: dystrobrevin binds to the intermediate filament protein syncoilin, and in addition to the spatial organization of proteins involved in signaling, also participates in the structural integrity of the cytoskeleton.[57] The mechanism of cardiac muscle progressive degeneration is believed to be similar to that of skeletal muscle: dystrophin deficiency leads to a disruption of the transmembrane complex, a loss in the integrity of the sarcolemma, and fiber necrosis. In the heart, this leads to the replacement of myocardium with connective tissue or fat. There does not seem to be evidence for a specific and early degeneration of the conduction system, and any evidence of conduction system disease seems to be limited to the final stages, when widespread fibrosis leads to systolic dysfunction and ventricular arrhythmias.[58,59]

Interestingly, other members of the dystrophin-glycoprotein complex have been implicated in several recessive forms of muscular dystrophy where prominent cardiac phenotypes are not observed.

PROTEIN KINASE DISORDERS

PRKAG2

Mutations PRKAG2 (R302Q, R531G, T172D), which encodes for a regulatory subunit of adenosine monophosphate-activated protein kinase, were found in association with Wolff-Parkinson-White syndrome.[60] The disorders are characterized by pseudohypertrophy of the left and right ventricles caused by glycogen deposition in cardiac muscle, and both accessory pathways and conduction system disturbances.[61] Although atrial fibrillation and atrial flutter are common, high-grade AV block is the dominant clinical arrhythmia.[62] Clinical studies suggest that in many cases, asymptomatic individuals are maximally pre-excited at rest, and so probably dependent on accessory AV connections from an early age. Syncope and sudden death are also reported in PRKAG2 families, but the mechanism is not always clear.

Patient's major complaints are atypical chest pain, palpitations, and exertional limitation. The index of suspicion for PRKAG2 disease is raised by massive LV wall thickening (>30 mm) and by the presence of high-grade AV block, because these features are rare in hypertrophic heart disease caused by sarcomere gene mutations. Of note, a mouse model carrying a mutation responsible for the human disease has been generated.[63] In this model the annulus fibrosis that normally insulates the atria and ventricles is penetrated by glycogen-filled cardiomyocytes that seem to be responsible for ventricular pre-excitation.

FATTY ACID OXIDATION DISORDERS

Fatty acid oxidation disorders are caused by enzymatic defects that affect normal transport and metabolism of fatty acids.[64] This may lead to cardiomyopathy with conduction and rhythm abnormalities, such as sinus node dysfunction, paroxysmal supraventricular arrhythmias, AV block, and intraventricular conduction abnormalities, without evident structural heart disease.[65,66] The defects are usually in enzymes that regulate mitochondrial transport of long-chain fatty acids (carnitine palmityltransferase type II, carnitine-acylcarnitine translocase). Accumulation of fatty acid metabolites results in conduction disorders. They have a direct toxic effect on the myocytes and could potentially affect ion channels, such as potassium, sodium, and calcium channels, in addition to gap-junctions.[65]

Refsum disease is an example for an inherited autosomal-recessive condition caused by defects in phytanic acid catabolism.[67,68] It presents with neurologic and cardiac symptoms, including CDs, mostly before the age of 20 but may present as late as the fifth decade.[69,70] Mutations in phytanoyl-CoA hydroxylase, the enzyme that catalyzes conversion of phytanoyl-CoA to 2-hydroxy-phytanoyl-CoA, are found in most patients. The downstream degradation pathway involves peroxisome function, and mutations in the peroxisomal matrix protein receptor PEX7 also have been found in patients.

Monnig and colleagues[71] characterize the electrophysiologic abnormalities they identified in a murine model of Refsum disease, using a knockout mouse for sterol carrier protein 2 (SCP2). They reported that SCP2−/− mice developed PR interval, QRS, and QTc prolongation consistent with delayed conduction when fed high-phytol diets. In addition, they developed heart block followed by asystole and death. Conduction defects were confirmed in vitro using programmed stimulation in Langendorff-perfused isolated heart preparations. No histologic or echocardiographic abnormalities were seen in SCP2−/− mice fed the high-phytol diet, and return to a low-phytol diet reversed the abnormalities. The changes seem specific to the conduction system.

It is difficult to make definitive correlations in such rare disorders, but there may be a propensity to specific arrhythmias with different defects. Although most fatty acid oxidation disorders are recognized in the first 2 to 3 years of life, there are well-documented cases that have presented in adulthood.[72]

CHANNELOPATHIES

SCN5A

Mutation in the SCN5A gene, which results in nonfunctional human cardiac sodium channels, was found to be involved with progressive CD and nonprogressive CD.[73] Compound heterozygotes for SCN5A alleles have been observed in a rare congenital form of sick sinus syndrome, with sinus bradycardia or sinus arrest. The relationship to adult forms of this disorder is unknown. Heterozygous SCN5A mutations have also been implicated in occasional families with sinoatrial disease, atrial fibrillation, AV block, and dilated cardiomyopathy. At present 11 SCN5A mutations have been published that seem to be causally related to inherited cardiac CD.[73–77] Interestingly, combinations of SCN5A mutations and degenerative abnormalities have also been reported.[78]

Remme and coworkers[79] generated a knock-in mouse carrying the mouse equivalent (1798insD) of the human SCN5A-1795insD mutation. Mice carrying the mutation display bradycardia, right ventricular conduction slowing, and QT prolongation, similar to the human phenotype. These results demonstrate that a single SCN5A mutation is sufficient to cause an overlap cardiac sodium channel disease, which may manifest with conduction disorders.

SCN1B

Recently, Watanabe and colleagues[80] investigated the SCN1B gene, which encodes the function-modifying sodium channel β1 subunit. They studied 282 probands with Brugada syndrome and 44 patients with CD, none of whom had SCN5A mutations. They identified two types of mutations that alter sodium current and consequently lead to a conduction delay. Interestingly, mutations in SCN1B have been previously reported in generalized epilepsy with febrile seizures,[81] and β1-null mice exhibit a severe seizure disorder and bradycardia and prolonged QT.[82,83]

KCNJ2

Another channelopathy that has been associated with conduction system disorders is the LQT7, known as the "Andersen-Tawil syndrome," caused by mutations in the KCNJ2 encoding an inward rectifier potassium channel, Kir2.1. This syndrome is manifest by potassium-sensitive periodic paralysis, ventricular arrhythmias, and dysmorphic features. Besides QT interval prolongation, Andersen-Tawil patients may present with conduction abnormalities, such as AV block, bundle branch block, and intraventricular conduction delay.[84]

HCN4

Sinus node dysfunction usually occurs secondary to acquired heart disease or during drug therapy. Recently, however, mutations in the hyperpolarization-activated cyclic nucleotide-gated channel 4 (HCN4) gene, which encodes for the pacemaker current I_f, have been identified in patients with idiopathic sinus node disease[85] and in patients with sinus node dysfunction combined with prolonged QT intervals and ventricular tachycardia.[86] HCN4-deficient mice die in utero and their hearts display slowed cardiac contraction and lack of pacemaker cells, which implies that HCN4 is has a pivotal role in functioning of the developing CD.[87]

CASQ2/RYR2

Mutation in these genes leads to catecholaminergic polymorphic ventricular tachycardia. Patients may suffer from sinus node dysfunction, although the pathophysiology is yet to be elucidated.[88] Autosomal-recessive catecholaminergic polymorphic ventricular tachycardia can be caused by mutations in the calsequestrin gene CASQ2,[88] whereas the autosomal-dominant form can be caused by mutations located in the ryanodine receptor 2 gene (RyR2).[89] These genes encode proteins that are involved in intracellular calcium homeostasis and excitation. Sinus node disease might be caused by altered intracellular calcium handling or calcium ion currents, influencing automaticity of SA nodal pacemaker cells.

CONNEXINS AND GAP JUNCTIONS

Connexin

Connexins constitute gap junction channels and are responsible for current conduction between neighboring myocytes.[3,90] Variations in connexin expression in different cardiac tissues might be responsible, at least partially, for the differences in intercellular resistance and conduction velocity. Conduction velocities are highest in the Purkinje network and slowest in the nodal tissue. Downregulation of the gap junction protein connexin 40 has been hypothesized to be responsible for the AV conduction defect in Nkx2.5, Tbx5, and HF-1b transcription factor mutations.[15,91] Furthermore, polymorphism in the atrial connexin 40 gene has been described in patients with familial atrial standstill and CD. These patients also carried an SCN5A mutation (D1275N) that reduced Na-current.[92] Recently, Lim and colleagues[93] have shown that the absence of coxsackievirus and adenovirus receptor in adult mouse hearts led to abnormal propagation of electrical conduction in the AV node. This protein is an adhesion molecule and its absence was associated with a decrease in connexin 45 expression. Because the latter is a prominent connexin expressed in the compact AV node,[94] the loss of connexin 45 in the cell-cell contacts of the AV node might explain why there is abnormal AV conduction in hearts that lack coxsackievirus and adenovirus receptor.

Connexin-deficient murine model allows understanding the molecular determinants of intercellular electrical communication. Modulation of specific connexin isoforms may lead to chamber-specific conduction defects.[95]

STORAGE DISORDERS

Many of the classic metabolic storage disorders are associated with cardiac involvement.[96] Neurologic or respiratory failure is often the cause of early death. Cardiac manifestations, including massive LV wall thickening (a combination of deposition and true hypertrophy) and valvular involvement, although present to some degrees in all cases, may manifest only later in life in those who survive as a result of therapeutic intervention or less penetrant alleles.[96,97] Prominent evidence of AV CD, often with ventricular preexcitation, is seen in all of these diseases. Atrial arrhythmias are also observed frequently.

Pompe Disease

This disease typically results in massive thickening of the ventricular wall in childhood, sometimes with endocardial fibroelastosis.[96,97] There is usually evidence of ventricular preexcitation and bizarre fractionation of the entire surface electrogram.[98] Although ectopy is commonly seen, arrhythmias do not dominate the clinical course and death is usually from cardiorespiratory failure.

Defects in glycogen phosporylase (McArdle disease), brancher, or debrancher enzymes all are reported to cause AV conduction system disease and dilated cardiomyopathy with disproportionate wall thickening.[96] In these disorders, heart failure and sudden death are seen occasionally.

Andersen-Fabry Disease

This is a rare inherited lysosomal storage disorder caused by the partial or complete deficiency of the lysosomal enzyme α-galactosidase A, resulting in excess cellular glycosphingolipid deposition. Cardiac involvement is usually part of the multisystem disorder and presents in the fourth decade with other organ manifestations.[99] A variant of Fabry disease with predominant cardiac manifestations has also been recognized.[100,101] Patients may present with angina pectoris, dyspnea, palpitations, or syncope, and these symptoms are caused by vascular, endothelial, myocardial (with increase in LV mass), and conduction system involvement. Advanced cardiac disease may require a permanent pacemaker and cardiac transplant. Substrate inhibition with enzyme replacement therapy and gene therapy instituted early in the disease course might slow progression of the cardiac manifestations.[96] Female heterozygotes often exhibit much less penetrant forms of the disease and cardiac-specific, late-onset variants exist.[102] Ventricular thickening is common especially in males, and correlates with the risk of nonsustained ventricular tachycardia.[103] Although atrial fibrillation is the most frequent arrhythmia, AV conduction system disease and preexcitation are less common.

Danon Disease

A rare X-linked genetic disorder caused by deficiency of lysosomal-associated membrane protein 2 (LAMP-2), a lysosomal membrane glycoprotein,[104–106] is characterized by skeletal muscle involvement with myopathy; often increased serum creatine kinase, aspartate transaminase, and alanine aminotransferase; variable mental retardation; ophthalmic abnormalities; and cardiac disease. The cardiac features include hypertrophic cardiomyopathy; preexcitation; heart failure; electrical conduction disorders; and sudden death, which is frequent.[107–110] The pathogenic mechanism leading to vacuolar formation in Danon disease is poorly understood. There is a LAMP2 knockout mouse model, which is known to have a reduced life expectancy and displays autophagic vacuoles in skeletal muscles, liver, pancreas, spleen, kidney, and heart.[111]

Cardiac involvement is the rule rather than an exception with a host of other rare storage disorders including mucopolysaccharidoses, mucolipidoses, gangliosidoses, and neuronal ceroid lipofuscinosis.[96] Most of these conditions are recessive and lethal in childhood. Reports of arrhythmias are rare, but are dominated by AV block.

MITOCHONDRIAL DISORDERS

Mitochondrial disorders comprise a group of diverse genetic diseases, with a large variety in clinical features. Although a large proportion of patients with mitochondrial disease cannot be classified according to specific disease entity, several syndromes have been described. Patients may have mutations in one of the nuclear-encoded genes that affect the oxidative phosphorylation pathway. Disorders may occur in any organ, at any age, and with any mode of inheritance.[112] The heart, being highly energy dependent, is particularly vulnerable to those defects and the most commonly encountered cardiac problems include hypertrophic cardiomyopathy, dilated cardiomyopathy, LV noncompaction, and cardiac conduction defects.[113–116] The incidence of cardiomyopathy ranges from 17% to 40% in patients with respiratory chain disorders.[113,114,117] Cardiac conduction defects are also reported in up to 40% of the patients,[113] although some have observed them in fewer than 12%.[114]

Interestingly, conduction disturbances have been reported in Kearns-Sayre syndrome (KSS) with large mitochondrial DNA deletions.[62] This syndrome was first described in 1958 and consists of the triad of complete AV block, chronic progressive external ophthalmoplegia, and pigmentary degeneration of the retina.[118] It can present with muscle weakness, dysfunction of the central nervous system, endocrinopathies, or cardiac abnormalities including AV block and dilated cardiomyopathy and Stokes-Adam syncope. Sudden death is reported in 20% of the cases.[118]

The conduction defects typically involve the distal His bundle, bundle branches, and infranodal conduction.[119,120] Electrophysiologic investigations have shown an increase in the H-V interval at rest that further lengthens on atrial pacing.[121] The ECG changes typically found in KSS are PR interval prolongation preceding second or third degree AV block. The development of heart block is not predicted, however, by a prolonged PR interval. This phenomenon has been explained by the finding on intracardiac electrophysiologic studies that the primary abnormalities in individuals with KSS are concentrated in the AV node-His-Purkinje system with shortened atrial-His conduction but prolonged H-V intervals.[121] The accelerated and unpredictable rate of progression to complete AV block, together with an associated mortality of up to 20%,[122] should lead to a routine and regular evaluation of patients for AV conduction disturbances. Screening of family members should be performed with routine ECGs.[118] A recent study supports the need to pace KSS patients with ECG changes indicative of conduction defects. In this cohort there was a 32% likelihood of sustaining cardiac conduction defects, a 12% likelihood of having a pacemaker implanted, and a 5% likelihood of sudden death.[118] The 2008 American College of Cardiology–American Heart Association guidelines for pacemaker implantation included neuromuscular diseases with AV block including KSS as a Class I indication. It is also recommended that pacing be considered in patients with neuromuscular diseases with AV block, such as KSS, with or without symptoms, because of their unpredictable progression of AV CD.[123]

Another example of mitochondrial disease known to affect the conduction system is the "MELAS" syndrome. This relates to a clinical syndrome manifested by mitochondrial encephalomyopathy, lactic acidosis, and recurrent stroke-like episodes.[124] This disease is caused by several gene mutations including mitochondrial adenine-to-guanine transition at nucleotide pair 3243 (m.3243A>G),[125,126] a mitochondrial thymine to cytosine transition at nucleotide pair 3271,[127] a T-to-C transition mutation at nucleotide position 3250,[128] and mutations in the MTND5 gene.[129] The cardiac manifestations include hypertrophic, dilated cardiomyopathy,[130,131] and preexcitation and AV heart block.[117,132,133]

MICRORNAS

MicroRNAs are genomically encoded small RNAs used by organisms to regulate the expression of proteins generated from messenger RNA transcripts. They play an important role in a wide range of biologic processes, including cell proliferation, differentiation, and apoptosis.[134–136] MicroRNAs are expressed in cardiac and skeletal muscle, and genetic studies have shown their importance during heart development, cardiac hypertrophy, and electrical conduction.

The miR-1 and miR-133 have been shown to regulate the development of cardiac conduction-system components and may contribute to arrhythmias in the adult heart.[137,138] Recently, Zaho and colleagues[139] studied the electrocardiography in miR-1-2 homozygous mutant mice. They found that the average heart rate of mutants was significantly lower than that of wild-type littermates and the PR interval was shortened. In addition, the QRS complex was significantly prolonged in the mutant hearts. Furthermore, Yang and colleagues[138] have shown that the injection of miR-1 into infarcted myocardium causes cardiac conduction disturbances and finally leads to arrhythmias. In contrast, the knockdown of miR-1 inhibits arrhythmogenesis. The miR-1 might have a role in electrical remodeling and arrhythmias. This is mediated through the repression of the KCNJ2 and GJA1 genes, which encode inward rectifying K+ channel[140] and cardiac gap-junction channel protein,[3] respectively.

The miR-133 has a role in cardiac conductance abnormalities through the repression of KNCH2, which encodes a cardiac K+ channel that is important for myocyte repolarization and is associated with congenital arrhythmias.[137] Interestingly, the introduction of miR-133 into isolated cardiomyocytes caused a delay in myocyte repolarization. There is increasing evidence that miRNAs play key roles as regulators of conduction system development and function.

MISCELLANEOUS

Klotho

This gene, which encodes a membrane protein that shares sequence similarity with the β-glucosidase, has been shown to be involved in the suppression of several ageing phenotypes. In 1997, Kuro-o and colleagues[141] showed that a defect in klotho gene expression in a mouse results in a syndrome that resembles human ageing. Later, Takeshita and colleagues[142] found that homozygous mutant mice with a defect of klotho gene expression develop sinus node dysfunction under stress conditions. In addition they found that in the heart, klotho is expressed solely in the sinoatrial node. They concluded that the sinoatrial node may require klotho expression for its normal and robust pacemaking activity in the heart under a variety of pathophysiologic conditions.

SPECIFIC LOCI FOR WHICH THE DISEASE GENES ARE NOT YET KNOWN

There are several disorders where CD is a prominent feature and genetic analyses have identified a unique genomic locus, but to date the causal gene has not been identified. These include the progressive familial heart blocks, forms of isolated AV CD, and CD found in association with congenital heart disease.

There are also additional loci yet to be discovered for many forms of CD. Families exist with sick sinus syndrome, AV CD, isolated bundle branch blocks, and autosomal-dominant EDMD, which do not map to any of the known loci for each of these conditions. The tremendous genetic heterogeneity seen in other inherited cardiac disorders is likely to be present in CD, and a concerted effort in clinical and molecular genetics is required to unravel the genetic contribution to CD.

COMMON FORMS OF CD

In most human CD there is no obvious inherited contribution. Sinoatrial disease and some degree of AV CD are common in aging populations, and in most instances it is assumed that this is a reflection of long-term degenerative processes. These features do not exclude an inherited component to the etiology, and the absence of symptoms in all but the latest stages of CD or the paroxysmal nature of atrial arrhythmias may lead to significant difficulties in the detection of any heritability should it exist. There is sufficient evidence from isolated families and population studies of heart rate, QRS duration, and other forms of CD that systematic approaches to the genetic architecture of CD are warranted. Some insights may be gained from the ongoing genome-wide association studies for a range of electrocardiographic parameters including heart rate and QRS duration.

CLINICAL IMPLICATIONS

The current understanding of the genetic contribution to CD is in its infancy, and the major clinical use of these insights at present serves to inform diagnosis and to aid in the identification of patient subsets that may benefit from additional therapy and prognosis.

Cell- and gene-based therapies are an expanding research field that promises to provide more elegant therapeutic alternatives for CD. Currently, electronic pacemakers are the mainstay of therapy for heart block and sinus node dysfunction, but particularly in the pediatric population they are problematic because of the size of the patients and their continued growth and activity. So far, several gene therapy and cell-based therapies are being explored as potential alternatives.[143–146]

Gene Therapy

IK1 knockout therapy is based on the observation that ventricular myocardium is capable of pacemaking but is normally suppressed by ionic currents, such as the inward rectifier potassium current (IK1). This channel is expressed widely but not in nodal pacemaker cells. It is encoded by the Kir2 gene family and causes a negative resting potential, suppressing excitability. Miake and colleagues[144] demonstrated that dominant-negative suppression of Kir2-encoded inward rectifier potassium channels in the ventricle causes spontaneous rhythmic electrical activity both in vitro and in vivo. This spontaneous activity was responsive to β-adrenergic stimulation (isoproterenol) just as are sinoatrial nodal cells with increases in pacing rate.[147] The suppression of Kir2 channels enables the pacemaker activity in ventricular myocytes.

Biologic Pacemaker Derived from Human Embryonic Stem Cells

Previous studies have demonstrated that spontaneously beating aggregates of myocytes could be generated from human embryonic stem cells.[148–151] These cells can integrate with host tissues to create biologic pacemakers.[148,152] Their spontaneous electrical depolarizations are conducted to neighboring cells through gap junctions. Optical mapping of the epicardial surface of guinea pig hearts transplanted with human embryonic stem cells–derived cardiomyocytes confirmed the spread of membrane depolarization from the site of injection to the surrounding myocardium.[153] These studies demonstrate that biologic pacemakers derived from human embryonic stem cells are capable of pacing recipient ventricular cardiomyocytes.

Human mesenchymal stem cells have also been used to create biologic pacemakers.[154,155] Injection of mouse HCN2-transfected human mesenchymal stem cells in the canine LV wall developed spontaneous ventricular rhythms of left-sided origin during sinus arrest. A requirement for this technique is the establishment of gap-junctional coupling between the human mesenchymal stem cells and the host tissue. The longevity of such connections remains to be determined. Recently, Cho and colleagues[156] explored the feasibility of converting normally quiescent ventricular myocytes into pacemakers by somatic cell fusion. The authors showed that a simple intracardiac, focal injection of HCN1-fibroblasts into the apex of guinea-pig hearts caused in vivo fusion events. Fusion of myocytes and HCN1-fibroblasts resulted in pacemaker function manifest by spontaneous action potentials with a slow phase-4 depolarization. In vivo biologic pacemaker activities were also confirmed by electrocardiography.

One of the major disadvantages in gene therapy is the current reliance on viruses to deliver the genes. It might induce inflammatory responses that may limit the therapeutic effect or even be proarrhythmic.[155]

SUMMARY

This article provides a brief overview of the major genetic causes of CD. Unfortunately, the lack of systematic data on prognosis and the absence of specific therapies currently preclude the use of genetic insights over traditional clinical parameters, such as standard electrocardiographic indications for permanent pacing, in most cases. At present, there is no clear role for genetic testing in most forms of conduction system disease.

A host of questions remain in the genetics of inherited CD. The role of major gene effects in late-onset forms of CD requires extensive clinical studies and family collections, as do approaches to the genetic architecture of CD. Understanding the genetic basis and pathophysiology of inherited forms of CD enables clinical or even genetic prediction of the need for pacing or other therapies, and aids the development of novel therapies for CD and its associated phenotypes.

Inherited conduction disorders are group of diseases that have a wide spectrum of presentation ranging from isolated sinoatrial or AV nodal defects to diffuse conduction system diseases associated with congenital heart diseases, neuromuscular disorders, and cardiomyopathies. Disease severity may be affected by environmental and other factors. The biologic mechanisms include early developmental transcription factor mutations, ion channelopathies, mutations in genes regulating energy metabolism, gap junctions, and other structural proteins. Based on the ever increasing understanding of the pathophysiology of conduction system disease, alternative diagnostic methods and new therapeutic strategies continue to evolve.

REFERENCES

1. Roden DM, Balser JR, George AL Jr, et al. Cardiac ion channels. Annu Rev Physiol 2002;64:431–75.
2. Roden DM, George AL Jr. Structure and function of cardiac sodium and potassium channels. Am J Physiol 1997;273:H511–25.
3. Jongsma HJ, Wilders R. Gap junctions in cardiovascular disease. Circ Res 2000;86:1193–7.
4. Schott JJ, Benson DW, Basson CT, et al. Congenital heart disease caused by mutations in the transcription factor NKX2-5. Science 1998;281:108–11.
5. Benson DW, Silberbach GM, Kavanaugh-McHugh A, et al. Mutations in the cardiac transcription factor NKX2.5 affect diverse cardiac developmental pathways. J Clin Invest 1999;104:1567–73.
6. Hosoda T, Komuro I, Shiojima I, et al. Familial atrial septal defect and atrioventricular conduction disturbance associated with a point mutation in the cardiac homeobox gene CSX/NKX2-5 in a Japanese patient. Jpn Circ J 1999;63:425–6.
7. Kasahara H, Lee B, Schott JJ, et al. Loss of function and inhibitory effects of human CSX/NKX2.5 homeoprotein mutations associated with congenital heart disease. J Clin Invest 2000;106:299–308.
8. Vaughan CJ, Basson CT. Molecular determinants of atrial and ventricular septal defects and patent ductus arteriosus. Am J Med Genet 2000;97:304–9.
9. Gutierrez-Roelens I, Sluysmans T, Gewillig M, et al. Progressive AV-block and anomalous venous return among cardiac anomalies associated with two novel missense mutations in the CSX/NKX2-5 gene. Hum Mutat 2002;20:75–6.
10. McElhinney DB, Geiger E, Blinder J, et al. NKX2.5 mutations in patients with congenital heart disease. J Am Coll Cardiol 2003;42:1650–5.
11. Basson CT, Cowley GS, Solomon SD, et al. The clinical and genetic spectrum of the Holt-Oram syndrome (heart-hand syndrome). N Engl J Med 1994;330:885–91.
12. Li QY, Newbury-Ecob RA, Terrett JA, et al. Holt-Oram syndrome is caused by mutations in TBX5, a member of the Brachyury (T) gene family. Nat Genet 1997;15:21–9.
13. Huang T. Current advances in Holt-Oram syndrome. Curr Opin Pediatr 2002;14:691–5.
14. Newbury-Ecob RA, Leanage R, Raeburn JA, et al. Holt-Oram syndrome: a clinical genetic study. J Med Genet 1996;33:300–7.
15. Bruneau BG, Nemer G, Schmitt JP, et al. A murine model of Holt-Oram syndrome defines roles of the T-box transcription factor Tbx5 in cardiogenesis and disease. Cell 2001;106:709–21.
16. Moskowitz IP, Pizard A, Patel VV, et al. The T-Box transcription factor Tbx5 is required for the patterning and maturation of the murine cardiac conduction system. Development 2004;131:4107–16.
17. Moskowitz IP, Kim JB, Moore ML, et al. A molecular pathway including Id2, Tbx5, and Nkx2-5 required for cardiac conduction system development. Cell 2007;129:1365–76.
18. Bjornstad PG, Leren TP. Familial atrial septal defect in the oval fossa with progressive prolongation of the atrioventricular conduction caused by mutations in the NKX2.5 gene. Cardiol Young 2009;19:40–4.
19. Wakimoto H, Kasahara H, Maguire CT, et al. Developmentally modulated cardiac conduction failure in transgenic mice with fetal or postnatal overexpression of DNA nonbinding mutant Nkx2.5. J Cardiovasc Electrophysiol 2002;13:682–8.

20. Jay PY, Harris BS, Maguire CT, et al. Nkx2-5 mutation causes anatomic hypoplasia of the cardiac conduction system. J Clin Invest 2004;113:1130–7.
21. Phillips MF, Harper PS. Cardiac disease in myotonic dystrophy. Cardiovasc Res 1997;33:13–22.
22. Fatkin D, MacRae C, Sasaki T, et al. Missense mutations in the rod domain of the lamin A/C gene as causes of dilated cardiomyopathy and conduction-system disease. N Engl J Med 1999; 341:1715–24.
23. Jakobs PM, Hanson EL, Crispell KA, et al. Novel lamin A/C mutations in two families with dilated cardiomyopathy and conduction system disease. J Card Fail 2001;7:249–56.
24. Arbustini E, Pilotto A, Repetto A, et al. Autosomal dominant dilated cardiomyopathy with atrioventricular block: a lamin A/C defect-related disease. J Am Coll Cardiol 2002;39:981–90.
25. Pelargonio G, Dello Russo A, Sanna T, et al. Myotonic dystrophy and the heart. Heart 2002;88: 665–70.
26. Charniot JC, Pascal C, Bouchier C, et al. Functional consequences of an LMNA mutation associated with a new cardiac and non-cardiac phenotype. Hum Mutat 2003;21:473–81.
27. Sebillon P, Bouchier C, Bidot LD, et al. Expanding the phenotype of LMNA mutations in dilated cardiomyopathy and functional consequences of these mutations. J Med Genet 2003;40:560–7.
28. Taylor MR, Fain PR, Sinagra G, et al. Natural history of dilated cardiomyopathy due to lamin A/C gene mutations. J Am Coll Cardiol 2003;41:771–80.
29. Ou Y, Strege P, Miller SM, et al. Syntrophin gamma 2 regulates SCN5A gating by a PDZ domain-mediated interaction. J Biol Chem 2003; 278:1915–23.
30. Srinivasan J, Schachner M, Catterall WA. Interaction of voltage-gated sodium channels with the extracellular matrix molecules tenascin-C and tenascin-R. Proc Natl Acad Sci U S A 1998;95: 15753–7.
31. Xiao ZC, Ragsdale DS, Malhotra JD, et al. Tenascin-R is a functional modulator of sodium channel beta subunits. J Biol Chem 1999;274:26511–7.
32. Malhotra JD, Kazen-Gillespie K, Hortsch M, et al. Sodium channel beta subunits mediate homophilic cell adhesion and recruit ankyrin to points of cell-cell contact. J Biol Chem 2000;275:11383–8.
33. Lynch HT, Mohiuddin S, Sketch MH, et al. Hereditary progressive atrioventricular conduction defect: a new syndrome? JAMA 1973;225:1465–70.
34. Surawicz B, Hariman RJ. Follow-up of the family with congenital absence of sinus rhythm. Am J Cardiol 1988;61:467–9.
35. Balderston SM, Shaffer EM, Sondheimer HM, et al. Hereditary atrioventricular conduction defect in a child. Pediatr Cardiol 1989;10:37–8.
36. Maltsev VA, Undrovinas AI. Cytoskeleton modulates coupling between availability and activation of cardiac sodium channel. Am J Physiol 1997; 273:H1832–40.
37. Ribaux P, Bleicher F, Couble ML, et al. Voltage-gated sodium channel (SkM1) content in dystrophin-deficient muscle. Pflugers Arch 2001;441: 746–55.
38. Aslanidis C, Jansen G, Amemiya C, et al. Cloning of the essential myotonic dystrophy region and mapping of the putative defect. Nature 1992;355: 548–51.
39. Brook JD, McCurrach ME, Harley HG, et al. Molecular basis of myotonic dystrophy: expansion of a trinucleotide (CTG) repeat at the 3′ end of a transcript encoding a protein kinase family member. Cell 1992;69:385.
40. Buxton J, Shelbourne P, Davies J, et al. Detection of an unstable fragment of DNA specific to individuals with myotonic dystrophy. Nature 1992;355:547–8.
41. Lazarus A, Varin J, Babuty D, et al. Long-term follow-up of arrhythmias in patients with myotonic dystrophy treated by pacing: a multicenter diagnostic pacemaker study. J Am Coll Cardiol 2002; 40:1645–52.
42. Schoser BG, Ricker K, Schneider-Gold C, et al. Sudden cardiac death in myotonic dystrophy type 2. Neurology 2004;63:2402–4.
43. Sovari AA, Bodine CK, Farokhi F. Cardiovascular manifestations of myotonic dystrophy-1. Cardiol Rev 2007;15:191–4.
44. Groh WJ, Groh MR, Saha C, et al. Electrocardiographic abnormalities and sudden death in myotonic dystrophy type 1. N Engl J Med 2008; 358:2688–97.
45. Berul CI, Maguire CT, Aronovitz MJ, et al. DMPK dosage alterations result in atrioventricular conduction abnormalities in a mouse myotonic dystrophy model. J Clin Invest 1999;103:R1–7.
46. Jacob KN, Garg A. Laminopathies: multisystem dystrophy syndromes. Mol Genet Metab 2006;87: 289–302.
47. Rankin J, Ellard S. The laminopathies: a clinical review. Clin Genet 2006;70:261–74.
48. Sylvius N, Tesson F. Lamin A/C and cardiac diseases. Curr Opin Cardiol 2006;21:159–65.
49. Zhang Q, Bethmann C, Worth NF, et al. Nesprin-1 and -2 are involved in the pathogenesis of Emery Dreifuss muscular dystrophy and are critical for nuclear envelope integrity. Hum Mol Genet 2007; 16:2816–33.
50. Pasotti M, Klersy C, Pilotto A, et al. Long-term outcome and risk stratification in dilated cardiolaminopathies. J Am Coll Cardiol 2008;52:1250–60.
51. Mounkes LC, Kozlov S, Hernandez L, et al. A progeroid syndrome in mice is caused by defects in A-type lamins. Nature 2003;423:298–301.

52. Novelli G, Muchir A, Sangiuolo F, et al. Mandibuloacral dysplasia is caused by a mutation in LMNA-encoding lamin A/C. Am J Hum Genet 2002;71:426–31.
53. De Sandre-Giovannoli A, Chaouch M, Kozlov S, et al. Homozygous defects in LMNA, encoding lamin A/C nuclear-envelope proteins, cause autosomal recessive axonal neuropathy in human (Charcot-Marie-Tooth disorder type 2) and mouse. Am J Hum Genet 2002;70:726–36.
54. Chen L, Lee L, Kudlow BA, et al. LMNA mutations in atypical Werner's syndrome. Lancet 2003;362: 440–5.
55. Shackleton S, Lloyd DJ, Jackson SN, et al. LMNA, encoding lamin A/C, is mutated in partial lipodystrophy. Nat Genet 2000;24:153–6.
56. Speckman RA, Garg A, Du F, et al. Mutational and haplotype analyses of families with familial partial lipodystrophy (Dunnigan variety) reveal recurrent missense mutations in the globular C-terminal domain of lamin A/C. Am J Hum Genet 2000;66: 1192–8.
57. Blake DJ, Martin-Rendon E. Intermediate filaments and the function of the dystrophin-protein complex. Trends Cardiovasc Med 2002;12:224–8.
58. Bushby K, Muntoni F, Bourke JP. 107th ENMC international workshop: the management of cardiac involvement in muscular dystrophy and myotonic dystrophy. 7th–9th June 2002, Naarden, the Netherlands. Neuromuscul Disord 2003;13: 166–72.
59. Finsterer J, Stollberger C. The heart in human dystrophinopathies. Cardiology 2003;99:1–19.
60. Gollob MH, Green MS, Tang AS, et al. Identification of a gene responsible for familial Wolff-Parkinson-White syndrome. N Engl J Med 2001;344:1823–31.
61. Arad M, Benson DW, Perez-Atayde AR, et al. Constitutively active AMP kinase mutations cause glycogen storage disease mimicking hypertrophic cardiomyopathy. J Clin Invest 2002;109:357–62.
62. MacRae CA, Ghaisas N, Kass S, et al. Familial Hypertrophic cardiomyopathy with Wolff-Parkinson-White syndrome maps to a locus on chromosome 7q3. J Clin Invest 1995;96:1216–20.
63. Arad M, Moskowitz IP, Patel VV, et al. Transgenic mice overexpressing mutant PRKAG2 define the cause of Wolff-Parkinson-White syndrome in glycogen storage cardiomyopathy. Circulation 2003;107:2850–6.
64. Rinaldo P, Matern D, Bennett MJ. Fatty acid oxidation disorders. Annu Rev Physiol 2002;64:477–502.
65. Bonnet D, Martin D, Pascale De L, et al. Arrhythmias and conduction defects as presenting symptoms of fatty acid oxidation disorders in children. Circulation 1999;100:2248–53.
66. Saudubray JM, Martin D, de Lonlay P, et al. Recognition and management of fatty acid oxidation defects: a series of 107 patients. J Inherit Metab Dis 1999;22:488–502.
67. Jansen GA, Waterham HR, Wanders RJ. Molecular basis of Refsum disease: sequence variations in phytanoyl-CoA hydroxylase (PHYH) and the PTS2 receptor (PEX7). Hum Mutat 2004;23:209–18.
68. Nguyen-Tran VT, Kubalak SW, Minamisawa S, et al. A novel genetic pathway for sudden cardiac death via defects in the transition between ventricular and conduction system cell lineages. Cell 2000; 102:671–82.
69. Skjeldal OH, Stokke O, Refsum S, et al. Clinical and biochemical heterogeneity in conditions with phytanic acid accumulation. J Neurol Sci 1987;77:87–96.
70. Leys D, Petit H, Bonte-Adnet C, et al. Refsum's disease revealed by cardiac disorders. Lancet 1989;1:621.
71. Monnig G, Wiekowski J, Kirchhof P, et al. Phytanic acid accumulation is associated with conduction delay and sudden cardiac death in sterol carrier protein-2/sterol carrier protein-x deficient mice. J Cardiovasc Electrophysiol 2004;15:1310–6.
72. Feillet F, Steinmann G, Vianey-Saban C, et al. Adult presentation of MCAD deficiency revealed by coma and severe arrythmias. Intensive Care Med 2003;29:1594–7.
73. Schott JJ, Alshinawi C, Kyndt F, et al. Cardiac conduction defects associate with mutations in SCN5A. Nat Genet 1999;23:20–1.
74. Kyndt F, Probst V, Potet F, et al. Novel SCN5A mutation leading either to isolated cardiac conduction defect or Brugada syndrome in a large French family. Circulation 2001;104:3081–6.
75. Tan HL, Bink-Boelkens MT, Bezzina CR, et al. A sodium-channel mutation causes isolated cardiac conduction disease. Nature 2001;409:1043–7.
76. Wang DW, Viswanathan PC, Balser JR, et al. Clinical, genetic, and biophysical characterization of SCN5A mutations associated with atrioventricular conduction block. Circulation 2002;105:341–6.
77. Bezzina CR, Rook MB, Groenewegen WA, et al. Compound heterozygosity for mutations (W156X and R225W) in SCN5A associated with severe cardiac conduction disturbances and degenerative changes in the conduction system. Circ Res 2003;92:159–68.
78. Probst V, Kyndt F, Potet F, et al. Haploinsufficiency in combination with aging causes SCN5A-linked hereditary Lenegre disease. J Am Coll Cardiol 2003;41:643–52.
79. Remme CA, Verkerk AO, Nuyens D, et al. Overlap syndrome of cardiac sodium channel disease in mice carrying the equivalent mutation of human SCN5A-1795insD. Circulation 2006;114: 2584–94.
80. Watanabe H, Koopmann TT, Le Scouarnec S, et al. Sodium channel beta1 subunit mutations

associated with Brugada syndrome and cardiac conduction disease in humans. J Clin Invest 2008;118:2260–8.
81. Wallace RH, Wang DW, Singh R, et al. Febrile seizures and generalized epilepsy associated with a mutation in the Na+-channel beta1 subunit gene SCN1B. Nat Genet 1998;19:366–70.
82. Chen C, Westenbroek RE, Xu X, et al. Mice lacking sodium channel beta1 subunits display defects in neuronal excitability, sodium channel expression, and nodal architecture. J Neurosci 2004;24:4030–42.
83. Lopez-Santiago LF, Meadows LS, Ernst SJ, et al. Sodium channel Scn1b null mice exhibit prolonged QT and RR intervals. J Mol Cell Cardiol 2007;43: 636–47.
84. Andelfinger G, Tapper AR, Welch RC, et al. KCNJ2 mutation results in Andersen syndrome with sex-specific cardiac and skeletal muscle phenotypes. Am J Hum Genet 2002;71:663–8.
85. Schulze-Bahr E, Neu A, Friederich P, et al. Pacemaker channel dysfunction in a patient with sinus node disease. J Clin Invest 2003;111:1537–45.
86. Ueda K, Nakamura K, Hayashi T, et al. Functional characterization of a trafficking-defective HCN4 mutation, D553N, associated with cardiac arrhythmia. J Biol Chem 2004;279:27194–8.
87. Stieber J, Herrmann S, Feil S, et al. The hyperpolarization-activated channel HCN4 is required for the generation of pacemaker action potentials in the embryonic heart. Proc Natl Acad Sci U S A 2003; 100:15235–40.
88. Lahat H, Eldar M, Levy-Nissenbaum E, et al. Autosomal recessive catecholamine- or exercise-induced polymorphic ventricular tachycardia: clinical features and assignment of the disease gene to chromosome 1p13-21. Circulation 2001;103: 2822–7.
89. Priori SG, Napolitano C, Tiso N, et al. Mutations in the cardiac ryanodine receptor gene (hRyR2) underlie catecholaminergic polymorphic ventricular tachycardia. Circulation 2001;103:196–200.
90. van Veen AA, van Rijen HV, Opthof T. Cardiac gap junction channels: modulation of expression and channel properties. Cardiovasc Res 2001;51:217–29.
91. Durocher D, Charron F, Warren R, et al. The cardiac transcription factors Nkx2-5 and GATA-4 are mutual cofactors. Embo J 1997;16:5687–96.
92. Groenewegen WA, Firouzi M, Bezzina CR, et al. A cardiac sodium channel mutation cosegregates with a rare connexin40 genotype in familial atrial standstill. Circ Res 2003;92:14–22.
93. Lim BK, Xiong D, Dorner A, et al. Coxsackievirus and adenovirus receptor (CAR) mediates atrioventricular-node function and connexin 45 localization in the murine heart. J Clin Invest 2008; 118:2758–70.
94. Severs NJ, Rothery S, Dupont E, et al. Immunocytochemical analysis of connexin expression in the healthy and diseased cardiovascular system. Microsc Res Tech 2001;52:301–22.
95. Thomas SA, Schuessler RB, Berul CI, et al. Disparate effects of deficient expression of connexin43 on atrial and ventricular conduction: evidence for chamber-specific molecular determinants of conduction. Circulation 1998;97:686–91.
96. Guertl B, Noehammer C, Hoefler G. Metabolic cardiomyopathies. Int J Exp Pathol 2000;81: 349–72.
97. Kelly DP, Strauss AW. Inherited cardiomyopathies. N Engl J Med 1994;330:913–9.
98. Moses SW, Wanderman KL, Myroz A, et al. Cardiac involvement in glycogen storage disease type III. Eur J Pediatr 1989;148:764–6.
99. Pierre-Louis B, Kumar A, Frishman WH. Fabry disease: cardiac manifestations and therapeutic options. Cardiol Rev 2009;17:31–5.
100. von Scheidt W, Eng CM, Fitzmaurice TF, et al. An atypical variant of Fabry's disease with manifestations confined to the myocardium. N Engl J Med 1991;324:395–9.
101. Chimenti C, Ricci R, Pieroni M, et al. Cardiac variant of Fabry's disease mimicking hypertrophic cardiomyopathy. Cardiologia 1999;44:469–73.
102. Chimenti C, Pieroni M, Morgante E, et al. Prevalence of Fabry disease in female patients with late-onset hypertrophic cardiomyopathy. Circulation 2004;110:1047–53.
103. Shah JS, Lee P, Hughes D, et al. The natural history of left ventricular systolic function in Anderson-Fabry disease. Heart 2005;91:533–4.
104. Danon MJ, Oh SJ, DiMauro S, et al. Lysosomal glycogen storage disease with normal acid maltase. Neurology 1981;31:51–7.
105. Mattei MG, Matterson J, Chen JW, et al. Two human lysosomal membrane glycoproteins, h-lamp-1 and h-lamp-2, are encoded by genes localized to chromosome 13q34 and chromosome Xq24-25, respectively. J Biol Chem 1990;265:7548–51.
106. Nishino I, Fu J, Tanji K, et al. Primary LAMP-2 deficiency causes X-linked vacuolar cardiomyopathy and myopathy (Danon disease). Nature 2000;406: 906–10.
107. Tripathy D, Coleman RA, Vidaillet HJ Jr, et al. Complete heart block with myocardial membrane-bound glycogen and normal peripheral alpha-glucosidase activity. Ann Intern Med 1988;109:985–7.
108. Charron P, Villard E, Sebillon P, et al. Danon's disease as a cause of hypertrophic cardiomyopathy: a systematic survey. Heart 2004;90: 842–6.
109. Arad M, Maron BJ, Gorham JM, et al. Glycogen storage diseases presenting as hypertrophic cardiomyopathy. N Engl J Med 2005;352:362–72.

110. Nadeau A, Therrien C, Karpati G, et al. Danon disease due to a novel splice mutation in the LAMP2 gene. Muscle Nerve 2008;37:338–42.
111. Tanaka Y, Guhde G, Suter A, et al. Accumulation of autophagic vacuoles and cardiomyopathy in LAMP-2-deficient mice. Nature 2000;406:902–6.
112. Munnich A, Rustin P. Clinical spectrum and diagnosis of mitochondrial disorders. Am J Med Genet 2001;106:4–17.
113. Holmgren D, Wahlander H, Eriksson BO, et al. Cardiomyopathy in children with mitochondrial disease: clinical course and cardiological findings. Eur Heart J 2003;24:280–8.
114. Scaglia F, Towbin JA, Craigen WJ, et al. Clinical spectrum, morbidity, and mortality in 113 pediatric patients with mitochondrial disease. Pediatrics 2004;114:925–31.
115. Yaplito-Lee J, Weintraub R, Jamsen K, et al. Cardiac manifestations in oxidative phosphorylation disorders of childhood. J Pediatr 2007;150: 407–11.
116. Gibson K, Halliday JL, Kirby DM, et al. Mitochondrial oxidative phosphorylation disorders presenting in neonates: clinical manifestations and enzymatic and molecular diagnoses. Pediatrics 2008;122:1003–8.
117. Lev D, Nissenkorn A, Leshinsky-Silver E, et al. Clinical presentations of mitochondrial cardiomyopathies. Pediatr Cardiol 2004;25:443–50.
118. Young TJ, Shah AK, Lee MH, et al. Kearns-Sayre syndrome: a case report and review of cardiovascular complications. Pacing Clin Electrophysiol 2005;28:454–7.
119. Roberts NK, Perloff JK, Kark RA. Cardiac conduction in the Kearns-Sayre syndrome (a neuromuscular disorder associated with progressive external ophthalmoplegia and pigmentary retinopathy): report of 2 cases and review of 17 published cases. Am J Cardiol 1979;44:1396–400.
120. Gallastegui J, Hariman RJ, Handler B, et al. Cardiac involvement in the Kearns-Sayre syndrome. Am J Cardiol 1987;60:385–8.
121. Polak PE, Zijlstra F, Roelandt JR. Indications for pacemaker implantation in the Kearns-Sayre syndrome. Eur Heart J 1989;10:281–2.
122. Charles R, Holt S, Kay JM, et al. Myocardial ultrastructure and the development of atrioventricular block in Kearns-Sayre syndrome. Circulation 1981;63:214–9.
123. Epstein AE, DiMarco JP, Ellenbogen KA, et al. ACC/AHA/HRS 2008 guidelines for device-based therapy of cardiac rhythm abnormalities: a report of the American College of Cardiology/American Heart Association Task Force on Practice Guidelines (Writing Committee to Revise the ACC/AHA/NASPE 2002 Guideline Update for Implantation of Cardiac Pacemakers and Antiarrhythmia Devices) developed in collaboration with the American Association for Thoracic Surgery and Society of Thoracic Surgeons. J Am Coll Cardiol 2008;51:e1–62.
124. Pavlakis SG, Phillips PC, DiMauro S, et al. Mitochondrial myopathy, encephalopathy, lactic acidosis, and strokelike episodes: a distinctive clinical syndrome. Ann Neurol 1984;16:481–8.
125. Goto Y, Nonaka I, Horai S. A mutation in the tRNA(Leu)(UUR) gene associated with the MELAS subgroup of mitochondrial encephalomyopathies. Nature 1990;348:651–3.
126. Vydt TC, de Coo RF, Soliman OI, et al. Cardiac involvement in adults with m.3243A>G MELAS gene mutation. Am J Cardiol 2007;99:264–9.
127. Goto Y, Nonaka I, Horai S. A new mtDNA mutation associated with mitochondrial myopathy, encephalopathy, lactic acidosis and stroke-like episodes (MELAS). Biochim Biophys Acta 1991; 1097:238–40.
128. Goto Y, Tojo M, Tohyama J, et al. A novel point mutation in the mitochondrial tRNA(Leu)(UUR) gene in a family with mitochondrial myopathy. Ann Neurol 1992;31:672–5.
129. Hirano M, Pavlakis SG. Mitochondrial myopathy, encephalopathy, lactic acidosis, and strokelike episodes (MELAS): current concepts. J Child Neurol 1994;9:4–13.
130. Wallace DC. Mitochondrial defects in cardiomyopathy and neuromuscular disease. Am Heart J 2000; 139:S70–85.
131. Okhuijsen-Kroes EJ, Trijbels JM, Sengers RC, et al. Infantile presentation of the mtDNA A3243G tRNA (Leu (UUR)) mutation. Neuropediatrics 2001;32: 183–90.
132. Anan R, Nakagawa M, Miyata M, et al. Cardiac involvement in mitochondrial diseases: a study on 17 patients with documented mitochondrial DNA defects. Circulation 1995;91:955–61.
133. Okajima Y, Tanabe Y, Takayanagi M, et al. A follow up study of myocardial involvement in patients with mitochondrial encephalomyopathy, lactic acidosis, and stroke-like episodes (MELAS). Heart 1998;80: 292–5.
134. Ambros V. The functions of animal microRNAs. Nature 2004;431:350–5.
135. Kloosterman WP, Plasterk RH. The diverse functions of microRNAs in animal development and disease. Dev Cell 2006;11:441–50.
136. Zhao Y, Srivastava D. A developmental view of microRNA function. Trends Biochem Sci 2007;32: 189–97.
137. Xiao J, Luo X, Lin H, et al. MicroRNA miR-133 represses HERG K+ channel expression contributing to QT prolongation in diabetic hearts. J Biol Chem 2007;282:12363–7.
138. Yang B, Lin H, Xiao J, et al. The muscle-specific microRNA miR-1 regulates cardiac arrhythmogenic

potential by targeting GJA1 and KCNJ2. Nat Med 2007;13:486–91.
139. Zhao Y, Ransom JF, Li A, et al. Dysregulation of cardiogenesis, cardiac conduction, and cell cycle in mice lacking miRNA-1-2. Cell 2007;129:303–17.
140. Diaz RJ, Zobel C, Cho HC, et al. Selective inhibition of inward rectifier K+ channels (Kir2.1 or Kir2.2) abolishes protection by ischemic preconditioning in rabbit ventricular cardiomyocytes. Circ Res 2004;95:325–32.
141. Kuro-o M, Matsumura Y, Aizawa H, et al. Mutation of the mouse klotho gene leads to a syndrome resembling ageing. Nature 1997;390:45–51.
142. Takeshita K, Fujimori T, Kurotaki Y, et al. Sinoatrial node dysfunction and early unexpected death of mice with a defect of klotho gene expression. Circulation 2004;109:1776–82.
143. Edelberg JM, Aird WC, Rosenberg RD. Enhancement of murine cardiac chronotropy by the molecular transfer of the human beta2 adrenergic receptor cDNA. J Clin Invest 1998;101:337–43.
144. Miake J, Marban E, Nuss HB. Biological pacemaker created by gene transfer. Nature 2002;419:132–3.
145. Qu J, Plotnikov AN, Danilo P Jr, et al. Expression and function of a biological pacemaker in canine heart. Circulation 2003;107:1106–9.
146. Plotnikov AN, Sosunov EA, Qu J, et al. Biological pacemaker implanted in canine left bundle branch provides ventricular escape rhythms that have physiologically acceptable rates. Circulation 2004;109:506–12.
147. Irisawa H, Brown HF, Giles W. Cardiac pacemaking in the sinoatrial node. Physiol Rev 1993;73:197–227.
148. Xu C, Police S, Rao N, et al. Characterization and enrichment of cardiomyocytes derived from human embryonic stem cells. Circ Res 2002;91:501–8.
149. Kehat I, Kenyagin-Karsenti D, Snir M, et al. Human embryonic stem cells can differentiate into myocytes with structural and functional properties of cardiomyocytes. J Clin Invest 2001;108:407–14.
150. He JQ, Ma Y, Lee Y, et al. Human embryonic stem cells develop into multiple types of cardiac myocytes: action potential characterization. Circ Res 2003;93:32–9.
151. Mummery C, Ward-van Oostwaard D, Doevendans P, et al. Differentiation of human embryonic stem cells to cardiomyocytes: role of coculture with visceral endoderm-like cells. Circulation 2003;107:2733–40.
152. Kehat I, Khimovich L, Caspi O, et al. Electromechanical integration of cardiomyocytes derived from human embryonic stem cells. Nat Biotechnol 2004;22:1282–9.
153. Xue T, Cho HC, Akar FG, et al. Functional integration of electrically active cardiac derivatives from genetically engineered human embryonic stem cells with quiescent recipient ventricular cardiomyocytes: insights into the development of cell-based pacemakers. Circulation 2005;111:11–20.
154. Plotnikov AN, Shlapakova I, Szabolcs MJ, et al. Xenografted adult human mesenchymal stem cells provide a platform for sustained biological pacemaker function in canine heart. Circulation 2007;116:706–13.
155. Potapova I, Plotnikov A, Lu Z, et al. Human mesenchymal stem cells as a gene delivery system to create cardiac pacemakers. Circ Res 2004;94:952–9.
156. Cho HC, Kashiwakura Y, Marban E. Creation of a biological pacemaker by cell fusion. Circ Res 2007;100:1112–5.

Heart Failure and Pulmonary Hypertension

Jordan T. Shin, MD, PhD[a,b,*], Marc J. Semigran, MD[b]

KEYWORDS

- Heart failure • Pulmonary hypertension
- Nitric oxide • PDE5 • BMPR2

Heart failure is a significant and growing problem in the United States, and is predicted to afflict 1 in 5 adults.[1] It represents the most common Medicare diagnosis at hospital discharge and will account for approximately $37.2 billion in healthcare expenditures in 2009.[2] Despite major advances in therapy over the past 2 decades, current treatment is often palliative and therapies are directed at symptom management and delay of disease progression. An improved understanding of the factors that modify prognosis and outcome would be beneficial in stratifying patient risk and developing novel therapeutic opportunities.

For any given myocardial insult, substantial variation is believed to exist in the susceptibility to developing heart failure, but the underlying factors responsible for this variation are only beginning to be understood. Interindividual differences in many components of the response to myocardial injury have been implicated, including local or remote myocardial remodeling. The impact of comorbid conditions, such as pulmonary hypertension (PH), is also believed to play a role in determining the course and prognosis of heart failure. The determinants and regulators of pulmonary vascular tone and the impact on heart failure are poorly characterized.

Increased pulmonary vascular tone and PH, together with consequent right ventricular dysfunction, are now known to be among the most significant modifiers of the natural history and prognosis of heart failure resulting from left ventricular disease. PH in heart failure is believed to result from congestion and chronic pulmonary venous hypertension. PH is associated with a negative impact on survival,[3] and reversibility of PH in response to pharmacologic or mechanical interventions is a predictor of improved heart failure outcomes.[4] PH in heart failure may begin as a passive process resulting from congestion and elevated filling pressures, and pulmonary venous hypertension. With chronic congestion, pulmonary vascular tone may be become irreversibly elevated. However, the fundamental mechanisms determining pulmonary vascular responses to heart failure and the development of PH remain incompletely understood.

Recently, advances have been made in understanding of the mechanisms underlying pulmonary arterial hypertension (PAH). In contrast to the substantial and growing burden of heart failure, primary PAH is a rare disease. Advances in dissecting the molecular pathogenesis of PAH have begun to illuminate some of the molecular pathways responsible for PH in its primary and secondary forms, and may help provide insights into the molecular and genetic factors regulating pulmonary vascular tone. Because pulmonary tone is a powerful determinant of outcomes in

Funding Disclosures: Dr Shin receives research support from the NIH.
[a] Cardiovascular Research Center, Department of Medicine, Massachusetts General Hospital and Harvard Medical School, 149 13th Street, Charlestown, MA 02129, USA
[b] Cardiology Division, Department of Medicine, Massachusetts General Hospital and Harvard Medical School, GRB 800, 55 Fruit Street, Boston, MA 02114, USA
* Corresponding Author. Cardiovascular Research Center, Department of Medicine, Massachusetts General Hospital and Harvard Medical School, 149 13th Street, Charlestown, MA 02129.
E-mail address: jshin1@partners.org

Heart Failure Clin 6 (2010) 215–222
doi:10.1016/j.hfc.2009.11.007
1551-7136/10/$ – see front matter

heart failure, this understanding may provide insights into the factors that determine prognosis and disease course.

CLASSIFICATION OF PULMONARY HYPERTENSION

PH represents a diverse spectrum of disease. PH is usually associated with an underlying primary diagnoses, such as congenital heart disease, scleroderma/CREST, thromboembolic disease, chronic hypoxia, chronic obstructive pulmonary disease, and left heart failure.[5] In the absence of an underlying cause, PAH is termed *idiopathic* or *primary*. Primary PAH is a rare disorder with an incidence of 1 to 2 cases per million in the United States,[6] but may offer insights into the cause of more general diathesis toward aberrant pulmonary vascular responses. Between 10% and 30% of cases of primary PAH cluster in familial cohorts. These cases are autosomal dominant with low penetrance; only 10% to 20% of patients harboring a mutation exhibit the overt disease phenotype.[7]

In 1998, the second World Symposium on Pulmonary Hypertension in Evian, France, represented the initial attempt to classify PH based on the underlying cause.[8] The spectrum of pulmonary hypertensive diseases was divided into five clinical categories, which were grouped according to therapeutic treatment interventions: (1) PAH; (2) pulmonary venous hypertension; (3) PH associated with disorders of the respiratory system; (4) PH caused by thrombotic or embolic disease; and (5) PH caused by diseases affecting pulmonary vasculature. The third World Symposium on Pulmonary Arterial Hypertension in Vienna held in 2003 revised and extended the Evian classification scheme.[5] As with the 1998 scheme, there were five categories but they were arranged somewhat differently: (1) PAH, (2) PH with left heart disease, (3) PH associated with lung diseases or hypoxemia, (4) PH caused by chronic thrombotic or embolic disease, and (5) miscellaneous. Important changes included the recognition of PH associated with left heart disease as a wholly distinct category (category 2).

THE CLINICAL DIAGNOSIS AND EVALUATION OF PULMONARY ARTERIAL HYPERTENSION

The clinical presentation of PH can be nonspecific and difficult to differentiate from other cardiopulmonary diseases. Based on national registry data, the most frequently recorded symptoms were dyspnea (60% of patients), fatigue (19%), and presyncope or syncope (13%). Other symptoms may include chest pain, palpitations, or edema. The lack of specific findings can delay identification of a definitive diagnosis; the average interval between onset of symptoms and diagnosis was 2 years.[9] Family history may offer little assistance given the relatively low prevalence and penetrance of identified mutations in PAH.

As pulmonary pressures rise and right heart failure ensues, the physical findings of PH become less subtle. Examination of the jugular pulsations can show elevated neck veins and prominent *v* waves. In the setting of more profound right ventricular dysfunction, hepatic enlargement, and pulsation, lower extremity edema and ascites may be found. Cardiac examination may also be notable for an right ventricular heave or lift. The classic auscultatory finding is of an accentuated pulmonic component of the second heart sound (P_2). Additionally, a systolic murmur of tricuspid regurgitation and a right-sided S_3 may also be heard. Other notable findings include Raynaud phenomenon in 10% of patients.[9]

No definitive set of laboratory tests confirm the diagnosis of PH. Testing for HIV, hepatic enzymes, thyroid function, and rheumatologic markers of autoimmune and connective tissue diseases are helpful in identifying secondary causes of PH. Measurement of serum brain natriuretic peptide levels may be a useful correlate of hemodynamics.[10]

Noninvasive testing can help raise PAH in the differential and in diagnosing PH. Although no pathognomonic EKG is available to diagnose PAH, common electrocardiographic findings include right atrial enlargement and prominent R wave voltages in the inferior leads, right-axis deviation, and right ventricular strain. The chest radiographic manifestations of PAH include pulmonary artery, right atrial, and ventricular enlargement. Ventilation/perfusion scans and CT angiography are useful in evaluating thromboembolic disease as the cause of dyspnea and pulmonary hypertension. Finally, transthoracic echocardiography can be used to confirm hypertrophy of the right-sided cardiac chambers and evaluate for structural defects, with the Doppler component of the echo serving as an important technique to evaluate right ventricular systolic pressure.[11]

Although noninvasive methods such as echocardiography can suggest elevated right- sided pressures, the gold standard for diagnosing PH remains the finding of elevated pressures in the pulmonary artery and on the right side of the heart through right heart catheterization. The clinical threshold for PH is crossed when the mean pulmonary artery pressure exceeds 25 mm Hg at rest or 30 mm Hg during exercise.[12]

PULMONARY ARTERIAL HYPERTENSION AND LEFT HEART FAILURE

Chronically elevated pulmonary venous pressures (reflected clinically as an elevation in pulmonary capillary wedge pressure [PCWP] on right heart catheterization) results from systolic and diastolic heart failure and mitral valvular disease and is the most common cause of PH.[13,14] Conversely, PH represents a common finding in heart failure, and portends a poorer prognosis and worse outcomes.

The work of Butler and colleagues[15] provides insight into the prevalence of PH in a cohort of patients who had advanced heart failure undergoing evaluation for heart transplantation. They studied 320 patients undergoing exercise testing with invasive hemodynamic monitoring for systolic heart failure. Overall, this was a relatively ill population that had a mean maximum oxygen consumption (Vo_2max) of 13 mL/kg per minute. Only 28% of their patients had a normal pulmonary vascular resistance (PVR) of less than 1.5 Woods units; the remaining 72% had elevated pulmonary vascular tone. Increased PVR negatively impacted peak exercise oxygen consumption per minute (Vo_2) and other indices of rest and exercise hemodynamics. No association was found between pulmonary vascular tone and ejection fraction, cause of the underlying cardiomyopathy, or functional status (according to New York Heart Association [NYHA] class). Similarly, Ghio and colleagues[3] found PH in more than 60% of the patients they studied. Although abnormal pulmonary vascular tone and PH are common in patients who have systolic heart failure, clinical characteristics do not predict the likelihood of developing PH.

More recently, heart failure with preserved ejection fraction (HFpEF), which accounts for nearly half of heart failure cases in the United States, has received considerable attention. PH also seems to be a common hemodynamic finding in this group. In a population of patients who had HFpEF in Olmstead County, Minnesota, pulmonary artery systolic pressure (PASP) and PCWP were estimated from echocardiography and compared with a control population who had no heart failure.[16] Although PH (defined here as PASP>35 mm Hg) was diagnosed in 8% of the control group, 83% of the HFpEF group had elevated pulmonary artery pressures. The median value in the hypertensive control group who had no heart failure was 28 mm Hg, whereas it was 48 mm Hg the HFpEF group.

Similar to systolic heart failure, PASP correlated with pulmonary venous pressures as determined by PCWP in HFpEF. PH also seems to impact survival when present in HFpEF, as the presence of PH was significantly associated with increased mortality. Hence, PH is both a prevalent comorbidity and poor prognostic finding in heart failure with either preserved or impaired left ventricular systolic function.

PH and abnormal pulmonary vascular tone may impact heart failure through affecting right ventricular function. The importance of right ventricular performance in predicting functional capacity and survival in heart failure was established by Di Salvo and colleagues,[17] who studied exercise capacity in patients who had advanced heart failure. Specifically, although left ventricular ejection fraction (LVEF) predicts prognosis in heart failure, the investigators found no association between LVEF and exercise capacity as determined by peak oxygen consumption. However, exercise capacity correlated with right ventricular ejection fraction (RVEF). Furthermore, better RVEF was a significant predictor of survival in the advanced heart failure population. Ghio and colleagues[3] examined the relationship between pulmonary artery pressures and right ventricular performance. Their analysis showed a significant inverse relationship between RVEF and pulmonary artery pressures, although they noted several clinically relevant exceptions to this finding (eg, normal pulmonary artery pressures with right ventricular dysfunction and PH with preserved RVEF). The combination of PH and heart failure is associated with an especially poor prognosis in the setting of concomitant right ventricular dysfunction. The authors speculate that the loss of right ventricular performance may represent a late finding in the setting of increased right ventricular afterload and PH, and that compromised RVEF may be a surrogate marker for the chronicity of heart failure. However, the determinants of right ventricular compromise in the setting of heart failure and PH remain unknown.

Recent studies support the notion that selective right ventricular afterload reduction using strategies to decrease PVR and treat PH may be beneficial in heart failure. Inhaled nitric oxide, a pulmonary specific vasodilator, has been shown to effectively decrease PVR in patients who have heart failure without lowering systemic vascular resistance or causing significant hypotension.[18] Koelling and colleagues[19] studied the impact of inhaled nitric oxide on exercise capacity in patients who had severe heart failure. In patients who had elevated pulmonary artery pressures, exercise capacity increased by 22% with treatment. Selective pulmonary vasodilation and right ventricular afterload reduction did not improve peak VO_2 in patients who had no PH. Thus, inhaled nitric oxide ameliorates exercise capacity only in patients who have PH.

Although administration of inhaled nitric oxide is not practical chronically, other strategies to augment its effects and preferentially reduce PVR have been attempted in heart failure. Specifically, pharmacologic agents such as sildenafil and tadalafil potentiate the endogenously produced nitric oxide through inhibiting type 5 phosphodiesterase (PDE5), resulting in intracellular accumulation of cGMP. Acutely, a single dose of sildenafil has been shown to decrease PVR and pulmonary artery pressures preferentially, compared with the systemic circulation, both at rest and with exercise in patients who have NYHA class III heart failure and PH.[20]

Moreover, the improvement in hemodynamics and measured peak oxygen consumption seems to be durable and generalizable to other indices of functional capacity. Lewis and colleagues[21] studied patients who had systolic heart failure and PH undergoing optimal medical therapy and randomized them to chronic treatment with either sildenafil or placebo. After 12-weeks of treatment, patients receiving sildenafil had significantly improved exercise time, VO_2max, 6-minute walk distance, and heart failure symptom scores. These findings have been substantiated in other trials of PDE5 inhibition in heart failure.[22,23] Therefore, decreasing pulmonary vascular tone and treating PH in heart failure with PDE5 inhibition seems to offer beneficial effects in terms of hemodynamics, symptoms of heart failure, and functional capacity. None of these studies has been sufficiently powered nor performed for sufficient duration to assess whether PDE5 inhibition might also impact survival in heart failure.

Although studies of sildenafil-induced right ventricular afterload reduction may provide enthusiasm for therapeutic strategies to treat PH and heart failure, earlier trials using the pulmonary vasodilators epoprostenol and endothelin antagonists in heart failure did not achieve positive primary end points,[24–27] suggesting that the functional benefits of inhaled nitric oxide and PDE5 inhibition may not result purely from the hemodynamic effects of these agents. Instead, activation of nitric oxide and cGMP signaling may have direct myocardial effects that at least may partly explain some of the beneficial effects of these agents.[28] A more detailed understanding of the basic biology of PH may help define the advantages and pitfalls and help in the development of novel treatment approaches.

THE BIOLOGY OF PULMONARY HYPERTENSION

Primary PAH is a rare disorder with an incidence of 1 to 2 cases per million in the United States.[6] However, it may offer insights into the cause of more general diathesis toward aberrant pulmonary vascular responses in the secondary PH encountered in heart failure. Familial PH is an autosomal dominant disease with low penetrance; only 10% to 20% of patients harboring a mutation exhibit the overt disease phenotype.[7]

The diathesis to PH seems to vary based on environmental and genetic factors. Acquired disorders and exposures serve as triggers for PH, including appetite suppressants (derivatives of fenfluramine and other anorexigens), toxins, and infection (eg, HIV[29]). However, only few individuals exposed to environmental triggers eventually develop PH, suggesting that the acquired exposure may trigger a genetic susceptibility. Gender clearly exerts an influence on the diathesis to PH; women are diagnosed two to five times more often than men.

Although several diverse causes of PH exist, shared pathologic findings are identified in lungs of affected patients, including (1) thickening of the walls of small pulmonary arteries with concomitant neointima formation and smooth muscle cell (SMC) proliferation in large and small pulmonary arteries, (2) the presence of plexiform endothelial cell lesions characterized by capillary-like channels near pulmonary arterioles (200–400 mM in diameter), and (3) the presence of thrombosis in situ. Tuder and colleagues[30,31] reported that these plexiform lesions are characterized by proliferating endothelial cells[30] and the abundant expression of angiogenesis-related molecules.[31] The same laboratory has also reported that endothelial cells in plexiform lesions of patients who have primary PH are monoclonal, but are not in those who have secondary PH.[32] Similarly, because patients who had PH associated with anorexigen use had monoclonal populations of endothelial cells in plexiform lesions, Tuder and colleagues[33] suggested that anorexigens may serve as an environmental cofactor that precipitates PAH in susceptible individuals.

The Role of BMP/BMPR2 Signaling in Disease Pathogenesis

The existence of familial forms of PH has offered a unique opportunity to define the cause of at least one form of pulmonary vascular disease. Using unbiased genetic approaches mutations in the bone morphogenetic protein (BMP) type 2 receptor (BMPR2) gene have been identified as the cause of approximately one third of familial PH.[34–36] *BMPR2* mutations characterized to date suggest that haploinsufficiency may be the primary mechanism of action in a proportion of these cases,[37] but detailed studies in tractable animal models will be required to establish this formally. *BMPR2* mutations also may have more pleiotropic cardiovascular effects than previously believed. In a detailed re-examination of families with PAH, Newman and colleagues[38] established that several families that were previously believed to be distinct were in fact distantly related and that several family members also harbored congenital cardiac abnormalities or developed cardiomyopathy. Therefore, in addition to their role in PH, heritable abnormalities in *BMPR2* may also be associated with congenital heart disease and cardiomyopathy.

Transforming growth factor β (TGF-β) family signal transduction has been implicated in other genetically mediated causes of PH in a separate but related condition called hereditary hemorrhagic telangiectasia (HHT). HHT is caused by mutations in *ACVRLK1/ALK1*, a type I TGF-β receptor, and endoglin, a TGF superfamily ligand.[39,40] These same pathways have been implicated in secondary forms of PH. Expression of *BMPR2* is diminished in patients who have PH; BMPR2 transcript is downregulated in the endothelium of patients who have PH who do not harbor a mutation in the gene. Acquired forms of PH have also been associated with attenuation of the BMPR2 coreceptor ALK3/BMPR1a, which may be mediated through angiopoietin-1.[41]

BMPR2 Signal Transduction

BMPs belong to a large family of proteins related to TGF-β. Proteins in this family have effects on various cell types, depending on the cell environment and developmental stage. The TGF- β family of peptides can modulate the function of vascular cells (endothelial cells and SMCs), including proliferation, migration, apoptosis, and secretion of extracellular cell matrix. BMPs are known to inhibit vascular SMC proliferation,[42,43] stimulate vascular SMC migration,[44] and inhibit neointima formation in balloon-injured rat carotid arteries.[43]

TGF-β family members bind to two different types of cell-surface receptors, referred to as type I and type II, both of which have intracellular serine-threonine kinase domains.[45] On ligand binding, type II receptors complex with type I receptors, leading to type I receptor phosphorylation and activation. The activated type I receptors subsequently phosphorylate receptor-regulated Smad proteins (R-Smads) that interact with common-mediator Smads (Co-Smads), leading to modulation of gene transcription (Smad-dependent signaling). TGF-β and BMPs have also been shown to activate mitogen-activated protein kinases, including ERK, SAPK/JNK, and p38 (Smad-independent signaling). As with all type 2 BMP receptors, BMPR2 consists of a ligand-binding (extracellular) domain, a transmembrane domain, a serine/threonine kinase domain, and a C-terminal cytoplasmic tail (a shorter splice variant was also found in humans).

All mammals, despite the large number of BMP ligands, have a limited repertoire of type I and II BMP receptors. Multiple combinations of type I and II receptors create ligand-binding preference for specific ligands, but also afford receptor redundancy within the same class of receptors. BMP binding activates a subset of R-Smads (Smad1, Smad5, and Smad8) that, together with the co-Smad (Smad-4) and other transcription factors, leads to BMP-responsive gene transcription. BMP (and TGF-β) signaling can be modulated by inhibitory Smads (I-Smads: Smad6 and Smad7), which compete with R-Smads for activated type I receptors and whose expression can be induced by TGF-β or BMPs in a negative feedback loop.

Abundant evidence has shown that TGF-β/BMP signaling is required for the normal development in several vertebrate model organisms, including chicken, mouse, frog, and zebrafish, in general and within the cardiovascular system specifically. BMPs can induce the expression of cardiac transcription factors such as Nkx2.5, GATA4, and TBX2 and -3.[46,47] Various cardiac phenotypes have been reported in mice carrying targeted deletions of the genes encoding members of the TGF-β/BMP family, including BMP2, -4, -5/7, -6/7, -10, and TGF-β2.[48] Investigations in Xenopus indicate that BMP signaling is required for late manifestation of cardiac development but not for early markers of cardiac specification.[49] Less is known about the contribution of specific receptors for BMP ligands and the roles played in cardiovascular development.

Signaling Defects Observed with BMPR2 Mutations

Signal transduction through BMPR2 is initiated by ligand binding to a receptor and activation of Smad-dependent and -independent intracellular signaling events. Although a relatively restricted set of type I and II receptors are known, heterodimerization enables potential combinatorial interactions between subunits. Hence, rather than interrupting BMP signaling altogether, nullification of one type II receptor may instead shift the balance of signaling through other receptor subtypes.

Yu and colleagues[50] investigated the impact of the loss of BMPR2 in pulmonary artery SMCs in vitro. Using cre-lox ex vivo inactivation and siRNA inactivation, they showed that, although some BMP ligands seemed to have attenuated intracellular signaling by way of the classic SMAD-1/5/8 pathway, others (specifically BMP6 and BMP7) exhibited augmented signaling through alternate use of the ActR-2a receptor. This finding suggests that the molecular defect in PH may result in augmented rather than attenuated BMP signaling. However, whether Smad activity is increased or decreased in vivo with PH is unclear.

ANIMAL MODELING OF PULMONARY HYPERTENSION WITH *BMPR2*

Transgenic mouse models have been used to dissect how *BMPR2* contributes to development. Knockout of both BMPR2 alleles showed that it is required for early development and led to complete involution and loss by embryonic day 9.5. Histologic analysis of homozygous embryos showed lack of mesoderm formation.[51] Mice heterozygous deficient for BMPR2, although grossly normal, exhibit increased mean PAH and PVR compared with their wild-type littermates. Quantitative histologic analysis shows that heterozygous mice have increased wall thickness in muscularized pulmonary arteries (<100 μm in diameter) and an increased number of alveolar–capillary units compared with wild-type mice.[52] These histologic findings parallel several pathologic findings in patients who had PH. Furthermore, under conditions of inflammatory stress, heterozygous mice are more likely to develop increased right-sided pressures and increased pulmonary vascular remodeling, consistent with the observation that environmental factors can exacerbate a genetic diathesis to PH.[53] Finally, transgenic mice with expression of a dominant-negative *BMPR2* in SMCs only have histologic findings of intimal proliferation and increased mural thickness in pulmonary arterioles.[54] The alveolar/capillary ratio was unchanged and abnormalities were not observed in the smallest vessels.

Thus, *BMPR2* is absolutely required in mammalian development. Germline heterozygous deficiency (ie, in all tissues) phenocopies many aspects of PH. Familial PH results from germline transmission to all cells rather than mosaic loss in one cell type, and observational in situ data suggest that PH is associated with greater loss of transcript in vascular endothelial cells rather than other cell types. Tissue specific interruption in the SMC of transgenic mice leads only to partial recapitulation of the observed pathologic deficits in PH.[54] Conditional deletion in other tissues with murine transgenics is an active area of investigation and anticipated to provide new insights into the ways BMP signaling is involved in the vascular abnormalities underlying PH.

These studies highlight the emerging understanding that the pathophysiologic abnormalities of PH may have their origin during ontogeny. Animal models such as transgenic mice and other vertebrate developmental systems should provide a suitable platform for discovering the molecular and cellular alterations that produce the structural and functional defects in primary and acquired forms of PH, as is seen in heart failure. The detailed exploration of these experimental systems will provide the opportunity to integrate the basic discoveries with the clinical observations and trial data reviewed earlier and inform strategies to treat the spectrum of pulmonary hypertensive diseases.

SUMMARY

When PH and right ventricular dysfunction accompany heart failure, the impact on functional capacity and prognosis are ominous. Newer clinical strategies to preferentially lower pulmonary pressures and pulmonary vascular tone improve functional performance and symptoms of heart failure by targeting the nitric oxide signal transduction pathways, as with PDE5 inhibition. Additional studies are needed to delineate if these therapies will impact long-term patient outcomes and elucidate the specific mechanisms whereby these treatments are effective. Furthermore, the recent finding that mutations in *BMPR2* cause familial forms of PAH and that *BMPR2* expression is decreased in secondary forms of PH strongly implicate BMP signaling in the underlying pathophysiology of PH. Translation of emerging basic science insights in the vascular biology of PH and BMP signaling will provide novel therapeutic strategies for the spectrum of pulmonary hypertensive diseases.

REFERENCES

1. Lloyd-Jones DM, Larson MG, Leip EP, et al. Lifetime risk for developing congestive heart failure: the Framingham Heart Study. Circulation 2002;106:3068.
2. Lloyd-Jones D, Adams R, Carnethon M, et al. Heart disease and stroke statistics—2009 update: a report from the American Heart Association Statistics Committee and Stroke Statistics Subcommittee. Circulation 2009;119:480.

3. Ghio S, Gavazzi A, Campana C, et al. Independent and additive prognostic value of right ventricular systolic function and pulmonary artery pressure in patients with chronic heart failure. J Am Coll Cardiol 2001;37:183.
4. Gavazzi A, Ghio S, Scelsi L, et al. Response of the right ventricle to acute pulmonary vasodilation predicts the outcome in patients with advanced heart failure and pulmonary hypertension. Am Heart J 2003;145:310.
5. Simonneau G, Galie N, Rubin LJ, et al. Clinical classification of pulmonary hypertension. J Am Coll Cardiol 2004;43:5S.
6. Rubin LJ. Primary pulmonary hypertension. N Engl J Med 1997;336:111.
7. Farber HW, Loscalzo J. Pulmonary arterial hypertension. N Engl J Med 2004;351:1655.
8. Fishman AP. Clinical classification of pulmonary hypertension. Clin Chest Med 2001;22:385.
9. Rich S, Dantzker DR, Ayres SM, et al. Primary pulmonary hypertension. A national prospective study. Ann Intern Med 1987;107:216.
10. Leuchte HH, Holzapfel M, Baumgartner RA, et al. Characterization of brain natriuretic peptide in long-term follow-up of pulmonary arterial hypertension. Chest 2005;128:2368.
11. Runo JR, Loyd JE. Primary pulmonary hypertension. Lancet 2003;361:1533.
12. Rubin LJ. Primary pulmonary hypertension. Chest 1993;104:236.
13. Rich S, Rabinovitch M. Diagnosis and treatment of secondary (non-category 1) pulmonary hypertension. Circulation 2008;118:2190.
14. Oudiz RJ. Pulmonary hypertension associated with left-sided heart disease. Clin Chest Med 2007;28:233.
15. Butler J, Chomsky DB, Wilson JR. Pulmonary hypertension and exercise intolerance in patients with heart failure. J Am Coll Cardiol 1999;34:1802.
16. Lam CS, Roger VL, Rodeheffer RJ, et al. Pulmonary hypertension in heart failure with preserved ejection fraction: a community-based study. J Am Coll Cardiol 2009;53:1119.
17. Di Salvo TG, Mathier M, Semigran MJ, et al. Preserved right ventricular ejection fraction predicts exercise capacity and survival in advanced heart failure. J Am Coll Cardiol 1995;25:1143.
18. Semigran MJ, Cockrill BA, Kacmarek R, et al. Hemodynamic effects of inhaled nitric oxide in heart failure. J Am Coll Cardiol 1994;24:982.
19. Koelling TM, Kirmse M, Di Salvo TG, et al. Inhaled nitric oxide improves exercise capacity in patients with severe heart failure and right ventricular dysfunction. Am J Cardiol 1998;81:1494.
20. Lewis GD, Lachmann J, Camuso J, et al. Sildenafil improves exercise hemodynamics and oxygen uptake in patients with systolic heart failure. Circulation 2007;115:59.
21. Lewis GD, Shah R, Shahzad K, et al. Sildenafil improves exercise capacity and quality of life in patients with systolic heart failure and secondary pulmonary hypertension. Circulation 2007;116:1555.
22. Behling A, Rohde LE, Colombo FC, et al. Effects of 5′-phosphodiesterase four-week long inhibition with sildenafil in patients with chronic heart failure: a double-blind, placebo-controlled clinical trial. J Card Fail 2008;14:189.
23. Guazzi M, Samaja M, Arena R, et al. Long-term use of sildenafil in the therapeutic management of heart failure. J Am Coll Cardiol 2007;50:2136.
24. Szokodi I, Piuhola J, Ruskoaho H. Endothelin receptor blockade and exacerbation of heart failure. Circulation 2003;107:e211.
25. Anand I, McMurray J, Cohn JN, et al. Long-term effects of darusentan on left-ventricular remodelling and clinical outcomes in the EndothelinA Receptor Antagonist Trial in Heart Failure (EARTH): randomised, double-blind, placebo-controlled trial. Lancet 2004;364:347.
26. Packer M, McMurray J, Massie BM, et al. Clinical effects of endothelin receptor antagonism with bosentan in patients with severe chronic heart failure: results of a pilot study. J Card Fail 2005;11:12.
27. Califf RM, Adams KF, McKenna WJ, et al. A randomized controlled trial of epoprostenol therapy for severe congestive heart failure: The Flolan International Randomized Survival Trial (FIRST). Am Heart J 1997;134:44.
28. Takimoto E, Champion HC, Li M, et al. Chronic inhibition of cyclic GMP phosphodiesterase 5A prevents and reverses cardiac hypertrophy. Nat Med 2005;11:214.
29. Archer S, Rich S. Primary pulmonary hypertension: a vascular biology and translational research "Work in progress. Circulation 2000;102:2781.
30. Tuder RM, Groves B, Badesch DB, et al. Exuberant endothelial cell growth and elements of inflammation are present in plexiform lesions of pulmonary hypertension. Am J Pathol 1994;144:275.
31. Tuder RM, Chacon M, Alger L, et al. Expression of angiogenesis-related molecules in plexiform lesions in severe pulmonary hypertension: evidence for a process of disordered angiogenesis. J Pathol 2001;195:367.
32. Lee SD, Shroyer KR, Markham NE, et al. Monoclonal endothelial cell proliferation is present in primary but not secondary pulmonary hypertension. J Clin Invest 1998;101:927.
33. Tuder RM, Radisavljevic Z, Shroyer KR, et al. Monoclonal endothelial cells in appetite suppressant-associated pulmonary hypertension. Am J Respir Crit Care Med 1998;158:1999.
34. Deng Z, Morse JH, Slager SL, et al. Familial primary pulmonary hypertension (gene PPH1) is caused by mutations in the bone morphogenetic protein receptor-II gene. Am J Hum Genet 2000;67:737.

35. Lane KB, Machado RD, Pauciulo MW, et al. Heterozygous germline mutations in BMPR2, encoding a TGF-beta receptor, cause familial primary pulmonary hypertension. The International PPH Consortium. Nat Genet 2000;26:81.
36. Thomson JR, Machado RD, Pauciulo MW, et al. Sporadic primary pulmonary hypertension is associated with germline mutations of the gene encoding BMPR-II, a receptor member of the TGF-beta family. J Med Genet 2000;37:741.
37. Machado RD, Pauciulo MW, Thomson JR, et al. BMPR2 haploinsufficiency as the inherited molecular mechanism for primary pulmonary hypertension. Am J Hum Genet 2001;68:92.
38. Newman JH, Wheeler L, Lane KB, et al. Mutation in the gene for bone morphogenetic protein receptor II as a cause of primary pulmonary hypertension in a large kindred. N Engl J Med 2001;345:319.
39. McAllister KA, Grogg KM, Johnson DW, et al. Endoglin, a TGF-beta binding protein of endothelial cells, is the gene for hereditary haemorrhagic telangiectasia type 1. Nat Genet 1994;8:345.
40. Johnson DW, Berg JN, Baldwin MA, et al. Mutations in the activin receptor-like kinase 1 gene in hereditary haemorrhagic telangiectasia type 2. Nat Genet 1996;13:189.
41. Du L, Sullivan CC, Chu D, et al. Signaling molecules in nonfamilial pulmonary hypertension. N Engl J Med 2003;348:500.
42. Dorai H, Vukicevic S, Sampath TK. Bone morphogenetic protein-7 (osteogenic protein-1) inhibits smooth muscle cell proliferation and stimulates the expression of markers that are characteristic of SMC phenotype in vitro. J Cell Physiol 2000;184:37.
43. Nakaoka T, Gonda K, Ogita T, et al. Inhibition of rat vascular smooth muscle proliferation in vitro and in vivo by bone morphogenetic protein-2. J Clin Invest 1997;100:2824.
44. Willette RN, Gu JL, Lysko PG, et al. BMP-2 gene expression and effects on human vascular smooth muscle cells. J Vasc Res 1999;36:120.
45. Miyazono K, Kusanagi K, Inoue H. Divergence and convergence of TGF-beta/BMP signaling. J Cell Physiol 2001;187:265.
46. Yamada M, Revelli JP, Eichele G, et al. Expression of chick Tbx-2, Tbx-3, and Tbx-5 genes during early heart development: evidence for BMP2 induction of Tbx2. Dev Biol 2000;228:95.
47. Brown CO III, Chi X, Garcia-Gras E, et al. The cardiac determination factor, Nkx2-5, is activated by mutual cofactors GATA-4 and Smad1/4 via a novel upstream enhancer. J Biol Chem 2004;279: 10659.
48. Zhao GQ. Consequences of knocking out BMP signaling in the mouse. Genesis 2003;35:43.
49. Walters MJ, Wayman GA, Christian JL. Bone morphogenetic protein function is required for terminal differentiation of the heart but not for early expression of cardiac marker genes. Mech Dev 2001;100:263.
50. Yu PB, Beppu H, Kawai N, et al. Bone morphogenetic protein (BMP) type II receptor deletion reveals BMP ligand-specific gain of signaling in pulmonary artery smooth muscle cells. J Biol Chem 2005;280: 24443.
51. Beppu H, Kawabata M, Hamamoto T, et al. BMP type II receptor is required for gastrulation and early development of mouse embryos. Dev Biol 2000;221: 249.
52. Beppu H, Ichinose F, Kawai N, et al. BMPR-II heterozygous mice have mild pulmonary hypertension and an impaired pulmonary vascular remodeling response to prolonged hypoxia. Am J Physiol Lung Cell Mol Physiol 2004;287:L1241.
53. Song Y, Jones JE, Beppu H, et al. Increased susceptibility to pulmonary hypertension in heterozygous BMPR2-mutant mice. Circulation 2005;112: 553.
54. West J, Fagan K, Steudel W, et al. Pulmonary hypertension in transgenic mice expressing a dominant-negative BMPRII gene in smooth muscle. Circ Res 2004;94:1109.

The Genetics of Congestive Heart Failure

Calum A. MacRae, MD, PhD

KEYWORDS

- Congestive heart failure • Cardiomyopathies
- Genome-wide association studies
- Mendelian cardiomyopathy genetics

Congestive heart failure (CHF) remains the single most common cause of mortality and morbidity in the developed world.[1] With as many as 5 million hospitalizations annually, treating heart failure represents a major component of the health-care budget of every developed nation, and an increasing component of the health-care budgets in many developing nations. The heart failure syndrome is known to represent a final common pathway for a broad range of etiologies, but there is tremendous variation in the propensity to develop CHF after a given insult.[1,2] This variation is thought to result in part from inherited differences in myocardial, vascular, or systemic responses, but the nature of the underlying traits responsible ultimately for the development of heart failure has remained elusive. Other articles in this issue highlight the impressive advances in our understanding of the genetics of the cardiomyopathies, and more recently in the genetics of specific traits within the heart failure syndrome. However, there has been limited progress in the genetic exploration of the key clinical phenotype itself: heart failure. In this article, the author attempts to place the results of genetic studies of cardiomyopathy in the broader context of the clinical syndrome of heart failure, highlighting some of the key questions for future study.

THE COMPONENT PHENOTYPES OF HEART FAILURE

Several decades of investigation have led to an increased understanding of the mechanisms underlying the later stages of heart failure. Adult cardiac myocytes do not divide in any meaningful numbers, and as a result increased workload leads not to cardiomyocyte hyperplasia, but rather to cellular hypertrophy and increased ventricular mass.[3] This fundamental response occurs in the face of a broad range of stressors including hypertension, myocardial infarction, or myocardial dystrophy, and has increasingly been associated with energetic defects.[1,4] Although initially adaptive, in most situations the myocardial remodeling pathways eventually become maladaptive. At this stage progressive effects on ventricular shape, substantial changes in most aspects of systolic and diastolic myocardial function, and proarrhythmic effects on calcium cycling or membrane biology occur in a significant subset of patients.[5–7] The remodeling in heart failure is not confined to the myocardium and there is also evidence of profound changes in the biology of many other organ systems.[1]

Early in the development of heart failure, long before the emergence of any symptoms, activation of the sympathetic nervous system can be detected, and adrenergic humoral factors and many other compensatory pathways (labeled generally as neurohormonal activation) are upregulated.[8–11] The field has been dominated by studies of adrenergic and renin-angiotensin systems, and the natriuretic peptides, but recent work has implicated many other endocrine or paracrine effectors, such as apelin, a host of cytokines, parathyroid hormone, and related peptides.[8,10,11]

Extensive remodeling also occurs throughout the vascular system. Systemic arterial and venous biology is often abnormal as a result of the diffuse atherosclerosis that underlies the most common cause of heart failure: coronary artery disease. However, it is also clear that there are

Cardiovascular Division, Brigham and Women's Hospital and Harvard Medical School, 75 Francis Street, Boston, MA 02115, USA
E-mail address: camacrae@bics.bwh.harvard.edu

Heart Failure Clin 6 (2010) 223–230
doi:10.1016/j.hfc.2009.11.004
1551-7136/10/$ – see front matter

perturbations of arterial structure and function, as well as venous capacitance in all forms of heart failure.[12] Two vascular beds merit specific mention: the renal and pulmonary circulations. There is no doubt that once hypoperfusion supervenes, physiologic salt and water retention plays a major role in the genesis of progressive expansion of extracellular fluid volume, worsening elevation of intracardiac pressures, and ultimately the congestion of overt CHF.[1] Whether as a result of systemic abnormalities of vessel biology or as a consequence of other unknown factors, disproportionate renal dysfunction occurs in subset of those with heart failure. This so-called cardiorenal syndrome is a marker of adverse events and is currently the subject of intense investigation.[13–15] In the pulmonary vascular tree, there is also variation in the responses to abnormal myocardial function. For reasons that are obscure, a significant subset of those with elevated left ventricular end-diastolic pressures will develop disproportionate and irreversible pulmonary hypertension.[1,16] This pulmonary hypertension can adversely affect right ventricular function (which is usually also afflicted by diffuse myocardial processes), and is a marker for conspicuously worse outcomes.

Virtually every cell type and every organ has been implicated in heart failure and the picture that is emerging is of a systemic disorder where the entire organism is engaged in a chronic stress response, that encompasses every pathway from insulin regulation of energy balance to innate immunity. The control hierarchy, and in many instances the primary sensor or sensors, for the local and global responses characteristic of CHF are completely unknown. Multiple cellular pathways have been implicated in the myocardial biology of heart failure. Numerous murine models of heart failure have been generated, but few, other than those recapitulating human cardiomyopathy alleles, have shed light on human heart failure mechanisms.[17] At a cellular level a central role for calcineurin signaling has been debated, and several other calcium-regulated pathways have been implicated.[6,7] It has proven particularly difficult to identify the upstream factors responsible for heart failure, as the much of our understanding of the human syndrome has been garnered from symptomatic late-phase or end-stage disease.[1] It is for this reason that genetic approaches to CHF are particularly attractive.

GENETIC ARCHITECTURE OF HEART FAILURE

Variation in propensity to CHF has been attributed to differences in the extent of myocardial injury, but there is evidence that identical myocardial insults may lead to disparate outcomes, and also of major inherited and environmental contributions to the risk for heart failure.[1,2] The CHF syndrome is a final common pathway for a vast range of insults including ischemic injury, trypanosomal infection and the mutation of multiple genes.[1,2] Non-ischemic CHF exhibits evidence of familiarity in 30% to 50% of cases, and there are more than 30 known genetic loci, but few cloned genes.[18] In subclinically affected relatives what appears to be a predisposition to ventricular remodeling in response to many different stimuli has been observed.[19] Environmental variables compound the phenotypic pleiotropy seen in such single gene disorders and confound the hope of predictive genetic testing. Therapeutic modulation of neurohormonal abnormalities will delay progression, but often does not prevent the emergence of CHF. In addition to the evidence of a role for genetics, early environmental exposures are now also thought to pattern cardiac biology and responses to injury.[20] Recently, major roles for microRNAs and epigenetic factors have been identified, suggesting that at each step the pathophysiology may be substantially modified by prior environmental or even transgenerational exposures.[20,21] The powerful tools of modern genetics offer the possibility that by defining the inherited contribution we will obtain direct inroads into the environmental and epigenetic modifiers underlying this major cause of morbidity and mortality.

INSIGHTS INTO HEART FAILURE FROM MENDELIAN CARDIOMYOPATHY GENETICS

The current state of genetic insight into human cardiomyopathies and the component traits of heart failure are outlined in the articles of this issue. The primary causes of rare forms of increased myocardial mass, left and right ventricular dysfunction, and other components of CHF risk have been identified in elegant genetic work with Mendelian families.[2] Similarly, recent work in the epidemiology and genetics of atrial fibrillation has uncovered direct links between CHF and this arrhythmia, at a myocardial and endocrine level.[22–24] Although investigators have identified the primary causes in many instances, a comprehensive understanding of the mechanisms downstream from each of these genes is far from a reality.

A central question in the field is the role, in more common forms of heart failure, of the pathways implicated in single-gene disorders. The selection pressures operating against inherited diseases where reproductive efficiency is reduced would be predicted to result in high de novo mutation rates and tremendous allelic heterogeneity. Indeed, in most inherited human heart diseases this is exactly what has been observed.[2,25] Common forms of heart failure may be hypothesized to result from less penetrant, milder alleles of the cardiomyopathy genes found in extended kindreds with Mendelian disease; alleles that would not be subject to the same negative selection pressures. Large scale re-sequencing efforts for several cardiomyopathy genes have been undertaken in many hundreds of subjects with undifferentiated nonischemic heart failure to test this hypothesis. The results have been rather disappointing to date, and in most instances fewer than 1% of cases have evidence of mutations in the known genes. These data reflect not only the tremendous heterogeneity of inherited forms of heart failure but also serve to emphasize that the genes that result in primary forms of myocardial injury may play little or no role in more common forms of heart failure. It is also conceivable that although the specific genes mutated in rare (and extreme) forms of heart failure may not be mutated in more common variants, the functions of the relevant pathways may be mechanistically important.

Genome-Wide Association Studies

Genome-wide association studies (GWAS) offer complementary approaches to the dissection of the genetic basis of heart failure and address common, small effect size alleles at the other end of the spectrum from Mendelian disease. At the core of this technique is the assumption that common diseases result from aggregations of common ancestral gene variants. As the particular combinations of alleles will vary across each unrelated individual, this approach does not use transmission probability, but instead relies on simple association of genotypes with phenotypes within a population.[26,27] By their nature GWASs are designed to detect small population-wide effects operant irrespective of the primary etiology, but these same design features reduce the sensitivity for the detection of even major genetic effects in the face of etiologic heterogeneity. A second limitation of GWAS is population stratification, which can result in the spurious association of a polymorphism with disease, simply because the disease and the unlinked sequence variant are found in the same population subgroup. This limitation can be partly addressed by replicating the findings in large study cohorts drawn from genetically distinct populations. The prior probability that any observed effect is a result of the specific polymorphisms studied is usually extremely low, resulting in an unacceptably high false-positive rate (through Bayesian inference). Because of the absence of segregation information inherent in these studies, it is also impossible to causally relate specific variants or a definitively bounded segment of DNA to a phenotype. The phenotype in question may result from variations in linked genes, in so-called disequilibrium with the tested polymorphism. These issues are, at least in part, dealt with by using extended haplotypes of markers in large populations.

In the last few years, the completion of the Human Genome Project and the emergence of comprehensive haplotype maps (HapMap) have led to a proliferation of genome-wide association projects. The theoretic advantages of GWAS have all, to some extent, been confirmed including the unbiased assessment of the role of common alleles in disease, the detection of population-wide effects, and the potential for disease pathway entry. Among the most successful GWASs have been those focused on quantitative traits where the allelic architecture likely favors the success of the technique.[28] Many dichotomous traits have also been successfully approached, but here the resolution of the phenotype is emerging as an important variable in determining the power of GWAS. For some traits, particularly where there is little selection pressure on reproductive efficiency (eg, senile macular degeneration or atrial fibrillation), large effect sizes are observed and relatively small studies have sufficed for the detection of genetic loci in the GWAS framework.[23] However, for other traits where there is presumably considerable selection pressure (eg, hypertension) and likely greater genetic and allelic heterogeneity, GWAS have proven less successful despite studies of increasing power.

In heart failure, robust association studies have only just begun to emerge. The EchoGen consortium recently identified several interesting loci for left ventricular (LV) structure and function in a large scale GWAS of echocardiographic parameters in 12,612 subjects. Not all of these loci replicated at genome-wide significance in a replication cohort of 4094 individuals, but at least two novel loci for cardiac chamber dimensions were confirmed. Additional meta-analyses of GWAS data for incident CHF are pending, and larger cohorts may reveal additional loci.[29] The most robust GWAS data for CHF-related phenotypes have been observed for natriuretic peptide levels that are strongly associated with variation at the NPPA-NPPB locus in a population of 14,743 subjects. Specific alleles within the natriuretic peptide gene locus are associated with lower systolic and diastolic blood pressure and reduced odds of hypertension in a second cohort of 29,717 individuals.[30] These are the first data in humans linking these classic biomarkers of heart failure with variation in blood pressure, the major risk factor for CHF. However, even the NPPA-NPPB locus contains several other genes that may affect the CHF phenotype, including genes for angiotensin interacting proteins.

The results of this initial wave of GWAS for heart failure and related traits have raised several important challenges. The phenotypes in question include several quantitative traits: biomarker levels, LV structure and function, and the binary diagnosis of incident heart failure. The power of GWAS is most evident in the case of readily quantifiable biomarkers, yet these same phenotypes may be less specific for CHF.[31] In common with many of the most successful genome-wide association studies to date, those in CHF have explained only a small proportion of the heritability. The cost of increasing the size (and power) of many human CHF cohorts for secondary analyses of those loci of borderline statistical significance and for exploring gene-gene or gene-environment interactions is prohibitive.

Detecting Intermediate Effect Size Alleles

Heart failure, like many human disease syndromes, is highly heterogeneous. Traditional clinical entities often encompass many disorders with distinctive natural histories, environmental contributions, and therapeutic responses. This etiologic heterogeneity compromises epidemiologic investigation, drug trials, and all forms of genetic study. Given the absence of any familial information, GWAS are particularly susceptible to the problems of heterogeneity. Small effect sizes in common pathways far downstream of the causal genes dominate the results, whereas major alleles operant in a small minority are simply not detected. As noted earlier, one of the central barriers to efficient translation of genetic and genomic insights is the reliance on traditional clinical syndromes, a problem best recognized in psychiatric disease.[32] In several clinical fields, efforts have begun to define new phenotypes that resolve heterogeneity by adopting novel approaches to genetic study and to phenotyping.[33–35]

Genetic Approaches to Intermediate Effect Sizes

One solution to the problems of genetic and phenotypic heterogeneity is the so-called kin-cohort design, which allows the detection of gene effects of a broad range of magnitudes in a single systematic ascertainment, using proband-based family collections.[36] In this way, the genetic epidemiology of a disorder may be defined; monogenic forms of the disorder identified; and homogeneous populations suitable for other genetic approaches, including nonparametric mapping and association studies, can be collected. This design allows the characterization of family-specific disease features, prioritizes genetic investigation of a condition by the magnitude of the effect, facilitates study of gene-gene or gene-environment interactions, and allows pathophysiologic insights to be gained irrespective of the role of any heritable factors.[36]

This approach has been used to address the genetic basis of atrial fibrillation (AF), a usually paroxysmal arrhythmia known to be a risk factor for CHF. Evidence of a substantial heritable contribution was detected, consistent with a major gene effect in each family, but with markedly reduced penetrance.[37] Multiple genes were mapped (on Chromosomes 3, 11, and 18), and sufficient probands were collected for one of the first GWASs for this condition, which identified a locus on Chromosome 4 in an intergenic region adjacent to the transcription factor Pitx2 and other candidate genes. In common with similar GWAS for other diseases, this latest locus explains less than 10% of the heritable contribution to AF confirming there are larger heritable effects at work. The biologic mechanism is obscure, but may reflect abnormal atrial patterning.[38]

NEW PHENOTYPES FOR HEART FAILURE

Although much of the focus in human genetics over the last two decades has been on the genetic contributors to complexity, there has been little work to improve the granularity of clinical phenotypes.[32,35,39] Many disease syndromes are rooted in the late 19th century, and the success of randomized controlled trials, although a major advance, has acted as a "lumping" influence over the last two decades. As we begin to explore interindividual variation in the natural history of disease, in drug responses and in drug toxicities (each in the context of the completion of the Human Genome Project), the concept of personalized medicine has emerged.[40,41] Implicit in this construct is a dramatic change in our understanding of the relationship between genotype and phenotype, including quantitative comprehension of gene-gene, gene-environment, and gene-drug interactions. New diagnostic tools are required to discriminate homogeneous disease subsets and to identify causally related, more penetrant endophenotypes. Similarly, a new scale of drug discovery will be necessary.[39] Formal phenome projects are being proposed for many human clinical syndromes, but the way forward in heart failure, as in other clinical entities, is not clear.

In most cases we are studying heart failure at rather limited resolution. Detailed cell biology, or even histology, is rarely available and current clinical classifications are based on chamber dimensions and wall thicknesses. Although these phenotypes have been extremely useful in clinical management and in the study of Mendelian disorders, there is extensive heterogeneity in clinical outcomes and in drug responses. Even in single gene disorders, the existence of overlap syndromes where families contain members who are each affected with a different morphologic class of cardiomyopathy (hypertrophic, restrictive, dilated or right ventricular) suggests that our current classification schemes cross important biologic boundaries. Individual genes or pathways may be causally involved in one form of heart failure, yet irrelevant in other forms of the same syndrome that are indistinguishable using current clinical techniques. To move beyond this impasse, novel phenotypic classifiers of heart failure and rigorous genetic approaches to identify genes across the entire range of effect size are required. Ultimately, much more powerful strategies than those currently employed will be necessary if we are to reach a quantitative understanding of disease etiology, far less than the gene-gene, gene-environment, or pharmacogenetic interactions implicit in personalized medicine.

EXAMPLES OF RATIONAL PHENOTYPE EXPLORATION IN HUMANS

There are many potential approaches to the definition of robust quantitative phenotypes in the causal chain leading to heart failure. Even a reevaluation of traditional clinical phenotypes can result in new insights. For example, characteristic EKG features of the major long QT loci were uncovered only as the genes were being cloned, approximately 50 years after the description of the original syndrome,[42] while the subtle EKG phenotypes of the Brugada syndrome went unnoticed until families were studied.[43] Similarly, evaluation of other phenotypes in the context of an extended family can offer novel insights. Tissue Doppler has proven useful in identifying pre-clinically affected individuals with hypertrophic cardiomyopathy, but has not been systematically explored in the relatives of those with other forms of inherited heart failure.[19,44] The neurohormones of the renin-angiotensin system and the natriuretic peptides are perturbed late in CHF, but other biomarkers may be discriminating in the appropriate context. For example, specific biomarkers of anabolic-catabolic balance, such as parathyroid hormone (PTH), PTH-related peptide (PTHrP), leptin, or ghrelin may be perturbed in discrete CHF subsets before any other abnormalities. These are but speculative examples of phenotypes that may be useful. Exploring the pathways already implicated in specific cardiomyopathies with innovative functional genomics, metabolomics, or other technologies will be a vital part of broadening the phenome of human heart failure. For example, unbiased metabolomics and small molecule profiling of patient-derived cellular samples (endothelial, fibroblast, and skeletal muscle) are already feasible.[45,46]

Novel endophenotypes not only enable the identification of distinctive disease subsets but also open the potential to detect abnormalities that might antedate, by many years, the onset of heart failure. The evaluation of endophenotypes requires strategies designed to reduce the influence of etiologic heterogeneity, because the specific subclinical traits of interest may vary widely across a single disease entity and from family to family. The kin-cohort design offers a robust assessment of candidate endophenotypes of any sort.[36] It is possible to validate such endophenotypes in at-risk relatives of those with inherited heart failure, and then apply such quantitative metrics not only as a means of extending Mendelian kindred for mapping and cloning the responsible genes but also to resolve heterogeneity.

INTEGRATIVE BIOLOGY

To define all of the major genetic and epigenetic contributors to the etiology of heart failure, systematic strategies to resolve distinctive forms of the syndrome, to identify the causal genes, and to explore new phenotypes must be deployed. Fortunately, many of these efforts are entirely complementary. Known human heart-failure genes offer inroads into the genetic pathways that might be perturbed, and animal modeling of these specific mutations is leading to the discovery of major modifier genes. New quantitative phenotypes, once rigorously validated, will be the focus of next generation human GWAS and will also be accessible in genetic model organisms. Screenable animal or cellular models of human heart failure could be used to systematize the discovery of new phenotypes. Ideally this effort would encompass unbiased assessment of multiple phenotypic axes including diverse organ systems or tissues.[32,35,39,47] Recently, the zebra fish has emerged as a screenable vertebrate, but at present the detection of basal phenotypes requires careful observation or directed rational assay design.[35] Modeling genetic defects, such as the dystrophin mutations causing X-linked dilated cardiomyopathy, not only allows surrogate fish phenotypes to be defined but might also detect new aspects of the disease.[48,49] Combining in vivo screening of existing drugs with such faithful animal models is one potential approach to the systematic discovery of pathway probes and could lead to the development of provoked phenotypes.

The explosion of genomic and post-genomic technologies (eg,transcript profiling, proteomics, and metabolomics), when combined with the challenges of interpreting the resultant large-scale datasets, has led to the reemergence of the concept of the organism as a system.[50–53] This reemergence has not only fostered a resurgence in classical integrative fields, such as physiology, but the sheer size and diversity of the available datasets have forced the development of new analytic strategies. These computational algorithms must define the basic relationships between disparate types of data, characterize the hierarchies of these relationships, and ultimately generate quantitative models to simulate and predict cellular or organismal phenotypes. Computational approaches have been developed to enable the identification of groups of variables that change as clusters, the functional annotation of genes, metabolites or proteins, and the classification of interactions based on shared phenotypes across multiple assays. The combination of such analytic strategies with large empiric datasets is beginning to revolutionize the rate of biologic discovery. In many instances, such systems approaches have not only validated established interactions but have predicted quite unsuspected behaviors. Taken together, these data outline how systematic approaches to a human phenotype, even if it is paroxysmal, can begin to unravel apparent complexity.[35,47]

SUMMARY

Genetic analyses to date suggest there may be substantial unidentified etiologic heterogeneity underlying many common disorders, and that this heterogeneity must be resolved if the genetic basis of these traits is to be understood. These challenges have emerged at a time when systematic functional genomics analyses are changing our approach to biologic problems. Although the application of such techniques to GWAS interpretation remains limited, work to date has been promising. The relationship between common alleles and disease is complex. However, initial efforts suggest that combining traditional genetics with higher-resolution phenotypes, implementing tissue-specific functional genomics in an approach known as *integrative genomics*, may elucidate not only the genes responsible at individual GWAS loci but also offer pathway entry points. The pathways can then be explored for further mechanistic insights and ultimately for drug discovery. Phenotype-driven modeling in model organisms has proven powerful for pathway dissection, and unbiased phenotypes are emerging in these fields. Large-scale in vivo modeling of vertebrate phenotypes is now feasible in the zebra fish. For each phenotype or disease entity, modeling must seek a compromise with robust recapitulation of complex vertebrate biology and accessibility to functional genomics for different tissues or organs, but with the scalability necessary for rigorous exploration of gene-gene and gene-environment analyses.

New diagnostic resolution might lead immediately to earlier diagnosis, introducing the possibility of screening for an underlying diathesis toward CHF, and possibly the preventative use of agents, such as beta-blockers, angiotensin-converting enzyme inhibitors, or angiotensin receptor blockers. Comparative biology and integrative approaches in humans will lead to new rational candidate approaches to diagnosis and therapy,[54] and even to empiric screening for disease markers or provoked phenotypes. New disease subsets would offer the potential for improved resolution in genetic and pharmacogenetic studies, as a result of larger effect sizes.[55] By analogy with recent work in oncology (though the clonality of neoplasia may be a unique advantage), new drug-response classifiers could lead to smaller, less expensive drug trials. The discovery of provoked, functional endophenotypes that integrate not only genetic but also epigenetic and environmental factors, may offer better disease or drug-response classifiers than genetics alone.[32,34]

REFERENCES

1. Mann DL, Bristow MR. Mechanisms and models in heart failure: the biomechanical model and beyond. Circulation 2005;111(21):2837–49.
2. Seidman JG, Seidman C. The genetic basis for cardiomyopathy: from mutation identification to mechanistic paradigms. Cell 2001;104(4):557–67.
3. Parmacek MS, Epstein JA. Pursuing cardiac progenitors: regeneration redux. Cell 2005;120(3): 295–8.

4. Pfeffer JM, Pfeffer MA, Fletcher PJ, et al. Progressive ventricular remodeling in rat with myocardial infarction. Am J Phys 1991;260(5 Pt 2):H1406–14.
5. Schmitt JP, Kamisago M, Asahi M, et al. Dilated cardiomyopathy and heart failure caused by a mutation in phospholamban. Science 2003;299(5611):1410–3.
6. Berridge MJ, Bootman MD, Roderick HL. Calcium signaling: dynamics, homeostasis and remodelling. Nat Rev Mol Cell Biol 2003;4(7):517–29.
7. Molkentin JD. Dichotomy of Ca2+ in the heart: contraction versus intracellular signaling. J Clin Invest 2006;116(3):623–6.
8. Mehra MR, Uber PA, Potluri S. Renin angiotensin aldosterone and adrenergic modulation in chronic heart failure: contemporary concepts. Am J Med Sci 2002;324(5):267–75.
9. Teerlink JR. Recent heart failure trials of neurohormonal modulation (OVERTURE and ENABLE): approaching the asymptote of efficacy? J Card Fail 2002;8(3):124–7.
10. Arnlov J, Vasan RS. Neurohormonal activation in populations susceptible to heart failure. Heart Fail Clin 2005;1(1):11–23.
11. Tang WH, Francis GS. Neurohormonal upregulation in heart failure. Heart Fail Clin 2005;1(1):1–9.
12. Balmain S, Padmanabhan N, Ferrell WR, et al. Differences in arterial compliance, microvascular function and venous capacitance between patients with heart failure and either preserved or reduced left ventricular systolic function. Eur J Heart Fail 2007;9(9):865–71.
13. Heywood JT. The cardiorenal syndrome: lessons from the ADHERE database and treatment options. Heart Fail Rev 2004;9(3):195–201.
14. Bongartz LG, Cramer MJ, Doevendans PA, et al. The severe cardiorenal syndrome: 'Guyton revisited'. Eur Heart J 2005;26(1):11–7.
15. Ronco C, Cruz DN, Ronco F. Cardiorenal syndromes. Curr Opin Crit Care 2009.
16. Delgado JF, Conde E, Sanchez V, et al. Pulmonary vascular remodeling in pulmonary hypertension due to chronic heart failure. Eur J Heart Fail 2005;7(6):1011–6.
17. Molkentin JD, Robbins J. With great power comes great responsibility: using mouse genetics to study cardiac hypertrophy and failure. J Mol Cell Cardiol 2009;46(2):130–6.
18. Baig MK, Goldman JH, Caforio AL, et al. Familial dilated cardiomyopathy: cardiac abnormalities are common in asymptomatic relatives and may represent early disease. J Am Coll Cardiol 1998;31(1):195–201.
19. Mahon NG, Murphy RT, MacRae CA, et al. Echocardiographic evaluation in asymptomatic relatives of patients with dilated cardiomyopathy reveals preclinical disease. Ann Intern Med 2005;143(2):108–15.
20. Wagner KD, Wagner N, Ghanbarian H, et al. RNA induction and inheritance of epigenetic cardiac hypertrophy in the mouse. Dev Cell 2008;14(6):962–9.
21. Divakaran V, Mann DL. The emerging role of microRNAs in cardiac remodeling and heart failure. Circ Res 2008;103(10):1072–83.
22. Ellinor PT, Low AF, Macrae CA. Reduced apelin levels in lone atrial fibrillation. Eur Heart J 2006;27(2):222–6.
23. Gudbjartsson DF, Arnar DO, Helgadottir A, et al. Variants conferring risk of atrial fibrillation on chromosome 4q25. Nature 2007.
24. Wang TJ, Larson MG, Levy D, et al. Temporal relations of atrial fibrillation and congestive heart failure and their joint influence on mortality: the Framingham Heart Study. Circulation 2003;107(23):2920–5.
25. Keating MT, Sanguinetti MC. Molecular and cellular mechanisms of cardiac arrhythmias. Cell 2001;104(4):569–80.
26. Lander ES, Schork NJ. Genetic dissection of complex traits. Science 1994;265(5181):2037–48.
27. Risch NJ. Searching for genetic determinants in the new millennium. Nature 2000;405(6788):847–56.
28. Arking DE, Pfeufer A, Post W, et al. A common genetic variant in the NOS1 regulator NOS1AP modulates cardiac repolarization. Nat Genet 2006;38(6):644–51.
29. Vasan RS, Glaze NL, Felix JF, et al. Genetic variants associated with cardiac structure and function: a meta-analysis and replication of genome-wide association data. JAMA 2009;302:168–78.
30. Newton-Cheh C, Larson MG, Vasan RS, et al. Association of common variants in NPPA and NPPB with circulating natriuretic peptides and blood pressure. Nat Genet 2009;41(3):348–53.
31. Gerszten RE, Wang TJ. Challenges in translating plasma proteomics from bench to bedside: update from the NHLBI Clinical Proteomics Programs. Am J Physiol Lung Cell Mol Physiol 2008;295(1):L16–22.
32. Freimer N, Sabatti C. The human phenome project. Nat Genet 2003;34(1):15–21.
33. Cannon TD. The inheritance of intermediate phenotypes for schizophrenia. Curr Opin Psychiatry 2005;18(2):135–40.
34. Garver DL, Holcomb JA, Christensen JD. Heterogeneity of response to antipsychotics from multiple disorders in the schizophrenia spectrum. J Clin Psychiatry 2000;61(12):964–72 [quiz: 973].
35. Rual JF, Ceron J, Koreth J, et al. Toward improving Caenorhabditis elegans phenome mapping with an ORFeome-based RNAi library. Genome Res 2004;14(10B):2162–8.
36. Gabriel SB, Salomon R, Pelet A, et al. Segregation at three loci explains familial and population risk in Hirschsprung disease. Nat Genet 2002;31(1):89–93.

37. Ellinor PT, Yoerger DM, Ruskin JN, et al. Familial aggregation in lone atrial fibrillation. Hum Genet 2005;118(2):179–84.
38. Franco D, Campione M. The role of Pitx2 during cardiac development. Linking left-right signaling and congenital heart diseases. Trends Cardiovasc Med 2003;13(4):157–63.
39. Singer E. "Phenome" project set to pin down subgroups of autism. Nat Med 2005;11(6):583.
40. Roden DM, George AL Jr. The genetic basis of variability in drug responses. Nat Rev Drug Discov 2002;1(1):37–44.
41. Lin M, Aquinlante C, Johnson JA, et al. Sequencing drug response with HapMap. Pharmacogenomics J 2005;5(3):149–56.
42. Allessie MA, Boyden PA, Camm AJ, et al. Pathophysiology and prevention of atrial fibrillation. Circulation 2001;103(5):769–77.
43. Antzelevitch C, Fish J. Electrical heterogeneity within the ventricular wall. Basic Res Cardiol 2001;96(6): 517–27.
44. Ho CY, Sweitzer NK, McDonough B, et al. Assessment of diastolic function with Doppler tissue imaging to predict genotype in preclinical hypertrophic cardiomyopathy. Circulation 2002;105(25):2992–7.
45. Shaw SY, Westly EC, Pitter MJ, et al. Perturbational profiling of nanomaterial biologic activity. Proc Natl Acad Sci U S A 2008;105(21):7387–92.
46. Lewis GD, Asnani A, Gerszten RE, et al. Metabolite profiling of blood from individuals undergoing planned myocardial infarction reveals early markers of myocardial injury. J Clin Invest 2008;118(10):3503–12.
47. Walhout AJ, Reboul J, Shtanko O, et al. Integrating interactome, phenome, and transcriptome mapping data for the C. elegans germline. Curr Biol 2002; 12(22):1952–8.
48. Plaster NM, Tawil R, Tristani-Firouzi M, et al. Mutations in Kir2.1 cause the developmental and episodic electrical phenotypes of Andersen's syndrome. Cell 2001;105(4):511–9.
49. Splawski I, Timothy KW, Sharpe LM, et al. Ca(V)1.2 calcium channel dysfunction causes a multisystem disorder including arrhythmia and autism. Cell 2004;119(1):19–31.
50. Li S, Armstrong CM, Bertin N, et al. A map of the interactome network of the metazoan C. elegans. Science 2004;303(5657):540–3.
51. Tong AH, Lesage G, Bader GD, et al. Global mapping of the yeast genetic interaction network. Science 2004;303(5659):808–13.
52. Rual JF, Venkatesan K, Hao T, et al. Towards a proteome-scale map of the human protein-protein interaction network. Nature 2005; 437(7062):1173–8.
53. Joyce AR, Palsson BO. The model organism as a system: integrating 'omics' data sets. Nat Rev Mol Cell Biol 2006;7(3):198–210.
54. Schadt EE, Lamb J, Yang X, et al. An integrative genomics approach to infer causal associations between gene expression and disease. Nat Genet 2005;37(7):710–7.
55. Lusis AJ. Genetic factors in cardiovascular disease. 10 questions. Trends Cardiovasc Med 2003;13(8): 309–16.

Clinical Screening and Genetic Testing

Rahul C. Deo, MD, PhD[a], Calum A. MacRae, MD, PhD[b,*]

KEYWORDS

- Genetic screening • Penetrance
- Mendelian disorders • Genetic architecture

Clinical screening lies at the heart of preventive medicine, because identification of a disease in its earliest form offers an opportunity to intervene and disrupt its expected deleterious course. In cardiovascular medicine, clinical screening is most effective in diseases such as hypercholesterolemia, where the disease in its earliest form may not have symptoms or signs but can be readily diagnosed with an inexpensive, noninvasive test. Other aspects of a disease like hypercholesterolemia also make a systematic screening program successful: it is relatively common, it has serious consequences such as myocardial infarction, and it is treatable, with the likelihood of adverse sequelae being reduced significantly by treatment. These and other criteria are used by groups, such as the US Preventive Task Force, to develop recommendations for screening programs (http://www.ahrq.gov/clinic/USpstfix.htm).

Genetic screening is a form of screening used for diseases with a significant heritable component. It involves searching for a one or more DNA variants in individuals believed to be at risk for a disease, where the DNA variant is believed to contribute to disease incidence or progression. Before comparing genetic and clinical screening, it would be helpful to review some aspects of the genetic basis of disease.

Genetic diseases lie along a continuum ranging from mendelian disorders to complex diseases, which arise from the interaction of a number of genetic and environmental factors. Mendelian disorders typically arise from a mutation in a single gene and have a sufficiently dramatic effect in that those who inherit the genetic mutation typically inherit the disease. The concept of penetrance captures the distinction between genetic variants contributing to Mendelian disorders and complex disease traits. Penetrance for a genetic mutation is defined as the proportion of individuals carrying a particular genetic mutation who also demonstrate the disease phenotype. The mutations that lead to Mendelian disorders have very high penetrances (approaching 100%); whereas, for most variants contributing to complex disease, the penetrance is quite low. This concept has significant relevance in the discussion of the utility of genetic screening.

The concept of genetic architecture describes the number of genes contributing to a disease trait, the number of variants per gene, and the magnitude of effect that each variant has on development of the trait. Although Mendelian disorders usually arise from inheritance of a single genetic mutation, many different individual genes may, when mutated, lead to a common disease phenotype (genetic heterogeneity). Furthermore, for any gene, many different mutations may also lead to the same disease phenotype (allelic heterogeneity). Both genetic and allelic heterogeneity introduce complexity when one goes about designing a genetic screening program for cardiomyopathies. Furthermore, although the penetrance of a disorder may be high, the exact manifestation of disease may vary from individual to individual, despite inheriting the same mutation (variable expressivity). A final level of complexity arises from the fact that multiple distinct diseases may share a common "low-resolution" phenotype, but in fact have a different pathologic basis (termed phenocopies), with potentially different disease course and treatment.

[a] Cardiology Division, Massachusetts General Hospital, 55 Fruit Street, Boston, MA 02114, USA
[b] Cardiovascular Division, Brigham and Women's Hospital, 75 Francis Street, Boston, MA 02115, USA
* Corresponding author. Cardiovascular Division, Brigham and Women's Hospital, 75 Francis Street, Boston, MA 02115.
E-mail address: camacrae@bics.bwh.harvard.edu

Heart Failure Clin 6 (2010) 231–238
doi:10.1016/j.hfc.2009.11.002

Genetic screening differs from clinical screening in several regards. Rather than serving as a way of diagnosing disease in asymptomatic individuals, the identification of a risk variant in an individual can give the probability of disease risk in individuals who may not yet have disease. Acting on this information may not only allow prevention of disease progression, but also the prevention of disease incidence, the "holy grail" of medicine. A second difference is that discovering that individuals with subclinical disease have a genetic risk variant may provide insight into the biologic basis of disease for that individual. For clinically heterogeneous diseases, such as atherosclerosis or hypertension, understanding the driving pathophysiologic progress may allow targeted therapy that may surpass the efficacy of the "one treatment fits all" approach commonly used. Moreover, with some limitations, knowledge of the causal process may permit a more accurate prognosis of catastrophic outcomes, such as sudden cardiac death or stroke, and allow the focused implementation of screening or preventive therapeutic procedures that may be too costly or risky for the general population, but have high likelihood of benefit for a limited number of high-risk individuals.

When should genetic screening used? An example may help illustrate the approach used for potentially heritable disorders. Consider an individual with a disease that does not appear to be arising from any known environmental cause—in genetic studies, this individual is called the proband. An initial step should be to establish whether the disease is familial, as this has relevance to pursuing a genetic diagnosis for the individual and on managing risk within family members. In addressing familiality, one must construct a careful family pedigree, asking about the health and manner of death of every relative. One needs to be careful to distinguish two apparently similar situations with considerably different ramifications: one where detailed pedigree information is available and no disease is apparent versus another where there does not appear to be any other relative with the disorder but inadequate family history is obtained. Only in the former case could one conclude that the disease is not familial but, instead, sporadic or attributable to environmental factors. If the proband has multiple relatives with the disorder, one would consider it to be familial and consider genetic screening.

The next considerations are related to the likelihood of identifying a causal variant in the proband. If the genetic architecture of the disease is such that there are a relatively small number of genes (low genetic heterogeneity) involved and there are causal genetic variants of moderate-to-high penetrance, genetic screening can be useful. Because many Mendelian disorders show significant allelic heterogeneity, screening for a single mutation tends to be unsuccessful and sequencing of portions of the gene (exons, splice junctions) tend to be required to find likely causal variants. Several limitations exist with genetic testing of a single proband. Sequencing errors can occur, resulting in false positives and false negative results. Even with careful sequencing, a variant may be found in one of the candidate genes but not actually be causal for the disease. To establish a sequence variant as a potential mutation requires that it have the potential to have a deleterious effect (missense or nonsense) and lie within a protein domain previously attributed functional significance. A mutation that is falsely assigned causality and used for genetic screening in family members would lead to both false reassurance and false alarm, as the inheritance of the variant would have no bearing on the likelihood of developing the disease. This situation may be ameliorated if a large number of family members are available for genetic testing, as cosegregation of mutation with disease can be used to infer causality.

How useful would the identification of a genetic variant be? Because of the bewildering genetic and allelic heterogeneity of most Mendelian disorders, the individualized prognostication and treatment that was once hoped to follow genetic diagnoses has not materialized. There is simply not enough prognostic information for individual mutations to provide mutation-specific predictions with any accuracy. As a result, the current utility of identifying a causal mutation in a proband is almost exclusively limited to facilitating screening of family members. In particular, with the help of genetic screening, it can help identify affected individuals at a preclinical phase or those with ambiguous clinical screening results.

A "cascade screening" approach allows an efficient method of evaluating which family members carry the causal allele. Once a genetic diagnosis of the proband is made, all of the first-degree relatives of the proband are screened. One can limit further genetic screening to first-degree relatives of the proband's affect first-degree relatives. This process continues until no further affected individual is identified. Genetic diagnosis allows a considerable degree of reassurance to family members who are genotype-negative, as they no longer need clinical surveillance and need not worry that disease will be passed on to their progeny. Conversely, a positive diagnosis in a clinically unaffected individual may lead to initiation of more frequent surveillance, avoidance of high-risk behavior, implementation of preventive treatment, and potentially it may affect reproductive choices. Of course, as discussed above, the success of such an approach depends fully on confidence that the mutation used for screening is actually causal.

If a causal genetic variant cannot be definitively established for the proband, clinical screening should then be considered, as it can be useful in many of the same ways as genetic screening. Cascade screening, described above, cannot work for clinical screening because of incomplete age-dependent penetrance, which may lead to premature termination of screening if any individual failed to display features of the disease. Thus, all relatives of the proband should be screened, typically at least one level beyond the last affected generation. The age of screening typically depends on the range of age of onset for the disease.

One can apply the above considerations to any disease with a heritable component. Below, the authors will address the screening approaches to dilated cardiomyopathy (DCM), hypertrophic cardiomyopathy (HCM), arrhythmogenic right ventricular dysplasia (ARVD), and restrictive cardiomyopathy (RCM), highlighting how the known genetic architecture of the trait guides a genetic screening approach and how clinical characteristics of the disease influence a clinical screening approach.

HCM

The genetic architecture of hypertrophic cardiomyopathy (**Table 1**) makes it amenable to genetic diagnosis. HCM appears to be familial in approximately 50% of cases and the inheritance pattern in documented cases is almost always autosomal dominant with high penetrance.[1,2] There are 12 known genes responsible for this disorder (not including several phenotypic mimics),[3] and mutations in the exons or splice junctions of one of eight sarcomeric genes explain approximately 50% to 60% of cases.[4] There are now several academic or commercial tests available for genetic screening. The Center for Genetics and Genomics at Harvard Medical School offers a $3000 screening test for 106 exons and splice sites of five sarcomeric genes (MYH7, MYBPC3, TNNT2, TNNI3, TPM1), and an additional $1150 screening test for 19 exons and splice sites in three other genes (ACTC, MYL2, MYL3) (http://www.hpcgg.org/LMM/comment/HCM%20Info%20Sheet.htm). Similarly, several companies offer comparable services for a range of genetic conditions. Despite the availability of commercial sequencing services, the prevalence of HCM, which is 0.2% to 0.5% of the general population, is too low to justify screening of the general population.

The allelic heterogeneity of HCM, which includes over 400 causal mutations, makes individualization of treatment and prognosis based on genetics implausible. It is highly unlikely that for any mutation adequate samples will ever be assembled for a reliable estimate of risk. Furthermore, incomplete penetrance and variable expressivity within families further erode confidence in the predictive utility of mutations. Attempts to prognosticate on the basis of genetic mutations have been difficult to replicate and designations of mutations as benign or malignant are often based on observational studies in small numbers

Table 1
Genetic architecture of hypertrophic and dilated cardiomyopathies and arrhythmogenic right ventricular dysplasia

	HCM	DCM	ARVD
Prevalence	1/500	1/2500	1/1000–1/5000
Number of known causal genes	12	20	7
Number of known variants	>400	>50	>70
Familiality	50%	35%	30%–50%
Predominant patterns of inheritance	Autosomal dominant	Autosomal dominant, autosomal recessive, X-linked	Autosomal dominant, autosomal recessive
Potential preventive treatment	AICD	ACE-I, beta-blocker, AICD	Avoidance of exercise, AICD

Abbreviations: ACE, angiotensin-converting enzyme; AICD, automatic implantable cardio-defibrillator.

of families.[5] It is, of course, expected that some mutations will have a more deleterious impact on protein function than others—but to extrapolate the clinical impact of a single mutation from a small number of individuals to others with different genetic and environmental backgrounds should only be undertaken with caution.

Thus, at present, a genetic diagnosis is most useful for screening relatives of the proband, with a cascade-type approach, as described above. If a genetic diagnosis is not pursued or made, clinical screening can be performed using ECG and echocardiography. Echocardiography has greater specificity, although ECG findings may precede changes in left ventricular (LV) thickness. ECG abnormalities, even in the absence of LV hypertrophy on echocardiography are suggestive for affected status, especially given the high pretest probability of disease in first-degree relatives.

There is uncertainty as to the age at which clinical screening should be initiated or terminated. Given the concern for sudden death in child athletes, an early diagnosis of HCM in children has clear relevance to mitigating risk. Furthermore, as multiple HCM variants can show clinical onset late in life,[6] it is unclear if screening can be stopped confidently at any age. Maron and colleagues[6] have recommended optional screening for age less than12 years (unless family history of premature sudden death, symptoms, or plan to pursue strenuous sporting activity), 12 to 18 month screening intervals for children between 12 and 18 to 21 years old, and screening every 5 years for ages greater than 18 to 21 years. Although representing a rational approach, there have been no efforts to validate this strategy in any large population for cost-effectiveness or influence on morbidity or mortality.

A preclinical diagnosis of HCM, either through genetic or clinical screening, leaves one with the opportunity to make clinical decisions before disease onset. Unfortunately, there are no clear options for treatment to alter the course of disease. Sudden death in HCM is certainly the most dreaded sequelum and the possibility exists of implanting a defibrillator for primary prevention. Unfortunately, one cannot be confident which HCM patients will benefit most from this therapy. At present, just as with ischemic cardiomyopathy, the best predictor of sudden death in HCM patients is a personal history of cardiac arrest: 59% of individuals with one episode of cardiac arrest have a second one within 5 years.[7] However, in the absence of a prior cardiac arrest, the criteria for risk prediction become less clear. A personal history of unexplained syncope or a family history of sudden cardiac death[8] has modest additional predictive utility. The caveats described above that apply to establishing familiality also apply to establishing a family history for sudden death—one must be concerned if there are simply not enough family members on which to base a negative conclusion. In other studies, features such as LV wall thickness, nonsustained ventricular tachycardia, and abnormal blood pressure response in exercise have been implicated as potential predictors of sudden death, but these studies did not account for familiality and no formal validation of any of these prognostic models has occurred.

DCM

DCM is considerably more complex than HCM, both in terms of genetic architecture and known contributing environmental factors. Coronary artery disease, nutritional deficiency, viral infection, and toxins such as alcohol can cause DCM, though familial predisposition may continue to play a role in many of these cases. The prevalence of DCM may be as high as 1 in 2500 adults.[9] Given that the histologic findings of DCM are nonspecific with myocyte loss and interstitial fibrosis, a diagnosis of idiopathic DCM requires an extensive work-up to exclude other causes, some of which may prove to be reversible.[10]

Over 20 genes have been implicated in the pathogenesis of DCM, with autosomal dominant, recessive, and X-linked patterns of inheritance (see **Table 1**).[11] Penetrance is often low, and expressivity varies considerably from individual to individual. Dilated cardiomyopathy can be syndromic, with other accompanying systemic abnormalities such as the skeletal muscle dystrophies and retinal disease.[12] Given the fact that mutations in DCM are distributed widely over a large number of different potential causal genes, there is usually too low a likelihood of success to recommend genetic sequencing or genetic screening. It is the associated cardiac and noncardiac findings that can help narrow the diagnosis. For example, in one small study, if atrioventricular block accompanied DCM, there was a mutation found in the lamin A/C gene in one-third of cases.[13]

As with all cardiomyopathies, it is challenging to predict risk for particular mutations. One exception may be a tendency for DCM caused by lamin A/C mutations to demonstrate a high rate of malignant arrhythmias in patients with conduction abnormalities.[14] This finding has not been replicated.

Although the complexity of DCM precludes genetic screening, clinical screening can often be very useful. Moreover, an early diagnosis in asymptomatic family members of the proband allows the initiation of potentially disease-modifying agents such as angiotensin-converting enzyme (ACE)-inhibitors (see below). Clinical screening is performed by echocardiography and ECG. Individuals with ECG abnormalities or mild echocardiographic abnormalities (mildly depressed systolic ejection fraction or mild LV enlargement) should be followed with screening that is more frequent. As with HCM, there are no explicit evidence-based guidelines for screening, although it would be reasonable to begin in childhood and continue at periodic intervals into late adulthood. For every affected individual, care must be taken to exclude age-appropriate, potentially reversible causes (eg, tachyarrhythmia, coronary artery disease, alcohol) as these may contribute to disease even in the context of an inherited tendency.[15]

The forbidding genetic and phenotypic heterogeneity of DCM makes genotype-based treatment unlikely. Clinical guidelines recommend ACE-I and beta blocker use for all dilated cardiomyopathies, independent of cause,[16] and automatic implantable cardio-defibrillator implantation in symptomatic individuals with severe LV dysfunction. It is unclear if early initiation of ACE-I or beta blockers mitigates the disease course in individuals with mild echocardiographic abnormalities, or exclusively ECG abnormalities. The authors tend to favor the use of ACE-I in such cases, given the efficacy in asymptomatic LV dysfunction of all types.

ARVD

ARVD is a genetically heterogeneous disorder, with 12 current genetic loci (ARVD1-12) identified through linkage studies (see **Table 1**).[17] Causal genes corresponding to eight of these loci have been found, with five encoding desmosomal proteins. The prevalence of ARVD is unknown but has been estimated at 1:1000 to 1:5000 individuals.[18] ARVD is familial in nearly 50% of cases[19] and inheritance is usually autosomal dominant, with variable expressivity and incomplete penetrance.

The routine diagnostic workup of a patient suspected to have ARVD includes ECG, Holter monitor, signal-averaged ECG, echocardiogram, and potentially cardiac magnetic resonance.[20] If the clinical and family history and these initial studies raise a high suspicion for ARVD, endomyocardial biopsy can be performed for confirmation and an electrophysiology study may be useful to exclude benign right-ventricular outflow-tract tachycardia. The above diagnostic tests have been incorporated into task force criteria (TFC) for the diagnosis of ARVD (see **Table 1**).[21]

The frequency distribution of causal genes appears to vary with geography and demography although a large percentage (up to 43%) of cases can be explained by mutations in the plakophilin 2 (PKP2) gene.[22,23] As with HCM, allelic heterogeneity is present, with over 50 PKP2 mutations currently known.[17] The penetrance of ARVD mutations appears lower than HCM, potentially due to the insensitivity of the TFC.[19,24] Sequencing of the most commonly mutated genes may be useful in identifying family members of the proband who require long-term clinical follow-up, especially since correct identification of affected individuals may be useful in prevention of sudden cardiac death. Toward those ends, the Center for Genetics and Genomics at Harvard Medical School also offers sequencing of 69 exons and splice sites for the four most common genes mutated in ARVD (PKP2, desmoplakin, desmoglein 2, and desmocollin 2), for $3000. It is unclear what percentage of probands will be identified through this assay. Once a mutation is found, additional family members can be screened at a cost of $250 each.

As with HCM, the relevance of genetic diagnosis to prognostication or individualization of therapy is limited by the fact that most mutations identified to date are rare and "private" to individual families.[25] Futhermore, given incomplete penetrance and variable expressivity within families, it is unclear to what extent one can extrapolate the sudden-death risk from one family with a given mutation to another, even if they share the same mutation. Given the wide range of effects that mutations can have on protein function, ranging from little to no change in activity to severe dominant negative action, it is highly unlikely that investigators will be able to define a common risk profile for all mutations of a single gene, such has been proposed for desmoplakin[26] and PKP2.[27,28]

If a genetic diagnosis cannot be made for the proband, clinical screening of family members would occur initially by ECG and echocardiogram. Abnormalities on either of these would result in further testing as described above, with a low threshold for declaring a positive diagnosis even if formal TFC are not met, given the high prior probability of disease. As a result of early onset of disease and the potential hazards of exercise on disease progression, screening for ARVD should begin in childhood. For genetic screening, all first-degree relatives should be screened initially, with cascade screening, as described above. If clinical screening is being performed, individuals who appear "negative" for disease should continue to be screened at some regular interval.[29] The late appearance of ARVD in some individuals[30] requires that screening should continue throughout adult life. Nava and colleagues[29] used a systematic (but uncontrolled) screening and prevention approach in 37 families with ARVD and demonstrated that frequent screening, initiation of anti-arrhythmics as needed, and avoidance of exercise led to very low mortality among affected individuals. A similar approach could be extrapolated to asymptomatic individuals harboring a potential ARVD mutation.

Implantable cardio-defibrillator (ICD) implantation in patients with the diagnosis of ARVD remains an area of uncertainty. Piccini and colleagues[31] recommend ICDs for all ARVD patients meeting TFC, given the high risk of ventricular tachycardia, even in patients with no prior history of syncope or cardiac arrest. As with HCM, attempts have been made to identify high-risk diagnostic features with high positive predictive value for sudden cardiac death, such as right ventricular (RV) dysfunction, LV dysfunction and recurrent ventricular tachycardia.[32,33] A consensus on criteria for ICD implantation has yet to appear.

RCM

RCMs demonstrate several rare hereditary variants, including familial idiopathic restrictive cardiomyopathy and hereditary amyloidosis. Familial idiopathic RCM is extremely rare, with reports only in small case series.[34,35] No gene has yet been identified. Furthermore, in some families with HCM, individual members can show a pattern of restrictive filling with little or no LV hypertropy.[36,37] In a systematic analysis of 1226 relatives of HCM probands, this "restrictive phenotype" of HCM was seen in 1.5% of individuals and the diagnosis was accompanied by a high rate of dyspnea and mortality.

Hereditary amyloidosis represents a more common form of heritable RCM and typically involves a genetic defect in the transthyretin (TTR) protein or Apo AI protein leading to misfolded proteins and infiltration of the myocardium with amyloid fibrils. RCM shows allelic heterogeneity, with over 100 TTR mutations identified to date.[38] The inheritance pattern is usually autosomal dominant.

An RCM patient with evidence of a familial inheritance pattern should undergo right heart catheterization with RV biopsy to evaluate for infiltrative disease. If amyloid deposits are found, hereditary amyloidosis should be presumed and TTR sequencing performed to identify the causal variant. The identified variant can be used for genetic screening. If no amyloid deposits are seen, one should suspect an idiopathic variant, and clinical screening of family members by echocardiography and ECG should be performed.

Unfortunately, none of the treatment measures for RCM have shown to impact mortality. Loop diuretics, calcium channel blockers, beta-blockers, and ACE-inhibitors are commonly used for relief of symptoms.

SUMMARY

General principles of genetic disease architecture can guide screening and diagnostic approaches for all of the cardiomyopathies and, in fact, for all inherited diseases. At present, the primary benefit of identifying a causal mutation in a proband is to facilitate screening in family members. A preclinical diagnosis achieved through screening programs can allow initiation of further monitoring programs for disease development, avoidance of high-risk behaviors, and potential implementation of disease-mitigating therapies. Although there is considerable incentive to offer genotype-based forecasting for patients, allelic and genetic heterogeneity and variable expressivity have rendered such individualization of care highly unlikely. The ultimate desire for tailored prognostication and therapy is likely only to be realized when phenotypic profiles are generated that can integrate individual genotypic and environmental information, yet be common enough to allow accuracy in prediction and classification.

REFERENCES

1. Ho CY, Seidman CE. A contemporary approach to hypertrophic cardiomyopathy. Circulation 2006; 113:e858–62.
2. Ashrafian H, Watkins H. Reviews of translational medicine and genomics in cardiovascular disease: new disease taxonomy and therapeutic implications cardiomyopathies: therapeutics based on molecular phenotype. J Am Coll Cardiol 2007;49:1251–64.
3. Arad M, Maron BJ, Gorham JM, et al. Glycogen storage diseases presenting as hypertrophic cardiomyopathy. N Engl J Med 2005;352:362–72.
4. Richard P, Charron P, Carrier L, et al. Hypertrophic cardiomyopathy: distribution of disease genes, spectrum of mutations, and implications for a molecular diagnosis strategy. Circulation 2003;107:2227–32.
5. Ackerman MJ, VanDriest SL, Ommen SR, et al. Prevalence and age-dependence of malignant mutations in the beta-myosin heavy chain and troponin T genes in hypertrophic cardiomyopathy: a comprehensive outpatient perspective. J Am Coll Cardiol 2002;39:2042–8.

6. Maron BJ, Seidman JG, Seidman CE. Proposal for contemporary screening strategies in families with hypertrophic cardiomyopathy. J Am Coll Cardiol 2004;44:2125–32.
7. Elliott PM, Sharma S, Varnava A, et al. Survival after cardiac arrest or sustained ventricular tachycardia in patients with hypertrophic cardiomyopathy. J Am Coll Cardiol 1999;33:1596–601.
8. Elliott PM, Poloniecki J, Dickie S, et al. Sudden death in hypertrophic cardiomyopathy: identification of high risk patients. J Am Coll Cardiol 2000;36:2212–8.
9. Codd MB, Sugrue DD, Gersh BJ, et al. Epidemiology of idiopathic dilated and hypertrophic cardiomyopathy. A population-based study in Olmsted County, Minnesota, 1975–1984. Circulation 1989; 80:564–72.
10. Mestroni L, Maisch B, McKenna WJ, et al. Guidelines for the study of familial dilated cardiomyopathies. Collaborative Research Group of the European Human and Capital Mobility Project on Familial Dilated Cardiomyopathy. Eur Heart J 1999; 20:93–102.
11. Taylor MR, Slavov D, Ku L, et al. Prevalence of desmin mutations in dilated cardiomyopathy. Circulation 2007;115:1244–51.
12. Marshall JD, Hinman EG, Collin GB, et al. Spectrum of ALMS1 variants and evaluation of genotype-phenotype correlations in Alstrom syndrome. Hum Mutat 2007.
13. Arbustini E, Pilotto A, Repetto A, et al. Autosomal dominant dilated cardiomyopathy with atrioventricular block: a lamin A/C defect-related disease. J Am Coll Cardiol 2002;39:981–90.
14. Meune C, Van Berlo JH, Anselme F, et al. Primary prevention of sudden death in patients with lamin A/C gene mutations. N Engl J Med 2006;354:209–10.
15. Mahon NG, Murphy RT, MacRae CA, et al. Echocardiographic evaluation in asymptomatic relatives of patients with dilated cardiomyopathy reveals preclinical disease. Ann Intern Med 2005;143:108–15.
16. Hunt SA. ACC/AHA 2005 guideline update for the diagnosis and management of chronic heart failure in the adult: a report of the American College of Cardiology/American Heart Association Task Force on Practice Guidelines (Writing Committee to Update the 2001 Guidelines for the Evaluation and Management of Heart Failure). J Am Coll Cardiol 2005;46:e1–82.
17. van Tintelen JP, Hofstra RM, Wiesfeld AC, et al. Molecular genetics of arrhythmogenic right ventricular cardiomyopathy: emerging horizon? Curr Opin Cardiol 2007;22:185–92.
18. Peters S, Trummel M, Meyners W. Prevalence of right ventricular dysplasia-cardiomyopathy in a non-referral hospital. Int J Cardiol 2004;97:499–501.
19. Hamid MS, Norman M, Quraishi A, et al. Prospective evaluation of relatives for familial arrhythmogenic right ventricular cardiomyopathy/dysplasia reveals a need to broaden diagnostic criteria. J Am Coll Cardiol 2002;40:1445–50.
20. Calkins H. Arrhythmogenic right-ventricular dysplasia/cardiomyopathy. Curr Opin Cardiol 2006;21:55–63.
21. McKenna WJ, Thiene G, Nava A, et al. Diagnosis of arrhythmogenic right ventricular dysplasia/cardiomyopathy. Task Force of the Working Group Myocardial and Pericardial Disease of the European Society of Cardiology and of the Scientific Council on Cardiomyopathies of the International Society and Federation of Cardiology. Br Heart J 1994;71:215–8.
22. Dalal D, James C, Devanagondi R, et al. Penetrance of mutations in plakophilin-2 among families with arrhythmogenic right ventricular dysplasia/cardiomyopathy. J Am Coll Cardiol 2006;48:1416–24.
23. van Tintelen JP, Entius MM, Bhuiyan ZA, et al. Plakophilin-2 mutations are the major determinant of familial arrhythmogenic right ventricular dysplasia/cardiomyopathy. Circulation 2006;113:1650–8.
24. Kies P, Bootsma M, Bax JJ, et al. Serial reevaluation for ARVD/C is indicated in patients presenting with left bundle branch block ventricular tachycardia and minor ECG abnormalities. J Cardiovasc Electrophysiol 2006;17:586–93.
25. Wichter T, Breithardt G. Implantable cardioverter-defibrillator therapy in arrhythmogenic right ventricular cardiomyopathy: a role for genotyping in decision-making? J Am Coll Cardiol 2005;45: 409–11.
26. Bauce B, Basso C, Rampazzo A, et al. Clinical profile of four families with arrhythmogenic right ventricular cardiomyopathy caused by dominant desmoplakin mutations. Eur Heart J 2005;26:1666–75.
27. Dalal D, Molin LH, Piccini J, et al. Clinical features of arrhythmogenic right ventricular dysplasia/cardiomyopathy associated with mutations in plakophilin-2. Circulation 2006;113:1641–9.
28. Syrris P, Ward D, Asimaki A, et al. Clinical expression of plakophilin-2 mutations in familial arrhythmogenic right ventricular cardiomyopathy. Circulation 2006; 113:356–64.
29. Nava A, Bauce B, Basso C, et al. Clinical profile and long-term follow-up of 37 families with arrhythmogenic right ventricular cardiomyopathy. J Am Coll Cardiol 2000;36:2226–33.
30. Frigo G, Bauce B, Basso C, et al. Late-onset arrhythmogenic right ventricular cardiomyopathy. J Cardiovasc Med (Hagerstown) 2006;7:74–6.
31. Piccini JP, Dalal D, Roguin A, et al. Predictors of appropriate implantable defibrillator therapies in patients with arrhythmogenic right ventricular dysplasia. Heart Rhythm 2005;2:1188–94.
32. Roguin A, Bomma CS, Nasir K, et al. Implantable cardioverter-defibrillators in patients with arrhythmogenic right ventricular dysplasia/cardiomyopathy. J Am Coll Cardiol 2004;43:1843–52.

33. Lemola K, Brunckhorst C, Helfenstein U, et al. Predictors of adverse outcome in patients with arrhythmogenic right ventricular dysplasia/cardiomyopathy: long term experience of a tertiary care centre. Heart 2005;91:1167–72.
34. Fitzpatrick AP, Shapiro LM, Rickards AF, et al. Familial restrictive cardiomyopathy with atrioventricular block and skeletal myopathy. Br Heart J 1990;63:114–8.
35. Angelini A, Calzolari V, Thiene G, et al. Morphologic spectrum of primary restrictive cardiomyopathy. Am J Cardiol 1997;80:1046–50.
36. Kubo T, Gimeno JR, Bahl A, et al. Prevalence, clinical significance, and genetic basis of hypertrophic cardiomyopathy with restrictive phenotype. J Am Coll Cardiol 2007;49:2419–26.
37. Mogensen J, Kubo T, Duque M, et al. Idiopathic restrictive cardiomyopathy is part of the clinical expression of cardiac troponin I mutations. J Clin Invest 2003;111:209–16.
38. Hughes SE, McKenna WJ. New insights into the pathology of inherited cardiomyopathy. Heart 2005;91:257–64.

Genetics of Atrial Fibrillation

Steven A. Lubitz, MD[a,b], B. Alexander Yi, MD, PhD[c], Patrick T. Ellinor, MD, PhD[d,e,*]

KEYWORDS

- Atrial fibrillation • Arrhythmia
- Mutation • Gene • Genetics

Atrial fibrillation (AF) is the most common arrhythmia encountered in clinical practice, and is increasing in both incidence and prevalence.[1,2] More than 2 million Americans currently have AF, and estimates project that between 5 and 12 million will be affected by 2050.[1,2] AF is associated with substantial morbidity, including one third of all strokes in patients older than 65[3] and a twofold increased risk of mortality.[4,5] The costs attributable to the care of individuals with AF are in excess of $6.4 billion per year.[3]

AF is often associated with hypertension and structural heart disease, and traditionally has not been considered a genetic condition. However, a number of recent studies have demonstrated that AF and in particular, lone AF, have a substantial genetic basis.[6–9] Mutations in several ion channels have been identified in individuals with familial AF,[10–17] although they appear to be rare causes of the arrhythmia.[18,19] Recently, a genome-wide association study has led to the identification of genetic variants associated with common forms of AF. In the course of this review we will discuss the heritability of AF, the methods used to identify causal variants underlying AF, and our current understanding of genetic variation implicated in AF.

ATRIAL FIBRILLATION IS A HERITABLE CONDITION

While familial forms of AF have long been reported,[20] a genetic predisposition for more common forms of AF has only recently been recognized. In 2003, Fox and coworkers[8] studied more than 5000 individuals whose parents were enrolled in the original Framingham Heart Study. Over a 19-year follow-up period, they found that the development of AF in the offspring was independently associated with parental AF, particularly if the offspring cohort was restricted to those younger than 75 and without antecedent heart disease. Having a parent with AF approximately doubled the 4-year risk of developing AF, even after adjustment for risk factors such as hypertension, diabetes mellitus, and myocardial infarction.

Arnar and colleagues[6] similarly described a genetic predisposition to AF in a study of more than 5000 Icelanders in 2006. After assessing relatedness from a nationwide genealogical database, 80% of those with AF were related to another individual with AF. The relative risk of AF for first-degree relatives of a family member with AF was 1.77, when compared with individuals in

This article originally appeared in *Cardiology Clinics of North America*, Volume 27, Issue 1.

[a] Cardiovascular Institute, Mount Sinai School of Medicine, New York, NY 10029, USA
[b] Division of Preventive Medicine, Brigham and Women's Hospital, Boston, MA 02446, USA
[c] Cardiology Division, Massachusetts General Hospital and Harvard Medical School, Boston, MA 02114, USA
[d] Cardiac Arrhythmia Service, Massachusetts General Hospital and Harvard Medical School, Boston, MA 02114, USA
[e] Cardiovascular Research Center, Massachusetts General Hospital and Harvard Medical School, Boston, MA 02114, USA
* Corresponding author. Cardiac Arrhythmia Service, Massachusetts General Hospital and Harvard Medical School, Boston, MA 02114.
E-mail address: pellinor@partners.org

Heart Failure Clin 6 (2010) 239–247
doi:10.1016/j.hfc.2009.12.004
1551-7136/10/$ – see front matter

the general population. The relative risk for AF increased to 4.67 when the sample was restricted to individuals less than 60 years old.

Further evidence of the heritability of AF was demonstrated in a chart review of more than 2000 patients with AF referred for evaluation at the Mayo Clinic.[9] Five percent of subjects had a family history of AF, and the number was as high as 15% among those with lone AF. In 2005, we found that nearly 40% of individuals with lone AF referred to the Arrhythmia Service at Massachusetts General Hospital had at least one relative with the arrhythmia, and a substantial number reported having multiple affected relatives.[7] In over 90% of cases, AF in the relatives could be verified. To obtain a crude index of heritability, we determined the prevalence of AF among each class of relative compared with that among age- and sex-matched subjects. The relative risk of AF was increased among family members, and ranged from twofold in fathers to nearly 70 fold in male siblings.

GENETIC STUDIES IN ATRIAL FIBRILLATION

Once a condition is found to be heritable, there are several techniques that are commonly used to identify the genetic basis of a disease. These include linkage analysis, candidate gene resequencing, and association studies. We will discuss each of these methods in the context of their application to AF.

Linkage Analysis

The genes that underlie simple monogenic disorders with a Mendelian pattern of inheritance can be identified using linkage analysis. When passed from generation to generation, genetic markers that lie close together on the same chromosome are likely to be transmitted en bloc in proportion to their proximity to each other. A genome-wide search for groups of markers that co-segregate with the disease as it travels through a family tree is performed to identify the approximate location of a genetic disease locus. Linkage studies report a logarithm of the odds, or LOD score, that reflects the likelihood of two markers or a marker and disease co-segregating when compared to chance alone. A LOD score of 3 or more (or odds of >1000:1) is considered statistically significant. Traditionally, restriction enzyme sites and microsatellite repeats have been used as genetic markers, but more recently, it has become possible to use single nucleotide polymorphisms, or SNPs.[21] The ease of use in genotyping has made SNPs the most widely used genetic markers today.

Linkage analysis can be used to narrow the search for a causative gene to a chromosomal locus, or relatively small region of the human genome associated with disease. However, this limited region may still contain hundreds of genes spread over millions of base pairs. Once a genetic locus is identified, online data from human genome databases developed as a result of the Human Genome Project are used to identify candidate genes within the locus. These genes are then sequenced in affected individuals in an attempt to identify the sequence variants that correlate with the disease.

Once a base pair change is identified, it is important to differentiate between a mutation and a genetic polymorphism, or common variant in the genome. For a sequence alteration to be considered a mutation it must segregate with the disease, have a plausible mechanism, and not be found in healthy controls. Ultimately, the mutation should be sufficient to cause the phenotype, either in a human kindred or in a genetic model organism.

Although several genetic loci have been reported in kindreds with Mendelian AF in which specific genetic mutations have yet to be identified (**Table 1**),[22–25] linkage analysis has facilitated the identification of individual mutations in several cases of familial AF.[10,26]

In one such family of Chinese descent, Chen and coworkers[10] identified a mutation in *KCNQ1*, which encodes a potassium channel that underlies the slowly repolarizing current in cardiomyocytes known as I_{Ks} (**Fig. 1**). The investigators were able to map the disease locus to a 12-megabase region on the short arm of chromosome 11, in a four-generation family with AF. The *KCNQ1* gene was located within this region, and sequencing revealed a serine to glycine missense mutation at position 140 (S140G) in affected family members. The S140G mutation is located in the first transmembrane-spanning segment[27] at the outer edges of the voltage-sensing domain and far from the pore-forming region of the potassium channel structure. The S140G mutation results in a gain of channel function, in contrast to mutations in *KCNQ1* associated with the long QT syndrome that typically result in a loss of channel function. In cultured cells, expression of the S140G mutant channel resulted in dramatically enhanced potassium channel currents and markedly altered potassium channel gating kinetics, which would be predicted to increase I_{Ks}. Such an increase would be expected to lead to a shortening of the action potential duration and thus predispose atrial myocytes to reentry and subsequent AF (see **Fig. 1**).

Table 1
Genes and loci implicated in familial atrial fibrillation

		Genes		References
11p15.5	*KCNQ1/KvLQT1*	Increases I_{Ks}; expected to shorten APD	AD	10,14
21q22.1	*KCNE2/MiRP1*	Increases I_{Ks}	AD	11
17q23.1-24.2	*KCNJ2*	Increases I_{K1}; expected to shorten APD	AD	12
12p13	*KCNA5*	Loss of I_{Kur}; prolongs APD	AD	13
3p21	*SCN5A*	Hyperpolarizing shift of resting membrane potential; expected to prolong APD	AD	15–17
1p36-p35	*NPPA*	Results in mutant atrial natriuretic peptide; associated with shortened APD	AD	26
		Genetic Loci		
Chr	**Gene**	**Comments**	**Inheritance**	**References**
5p13	Unknown	Associated with sudden death	AR	24
6q14-q16	Unknown	Overlaps with locus for DCM	AD	23
10q22-q24	Unknown	Overlaps with locus for DCM	AD	22
10p11-q21	Unknown		AD	25

Abbreviations: AD, autosomal dominant; AR, autosomal recessive; Chr, Chromosome; DCM, dilated cardiomyopathy.

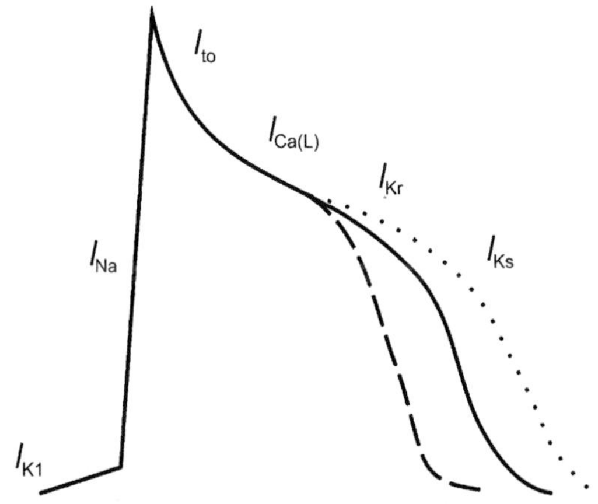

Fig. 1. Both gain of function and loss of function mutations in I_{Ks} have been associated with AF. Mutations in *KCNQ1* and *KCNE2* increase the current I_{Ks}, which is predicted to shorten the action potential (*dashed line*) in cardiac myocytes and render atrial myocytes susceptible to reentrant arrhythmias. Mutations in *KCNA5* (encodes Kv1.5) that are predicted to prolong the action potential duration (*dotted line*) have also been associated with AF.

While the identification of this mutation provided an initial inroad into the pathogenesis of AF, this family also illustrates our limited understanding of the role of the KCNQ1 channel in atrial versus ventricular repolarization. Specifically, it remains unclear why a mutation that results in an in vitro gain of function in KCNQ1 is associated with delayed ventricular repolarization, as manifested by a prolonged QT interval, in more than half of the individuals with the S140G mutation.

Other gain of function mutations in *KCNQ1* have been associated with the short QT syndrome.[28] Hong and colleagues[29] reported an unusual case of AF detected in utero and confirmed on electrocardiogram upon delivery of the newborn. The infant's electrocardiogram also displayed a short QT interval. Based on this association, they sequenced the *KCNQ1* gene and found a valine to methionine mutation in position 141 (adjacent to the mutated position found by Chen and colleagues). Like the S140G mutation, in vitro expression of V141M mutant channels displayed markedly enhanced current density and altered gating kinetics.

More recently, Hodgson-Zingman and colleagues[26] identified a frameshift mutation in *NPPA* in a family with AF. The mutation in *NPPA*, which encodes atrial natriuretic peptide, resulted in increased levels of a circulating mutant peptide. Electrophysiological assessment in a rat heart model revealed decreased action potential duration, consistent with known mechanisms of reentrant mediated AF.[30]

Candidate Gene Studies

A candidate gene can be any gene that is hypothesized to cause a disease. Based on the work relating *KCNQ1* to AF, investigators have considered other potassium channels as potential candidate genes for AF and screened for mutations in these genes in cohorts of subjects with AF.

Otway and colleagues[14] examined 50 kindreds with AF and amplified the genes for *KCNQ1* and *KCNE1-3*, which encode accessory subunits of KCNQ1. They found a single mutation in *KCNQ1* in only one family—an arginine to cysteine change at amino acid position 14 (R14C) in *KCNQ1*. Unlike the S140G mutation discovered by Chen and colleagues,[10] R14C had no significant effect on KCNQ1/KCNE1 current amplitudes in cultured cells at baseline. However, upon exposure to hypotonic solution, mutant channels exhibited a marked increase in currents compared with wild type channels. Interestingly, of those who carried the R14C mutation, only those with left atrial dilatation had AF, leading the authors to propose a "two-hit" hypothesis for AF. They also identified a mutation in *KCNE2* in two of the kindreds. Like the S140G mutation in *KCNQ1* the mutation in *KCNE2* (R27C) dramatically increased the amplitude of I_{Ks}.[11]

Finally, other work has suggested that the relationship between potassium channels and AF extends beyond I_{Ks}. The work of Xia and colleagues[12] may also implicate *KCNJ2* which encodes, an inward rectifier potassium channel that underlies the I_{K1} current, in AF. In their work, a V93I mutation was found in all affected members in one kindred with familial AF. The V93I also leads to gain of function KCNJ2 channels, which increase potassium current amplitudes. However, there is still an incomplete understanding of how an increase in the background current I_{K1} might lead to atrial arrhythmias.

We have screened our cohort with lone AF for mutations in *KCNQ1*, *KCNJ2* and *KCNE1-5* and were unable to find any mutations in these genes.[18] These findings suggest that potassium channels are an uncommon cause of AF and there is much more to be learned about the diversity of molecular pathways that lead to this arrhythmia.

The genes encoding connexins, gap-junction proteins that mediate the spread of action potentials between cardiac myocytes, have also been examined as potential candidates for AF. Prior work has shown that mice with null alleles of *GJA5*, the gene for connexin40, exhibit atrial reentrant arrhythmias.[31] From this work, Gollob and coworkers[32] considered this gene as a potential candidate in individuals with idiopathic AF who underwent pulmonary vein isolation surgery. An analysis of DNA isolated from their cardiac tissue showed that 4 of the 15 subjects had mutations in *GJA5* that markedly interfered with the electrical coupling between cells. In three of the patients, DNA isolated from their lymphocytes lacked the same mutation in *GJA5* indicating that the connexin40 mutations had been acquired after fertilization or was a somatic mutation. One of the four individuals carried the mutation in both cardiac tissue and lymphocytes consistent with a germline rather than somatic mutation. However, more information about the transmission of AF in relatives of these individuals was not available.

Association Studies

Although traditional methods such as linkage analysis can be applied to families where the phenotype and pattern of inheritance are consistent with a monogenic disorder, the mode of transmission for AF is less clear. Association studies have been used in an attempt to identify the genetic basis of AF and other apparently complex traits. In an association study the frequency of a genetic marker, such as a SNP, is compared between individuals with an outcome (cases) and those without an outcome (controls). Over the past 10 years, many case-control and cohort studies have been performed in subjects with AF, leading to the identification of variants associated with disease. These studies have typically tested a small number of variants and have been directed at candidate genes previously believed to be involved in AF. Examples include genes encoding products involved in regulation of the renin-angiotensin-aldosterone axis[33–40] and calcium handling,[41] as well as neurohormonal[39] and lipoprotein[42] pathways. Additionally, genes encoding gap junction proteins,[43,44] ion channels,[15,45–49] interleukins,[50,51] signaling molecules,[34,45,52] and mediators of other molecular pathways[53] have been examined (summarized in **Table 2**). Unfortunately, these studies have been limited by a low prior probability of any polymorphism truly being associated with AF. Further complicating these

Table 2
Polymorphisms associated with atrial fibrillation

Gene	Variant	Cases	Controls	OR	*P* Value	Replicated?	Comments	References
–	rs2200733	3913	22,092	1.72	3.3×10^{-41}	Yes	Identified in GWAS	62
–	rs10033464	3913	22,092	1.39	6.9×10^{-11}	Yes	Identified in GWAS	62
ACE	D/D	51	289	1.5	.016	Yes	In patients with CHF	34
ACE	D/D	404	520	1.89	<.001	Yes		36
CYP11B2	T-344C	63	133	2.65	.03	No	In patients with CHF	40
AGT	M235T	250	250	2.5	<.001	No		33
AGT	G-6A	250	250	3.3	.005	No		33
AGT	G-217A	250	250	2.0	.002	No		33
AGT	T174M	968	8267	1.2	.05	No		37
AGT	20 C/C	968	8267	1.5	.01	No		37
CETP	Taq1B	97	97	0.35	.05	No		42
GJA5	−44A	14	16	5.3	.0019	Yes		44
GJA5	−44A, +71G	173	232	1.514	< .006	Yes (for -44A only)		43
EDN2	A985G	26	84	5.89	.018	No	In patients with HCM	39
NOS3	894T/T	51	289	3.2	.001	No	In patients with CHF	34
NOS3	T-786C	331	441	1.4	.05	No		45
GNB3	C825T	291	292	0.46	.02	No		52
hsp70	Met439Thr	48	194	2.43	.016	No	In postoperative CABG patients	53
IL6	G-174C	26	84	3.25	.006	No	In postoperative CABG patients	50
IL10	A-592C	196	873	0.32	3.70×10^{-03}	No	Lone AF	51
KCNE4	E145D	142	238	1.66	.044	No		49
KCNE5	97T	158	96	0.52	.007	No		48
KCNH2	K897T	1207	2475	1.25	.00033	No		46
MinK/KCNE1	38G	108	108	1.8	.024	Yes		47
MinK/KCNE1	38G	331	441	1.73	<.005	Yes		45
MMP2	C1306T	196	873	8.1	1.26×10^{-02}	No	Lone AF	51
SLN	G-65C	147	92	1.98	.011	No		41

Abbreviations: ACE, Angiotensin I converting enzyme; AF, atrial fibrillation; AGT, Angiotensinogen; CABG, coronary artery bypass graft; CETP, cholesteryl ester transfer protein; CHF, congestive heart failure; CYP11B2, Aldosterone synthase; EDN2, endothelin 2; GJA5, connexin 40; GNB3, guanine nucleotide binding protein; GWAS, genome-wide association study; HCM, hypertrophic cardiomyopathy; hsp70, heat shock protein 70; IL6, interleukin 6; IL10, interleukin 10; NOS3, nitric oxide synthase 3;S LN, sarcolipin gene.

analyses are the small sample sizes and a lack of replication in distinct populations, as well as phenotypic and genetic heterogeneity.

In recent years, genome-wide association studies (GWAS) have been made possible by advancements in genotyping technology that allow investigators to assay hundreds of thousands of SNPs spread over the entire human genome. The studies are typically executed using a case-control study design.[54] GWAS attempt to identify novel genetic polymorphisms that are significantly more or less common in a group with a disease as compared with a control group. Since the markers are spread over the entire genome, these experiments give no weight to existing candidate genes. Such studies have been used successfully in the past several years to identify potential novel pathways for diabetes,[55] obesity,[56] coronary heart disease,[57,58] macular degeneration,[59] and repolarization.[60]

Although GWAS have the potential to identify new pathways for disease, they also have a number of limitations. In particular, with hundreds of thousands of individual associations being tested, these studies have a high likelihood of producing false-positive associations. There is still discussion within the field of what the threshold level should be for genome-wide significance.[61] False-positive results can also emerge from population stratification or the failure to properly control for ethnicity, thus resulting in over- or underrepresentation of spurious ethnic-specific markers. Although variations in study design have been proposed in an effort to eliminate false associations, ultimately replication of the associations in other populations is the best method of validation.[54]

The biological significance of the identified variants is another concern. Most variants found in genetic association studies have been associated with relatively weak effects, with typical odds ratios ranging from approximately 1.3 to 1.5. Although such variants may generate new ideas about disease pathogenesis, understanding the biological mechanisms by which the majority of variants confer disease susceptibility remains challenging.

Recently, a team led by the researchers at deCODE genetics have reported the results of a GWAS for AF. Gudbjartsson and colleagues[62] examined over 300,000 SNPs and identified two polymorphisms on the long arm of chromosome 4 (4q25) that were highly associated (rs2200733 and rs10033464, $P = 3.3 \times 10^{-41}$ and 6.9×10^{-11}, respectively) with AF or atrial flutter in a group of Icelanders. To improve both the validity and generalizability of the findings, the study was replicated in other populations in Iceland, Sweden, the United States, and Hong Kong. Neither variant was correlated with obesity, hypertension, or myocardial infarction suggesting that the genetic variants are not associated with AF by affecting those risk factors.

How do the variants on chromosome 4 lead to AF? At present, the mechanism of action of these variants is unclear. Interestingly, these SNPs lie upstream from a gene that could plausibly play a role in the pathogenesis of AF, the paired-like homeodomain transcription factor 2, *PITX2*. This gene is known to be critical in the development of the left atrium,[63–66] pulmonary myocardium,[67] and in the suppression of left atrial pacemakers cells in early development.[68] One can speculate that these variants may alter the function of PITX2 either in early development or in adulthood and thus predispose to AF. However, currently there is no direct link between the *PITX2* gene and these noncoding variants more than 50,000 base pairs away. Future work examining the correlation between these variants and PITX2 RNA levels, protein levels, or tissue specificity will hopefully clarify the mechanism underlying the association of these SNPs with AF.

REFINING GENETIC STUDIES OF ATRIAL FIBRILLATION

To continue to improve upon the utility of genetic studies for AF we will need to overcome a number of obstacles. A critical step in any genetic study is the ability to correctly assign the diagnosis. AF represents a particular challenge because many individuals are asymptomatic, some have paroxysmal disease, and yet others develop AF late in life. Genotypic and phenotypic heterogeneity further complicate the classification of AF. Rather than a single entity, AF may represent the final common pathway for a number of distinct pathogenic insults such as heart failure, hypertension, or thyroid abnormalities.

To address these challenges, we will have to continue to improve upon the characterization and classification of AF. The identification of endophenotypes, or subtle, heritable traits that cosegregate with AF, may help to refine ongoing genetic studies. For AF, endophenotypes such as specific P-wave morphologies, pulmonary venous anatomy as assessed by CT or MRI, or biomarkers that are heritable and easily detectable may be helpful.

SUMMARY

Recent studies of AF have identified mutations in a series of ion channels; however, these mutations appear to be relatively rare causes of AF. A genome-wide association study has identified novel variants on chromosome 4 associated with AF, although the mechanisms of action for these variants remain unknown. Ultimately, a greater understanding of the genetics of AF should yield insights into novel pathways, therapeutic targets, and diagnostic testing for this common arrhythmia.

ACKNOWLEDGMENTS

This work was supported by a grant from the Disque Deane Foundation to Dr Ellinor and a National Institutes of Health training grant (5T32HL007575) to Dr Lubitz.

REFERENCES

1. Miyasaka Y, Barnes ME, Gersh BJ, et al. Secular trends in incidence of atrial fibrillation in Olmsted County, Minnesota, 1980 to 2000, and implications on the projections for future prevalence. Circulation 2006;114(2):119–25.
2. Go AS, Hylek EM, Phillips KA, et al. Prevalence of diagnosed atrial fibrillation in adults: national implications for rhythm management and stroke prevention: the AnTicoagulation and Risk Factors in Atrial Fibrillation (ATRIA) study. JAMA 2001;285(18): 2370–5.
3. Coyne KS, Paramore C, Grandy S, et al. Assessing the direct costs of treating nonvalvular atrial fibrillation in the United States. Value Health 2006;9(5): 348–56.
4. Benjamin EJ, Wolf PA, D'Agostino RB, et al. Impact of atrial fibrillation on the risk of death: the Framingham heart study. Circulation 1998;98(10):946–52.
5. Gajewski J, Singer RB. Mortality in an insured population with atrial fibrillation. JAMA 1981;245(15): 1540–4.
6. Arnar DO, Thorvaldsson S, Manolio TA, et al. Familial aggregation of atrial fibrillation in Iceland. Eur Heart J 2006;27(6):708–12.
7. Ellinor PT, Yoerger DM, Ruskin JN, et al. Familial aggregation in lone atrial fibrillation. Hum Genet 2005;118(2):179–84.
8. Fox CS, Parise H, D'Agostino RB Sr, et al. Parental atrial fibrillation as a risk factor for atrial fibrillation in offspring. JAMA 2004;291(23):2851–5.
9. Darbar D, Herron KJ, Ballew JD, et al. Familial atrial fibrillation is a genetically heterogeneous disorder [comment]. J Am Coll Cardiol 2003;41(12):2185–92.
10. Chen YH, Xu SJ, Bendahhou S, et al. KCNQ1 gain-of-function mutation in familial atrial fibrillation. Science 2003;299(5604):251–4.
11. Yang Y, Xia M, Jin Q, et al. Identification of a KCNE2 gain-of-function mutation in patients with familial atrial fibrillation. Am J Hum Genet 2004;75(5):899–905.
12. Xia M, Jin Q, Bendahhou S, et al. A Kir2.1 gain-of-function mutation underlies familial atrial fibrillation. Biochem Biophys Res Commun 2005;332(4):1012–9.
13. Olson TM, Alekseev AE, Liu XK, et al. Kv1.5 channelopathy due to KCNA5 loss-of-function mutation causes human atrial fibrillation. Hum Mol Genet 2006;15(14):2185–91.
14. Otway R, Vandenberg JI, Guo G, et al. Stretch-sensitive KCNQ1 mutation A link between genetic and environmental factors in the pathogenesis of atrial fibrillation? J Am Coll Cardiol 2007;49(5):578–86.
15. Chen LY, Ballew JD, Herron KJ, et al. A common polymorphism in SCN5A is associated with lone atrial fibrillation. Clin Pharmacol Ther 2007;81(1): 35–41.
16. Darbar D, Kannankeril PJ, Donahue BS, et al. Cardiac sodium channel (SCN5A) variants associated with atrial fibrillation. Circulation 2008;117(15): 1927–35.
17. Ellinor PT, Nam EG, Shea MA, et al. Cardiac sodium channel mutation in atrial fibrillation. J Neurosci 2008;5(1):99–105.
18. Ellinor PT, Moore RK, Patton KK, et al. Mutations in the long QT gene, KCNQ1, are an uncommon cause of atrial fibrillation. Heart 2004;90(12):1487–8.
19. Ellinor PT, Petrov-Kondratov VI, Zakharova E, et al. Potassium channel gene mutations rarely cause atrial fibrillation. BMC Med Genet 2006;7:70.
20. Wolff L. Familial auricular fibrillation. N Engl J Med 1943;229:396–8.
21. Consortium TIH. A haplotype map of the human genome. Nature 2005;437(7063):1299–320.
22. Brugada R, Tapscott T, Czernuszewicz GZ, et al. Identification of a genetic locus for familial atrial fibrillation. N Engl J Med 1997;336(13):905–11.
23. Ellinor PT, Shin JT, Moore RK, et al. Locus for atrial fibrillation maps to chromosome 6q14-16. Circulation 2003;107(23):2880–3.
24. Oberti C, Wang L, Li L, et al. Genome-wide linkage scan identifies a novel genetic locus on chromosome 5p13 for neonatal atrial fibrillation associated with sudden death and variable cardiomyopathy. Circulation 2004;110(25):3753–9.
25. Volders PG, Zhu Q, Timmermans C, et al. Mapping a novel locus for familial atrial fibrillation on chromosome 10p11-q21. Heart Rhythm 2007;4(4):469–75.
26. Hodgson-Zingman DM, Karst ML, Zingman LV, et al. Atrial natriuretic peptide frameshift mutation in familial atrial fibrillation. N Engl J Med 2008;359(2): 158–65.
27. Schenzer A, Friedrich T, Pusch M, et al. Molecular determinants of KCNQ (Kv7) K+ channel sensitivity to the anticonvulsant retigabine. J Neurosci 2005; 25(20):5051–60.
28. Bellocq C, van Ginneken ACG, Bezzina CR, et al. Mutation in the KCNQ1 gene leading to the short QT-interval syndrome. Circulation 2004;109:2394–7.

29. Hong K, Piper DR, Diaz-Valdecantos A, et al. De novo KCNQ1 mutation responsible for atrial fibrillation and short QT syndrome in utero. Cardiovasc Res 2005;68(3):433–40.
30. Nattel S. New ideas about atrial fibrillation 50 years on. Nature 2002;415(6868):219–26.
31. Hagendorff A, Schumacher B, Kirchhoff S, et al. Conduction disturbances and increased atrial vulnerability in connexin40-deficient mice analyzed by transesophageal stimulation. Circulation 1999; 99:1508–15.
32. Gollob MH, Jones DL, Krahn AD, et al. Somatic mutations in the connexin 40 gene (GJA5) in atrial fibrillation. N Engl J Med 2006;354(25): 2677–88.
33. Tsai CT, Lai LP, Lin JL, et al. Renin-angiotensin system gene polymorphisms and atrial fibrillation. Circulation 2004;109(13):1640–6.
34. Bedi M, McNamara D, London B, et al. Genetic susceptibility to atrial fibrillation in patients with congestive heart failure. Heart Rhythm 2006;3(7): 808–12.
35. Yamashita T, Hayami N, Ajiki K, et al. Is ACE gene polymorphism associated with lone atrial fibrillation? Jpn Heart J 1997;38(5):637–41.
36. Fatini C, Sticchi E, Gensini F, et al. Lone and secondary nonvalvular atrial fibrillation: role of a genetic susceptibility. Int J Cardiol 2007;120(1): 59–65.
37. Ravn LS, Benn M, Nordestgaard BG, et al. Angiotensinogen and ACE gene polymorphisms and risk of atrial fibrillation in the general population. Pharmacogenet Genomics 2008;18(6):525–33.
38. Tsai CT, Hwang JJ, Chiang FT, et al. Renin-angiotensin system gene polymorphisms and atrial fibrillation: a regression approach for the detection of gene-gene interactions in a large hospitalized population. Cardiology 2008;111(1):1–7.
39. Nagai T, Ogimoto A, Okayama H, et al. A985G polymorphism of the endothelin-2 gene and atrial fibrillation in patients with hypertrophic cardiomyopathy. Circ J 2007;71(12):1932–6.
40. Amir O, Amir RE, Paz H, et al. Aldosterone synthase gene polymorphism as a determinant of atrial fibrillation in patients with heart failure. Am J Cardiol 2008; 102(3):326–9.
41. Nyberg MT, Stoevring B, Behr ER, et al. The variation of the sarcolipin gene (SLN) in atrial fibrillation, long QT syndrome and sudden arrhythmic death syndrome. Clin Chim Acta 2007;375(1–2):87–91.
42. Asselbergs FW, Moore JH, van den Berg MP, et al. A role for CETP TaqIB polymorphism in determining susceptibility to atrial fibrillation: a nested case control study. BMC Med Genet 2006;7:39.
43. Juang JM, Chern YR, Tsai CT, et al. The association of human connexin 40 genetic polymorphisms with atrial fibrillation. Int J Cardiol 2007;116(1):107–12.
44. Firouzi M, Ramanna H, Kok B, et al. Association of human connexin40 gene polymorphisms with atrial vulnerability as a risk factor for idiopathic atrial fibrillation. Circ Res 2004;95(4):e29–33.
45. Fatini C, Sticchi E, Genuardi M, et al. Analysis of minK and eNOS genes as candidate loci for predisposition to non-valvular atrial fibrillation. Eur Heart J 2006;27(14):1712–8.
46. Sinner MF, Pfeufer A, Akyol M, et al. The non-synonymous coding IKr-channel variant KCNH2-K897T is associated with atrial fibrillation: results from a systematic candidate gene-based analysis of KCNH2 (HERG). Eur Heart J 2008;7:907–14.
47. Lai LP, Su MJ, Yeh HM, et al. Association of the human minK gene 38G allele with atrial fibrillation: evidence of possible genetic control on the pathogenesis of atrial fibrillation. Am Heart J 2002; 144(3):485–90.
48. Ravn LS, Hofman-Bang J, Dixen U, et al. Relation of 97T polymorphism in KCNE5 to risk of atrial fibrillation. Am J Cardiol 2005;96(3):405–7.
49. Zeng Z, Tan C, Teng S, et al. The single nucleotide polymorphisms of I(Ks) potassium channel genes and their association with atrial fibrillation in a Chinese population. Cardiology 2007;108(2):97–103.
50. Gaudino M, Andreotti F, Zamparelli R, et al. The -174G/C interleukin-6 polymorphism influences postoperative interleukin-6 levels and postoperative atrial fibrillation. Is atrial fibrillation an inflammatory complication? Circulation 2003;108(Suppl 1):II195–9.
51. Kato K, Oguri M, Hibino T, et al. Genetic factors for lone atrial fibrillation. Int J Mol Med 2007;19(6): 933–9.
52. Schreieck J, Dostal S, von Beckerath N, et al. C825T polymorphism of the G-protein beta3 subunit gene and atrial fibrillation: association of the TT genotype with a reduced risk for atrial fibrillation. Am Heart J 2004;148(3):545–50.
53. Afzal AR, Mandal K, Nyamweya S, et al. Association of Met439Thr substitution in heat shock protein 70 gene with postoperative atrial fibrillation and serum HSP70 protein levels. Cardiology 2008;110(1):45–52.
54. Risch NJ. Searching for genetic determinants in the new millennium. Nature 2000;405(6788):847–56.
55. Saxena R, Voight BF, Lyssenko V, et al. Genome-wide association analysis identifies loci for type 2 diabetes and triglyceride levels. Science 2007; 316(5829):1331–6.
56. Frayling TM, Timpson NJ, Weedon MN, et al. A common variant in the FTO gene is associated with body mass index and predisposes to childhood and adult obesity. Science 2007;316(5826): 889–94.
57. McPherson R, Pertsemlidis A, Kavaslar N, et al. A common allele on chromosome 9 associated with coronary heart disease. Science 2007;316(5830): 1488–91.

58. Helgadottir A, Thorleifsson G, Manolescu A, et al. A common variant on chromosome 9p21 affects the risk of myocardial infarction. Science 2007; 316(5830):1491–3.
59. Dewan A, Liu M, Hartman S, et al. HTRA1 promoter polymorphism in wet age-related macular degeneration. Science 2006;314(5801):989–92.
60. Arking DE, Pfeufer A, Post W, et al. A common genetic variant in the NOS1 regulator NOS1AP modulates cardiac repolarization. Nat Genet 2006; 38(6):644–51.
61. Hunter DJ, Kraft P. Drinking from the fire hose—statistical issues in genomewide association studies. N Engl J Med 2007;357(5):436–9.
62. Gudbjartsson DF, Arnar DO, Helgadottir A, et al. Variants conferring risk of atrial fibrillation on chromosome 4q25. Nature 2007;448(7151):353–7.
63. Gage PJ, Suh H, Camper SA. Dosage requirement of Pitx2 for development of multiple organs. Development 1999;126(20):4643–51.
64. Campione M, Ros MA, Icardo JM, et al. Pitx2 expression defines a left cardiac lineage of cells: evidence for atrial and ventricular molecular isomerism in the iv/iv mice. Dev Biol 2001;231(1): 252–64.
65. Franco D, Campione M. The role of Pitx2 during cardiac development. Linking left-right signaing and congenital heart diseases. Trends Cardiovasc Med 2003;13:157–63.
66. Logan M, Pagan-Westphal SM, Smith DM, et al. The transcription factor Pitx2 mediates situs-specific morphogenesis in response to left-right asymmetric signals. Cell 1998;94(3):307–17.
67. Mommersteeg MT, Brown NA, Prall OW, et al. Pitx2c and Nkx2-5 are required for the formation and identity of the pulmonary myocardium. Circ Res 2007; 101(9):902–9.
68. Mommersteeg MT, Hoogaars WM, Prall OW, et al. Molecular pathway for the localized formation of the sinoatrial node. Circ Res 2007;100(3):354–62.

Genetic Basis of Ventricular Arrhythmias

Tim Boussy, MD[a,*], Gaetano Paparella, MD[a], Carlo de Asmundis, MD[a], Andrea Sarkozy, MD[a], Gian Battista Chierchia, MD[a], Josep Brugada, MD, PhD[b], Ramon Brugada, MD, PhD[c], Pedro Brugada, MD, PhD[a]

KEYWORDS

• Ventricular arrhythmia • Genetics • Channelopathy
• Brugada syndrome • Arrhythmogenic cardiomyopathy

Sudden cardiac death caused by malignant ventricular arrhythmias is the most important cause of death in the industrialized world. Most of these lethal arrhythmias occur in the setting of ischemic heart disease. A significant number of sudden deaths, especially in young individuals, are caused by inherited ventricular arrhythmic disorders, however. Genetically induced ventricular arrhythmias can be divided in two subgroups: the primary electrical disorders or channelopathies, in which no apparent structural heart disease can be identified, and the secondary arrhythmogenic cardiomyopathies. In these "single gene disorders," mutations are restricted to one gene, rendering a predictable mendelian fashion of transmission. The highly variable phenotypic expression of these monogenic mutations (even within the same family) makes risk assessment of a single individual difficult, if not impossible. This article focuses on the genetic background of these electrical disorders and the current knowledge of genotype-phenotype interactions.

MONOGENIC MODES OF TRANSMISSION

Protein-coding sequences comprise less than 1.5% of the human genome.[1] The rest contain RNA genes, regulatory sequences, introns, and so-called "junk DNA." Each individual has two copies of each gene (called alleles), which are localized along 23 chromosome pairs (22 pairs of autosomes, 1 pair of sex chromosomes). Each parent contributes one member of each chromosome pair, thus providing one copy of each gene. An individual is considered "homozygous" for a specific gene locus when both gene loci are occupied by two identical alleles or "heterozygous" when both alleles differ. According to Mendel's first law, each of the two alleles separates independently and is passed on to the next generation. Most of the single gene disorders are caused by point mutations (alteration of a single nucleotide), in which a nucleotide is substituted, resulting in formation of a different amino acid (missense mutation), a truncated protein (caused by mutation to a stop codon), or an elongated protein (caused by elimination of a stop codon). If the phenotype is expressed in the presence of only one mutated allele, the inheritance is called dominant. When phenotype expression requires both alleles to be mutant, the pattern of inheritance is called recessive (**Fig. 1**).

AUTOSOMAL DOMINANT INHERITANCE

The phenotype can be expressed in a heterozygous setting, in which only one of the two alleles

This article originally appeared in *Cardiology Clinics of North America*, Volume 26, Issue 3.
[a] Heart Rhythm Management Institute, University hospital Brussels, Belgium, Laarbeeklaan 101 - 1090 Brussels, Belgium
[b] Thorax Institute, Hospital Clinic, University of Barcelona, C. Villaroel, Barcelona, Spain
[c] Montreal Heart Institute, 5000 reu Belanger, Montreal QC HiT iC8, Canada
* Corresponding author.
E-mail address: tboussy@yahoo.com

Heart Failure Clin 6 (2010) 249–266
doi:10.1016/j.hfc.2009.12.005
1551-7136/10/$ – see front matter

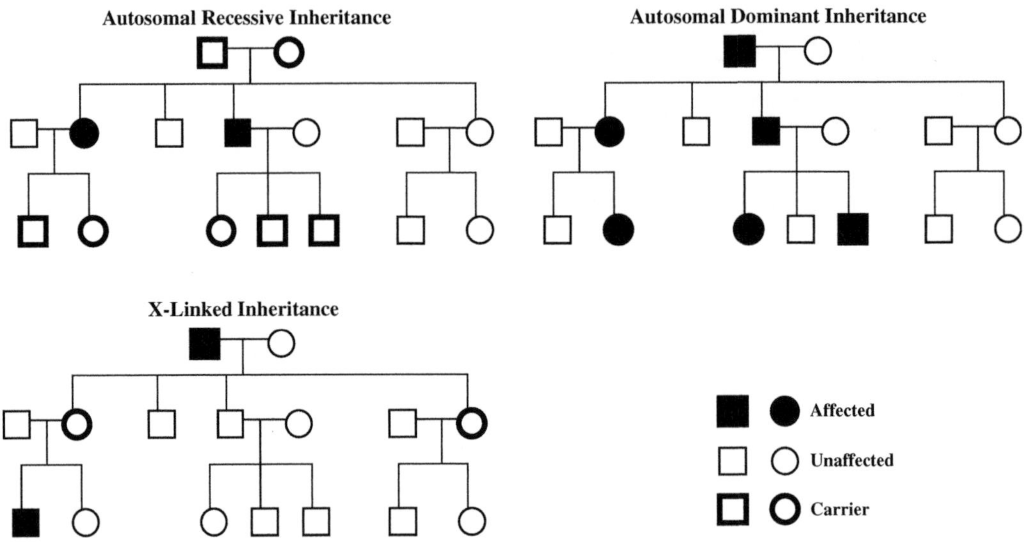

Fig. 1. Monogenic patterns of inheritance.

is affected. In the presence of identical mutations, different individuals may express different clinical features because of a different degree of expressivity, which is amenable to environmental and genetic factors. In an autosomal dominant trait, men and women are equally prone to inherit the mutation, and each child has a 50% chance of being affected by receiving the mutant allele. Each affected person has an affected parent. Normal children of an affected parent are noncarriers and cannot pass on the disease. In most autosomal dominant inherited diseases, the onset of the first phenotypic expression is delayed.

AUTOSOMAL RECESSIVE INHERITANCE

In autosomal recessive disorders, the phenotype can only manifest when both alleles are mutated at the locus responsible for the disease. Because 1 of the 22 autosomes is involved, there is an equal distribution between male and female subjects. Because of the early onset of expression, recessive disorders are mainly diagnosed during childhood. Each child has a 25% chance of being affected, and heterozygote parents are clinically normal.

X-LINKED INHERITANCE

Disorders caused by genes located on the sex chromosomes (X-linked) demonstrate a significantly different pattern of transmission with a different clinical outcome between both sexes. In women, one or both X chromosomes can be affected, with dominant or recessive properties. Because men only carry one X chromosome, the probability that the disease will manifest in the presence of a mutant gene is much higher. Mutant X genes can be received from the affected father or the homozygote (affected) or heterozygote mother. No male-to-male transmission is possible (genetic material from father to son is located on the Y chromosome), and all daughters of affected men are carriers.

CHANNELOPATHIES

The genetic background and detailed pathogenic mechanisms of these primary electrical disorders have been studied extensively in the last two decades.[2] At first, because of a lack of systematic investigation and low patient numbers, information was obtained from animal models, which were extrapolated to humans. Later, genetic linkage techniques and long-term information of multigenerational families increased our understanding of these relatively new diseases. Currently, several genes have been identified coding for the expression of ion channel proteins, located in the membrane of the cardiomyocyte. The principal function of these cardiac channels is the formation of an electrical potential. Ion currents are regulated by synchronized opening and closing of these channels. Gene mutations alter their pore-forming capacities and gate function, which results in an impaired depolarization or repolarization. This results in an increased vulnerability of the cardiomyocyte for dangerous arrhythmias. The channelopathies show a pronounced genetic heterogeneity, with dispersion of gene mutations within the affected gene.

VOLTAGE-GATED SODIUM CHANNELOPATHIES

The Cardiac Sodium Channel

Voltage-gated sodium channels are responsible for the upstroke of the action potential and play an important role in the propagation of the electrical impulse in all excitable tissues (eg, muscle, nerve, and heart). The opening of sodium channels in the heart underlies the QRS-complex on the electrocardiogram (ECG) and enables a synchronous ventricular ejection. Because the upstroke of the electrical potential primarily determines the speed of conduction between adjacent cells, sodium channels can be found in tissues in which speed is of importance.[3–5] Cardiac Purkinje cells contain up to 1 million sodium channels, which illustrates the importance of rapid conductance in the heart.

Sodium channels consist of a pore-forming α-subunit and one or two β-subunits (**Figs. 2** and **3**). The α-subunit is a large transmembrane protein encoded by nine genes, in which the SCN5A gene (chromosome 3p21) is the only one coding for the cardiac isoform (**Table 1**). Mutations in the Na-channel α-subunit gene SCN5A result in multiple cardiac arrhythmia syndromes.

Mutations leading to a voltage-gated sodium channel dysfunction can result in Brugada syndrome, progressive cardiac conduction disturbances (PCCD) or Lenègre disease, and long QT syndrome. Several different types of mutations have been identified, including missense, deletions, insertions, and splicing errors, resulting in a decreased or increased function of the sodium channel. Combinations of all three phenotypes have been documented.[6] Certain mutations may manifest different phenotypes in different individuals of the same family.

Loss of sodium channel function disorders

The Brugada syndrome Since 1992, Brugada syndrome (BS) has been known as one of the genetically transmittable cardiac channelopathies, characterized by a susceptibility for lethal ventricular arrhythmias in the presence of typical ST-segment changes in the right precordial leads.[7] In patients who have BS, no structural heart disease can be identified despite thorough invasive and noninvasive exploration. The baseline ECG deviations show a dynamic character, with possible transient normalization.[8] They seem to be based on an impaired function of cardiac sodium channels, creating an altered morphology of the cardiac action potential associated with increased arrhythmic vulnerability.

More than 70 gene mutations have been identified in only 20% to 25% of all patients who have BS (most are located in the cardiac SCN5A gene), which suggests that other gene mutations may be responsible.[9] All SCN5A mutations modify the sodium channel function by either creating a truncated protein or increasing the channel inactivation. This results in a shortening of the action potential because of faster phase 1 depolarization. In 2002, Weiss and colleagues[10] located a second locus linked to BS on chromosome 3, and recently the same group identified the causative mutation in the glycerol-3-phosphate dehydrogenase 1-like gene (GPD1L).[11] Patients who have BS, particularly with an SCN5A mutation, show clinical signs of slowed conduction by means of PR, HV, and QRS prolongation, which illustrates the overlap with Lenègres syndrome.

Recently, remarkable genetic data were published regarding the importance of single nucleotide polymorphisms, which might possibly

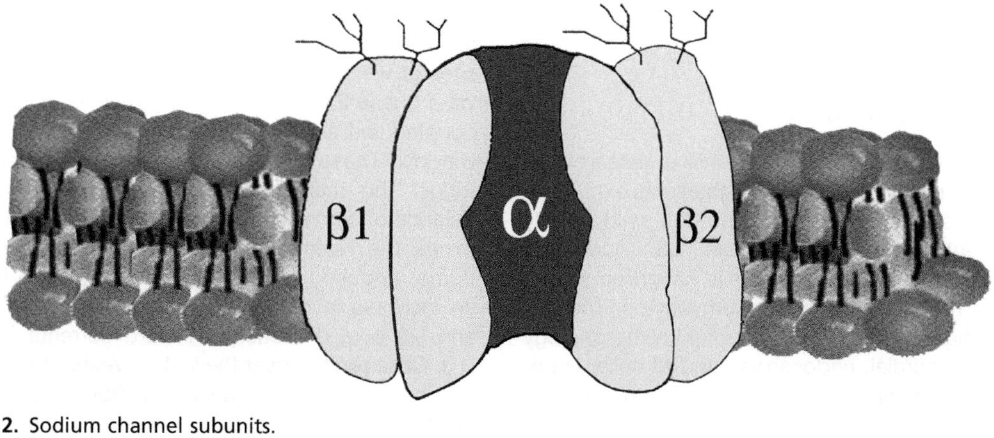

Fig. 2. Sodium channel subunits.

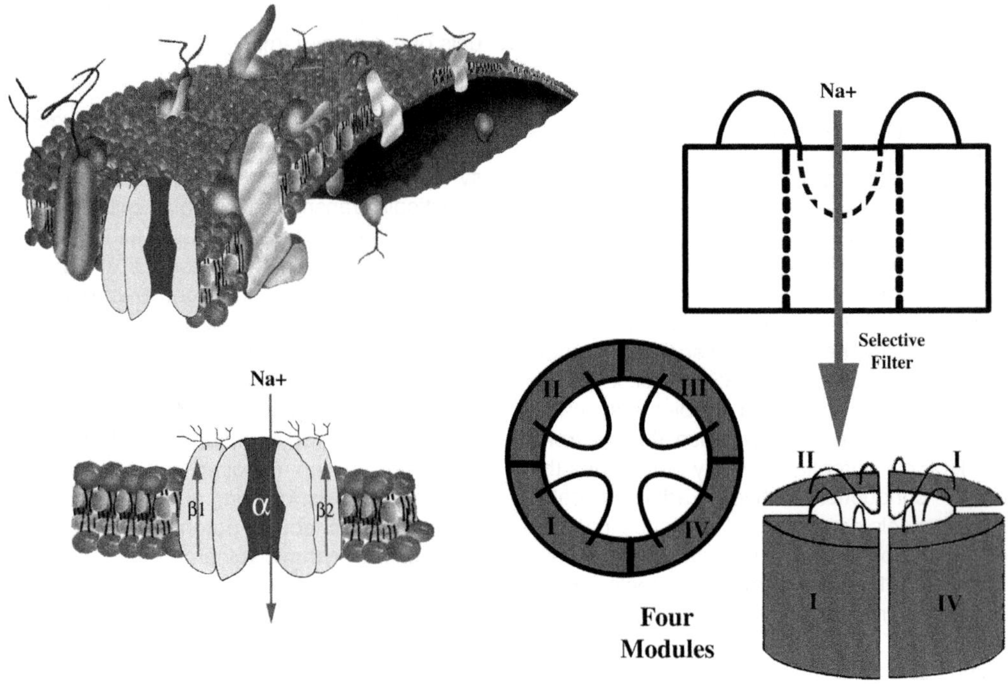

Fig. 3. Sodium channel.

explain the different clinical phenotypes and incidence of BS in diverse geographic regions.[12] Ethnic-specific single nucleotide polymorphism distributions in the SCN5A promoter region were reported. A certain combination of six single nucleotide polymorphisms (designated as haplotype B variant) only occurred in Asian subjects (at an allele frequency of 22%) and was absent in the other ethnic groups. This haplotype variant resulted in decreased sodium channel expression and function. In the last years, several case reports proved that certain SCN5A polymorphism in the presence of a BS-causing SCN5A mutation can influence the clinical phenotype and clinical consequences of the mutation. The polymorphism can rescue and restore or—by contrast—further worsen the sodium channel function.[13]

PATHOPHYSIOLOGY

Antzelevitch[14] performed extensive research on possible pathophysiologic mechanisms explaining the ST-segment changes and the vulnerability for ventricular arrhythmias in BS. According to their findings, the disorder is based on an impaired repolarization of cardiomyocytes. There is a striking difference in action potential morphology in the epicardial, endocardial, and M cells, especially during phases 2 and 3 of the action potential. Whereas the epicardial action potential shows a prominent notch and dome immediately after phase 0 depolarization, the endocardial action potential has a steadier shape during early repolarization. The transmural gradient that originates from this shape difference corresponds to the ST segment on the surface ECG. Alterations of spike and dome morphology (phase 1), in particular in the epicardium, are predominantly mediated by the transient outward current (I_{to}). In BS, the loss of right ventricular outflow tract (RVOT)-epicardial (not endocardial) action potential dome and plateau amplitude, caused by an increase in I_{to} and simultaneous decrease in (inward) I_{Na}, underlies the prominent J-wave and ST-segment elevation (mimicking right bundle branch block morphology). The conduction of the action potential dome from sites at which it is maintained to sites at which it is lost allows local pre-excitation via a phase 2 re-entry mechanism when a closely coupled extra systole occurs in the vulnerable window. These premature beats might eventually trigger the malignant arrhythmia. Because the balance of currents at the onset of phase 2 determines the maintenance of the action potential dome, acquired forms of BS can originate from an increase in outward currents (I_{to}, $I_{K\text{-}ATP}$, IKs, and I_{Kr}) or a decrease in inward currents ($I_{Ca\text{-}L}$, I_{Na}). Case reports over the last 13 years described ST changes as in BS caused by drugs, ischemia, electrolyte disturbances, hyper- and hypothermia,

Table 1
Overview of sodium channel genes, tissue specificity, and clinical features associated with channelopathies

Gene	Channel	Location	Tissue	Associated Disorders
SCN1A	$Na_v1.1$	2q24	Brain, CNS	Brain sodium channelopathies: epilepsy, familial hemiplegic migraine, familial autism
SCN2A	$Na_v1.2$	2q23–q24.3	Brain, CNS	Severe myoclonic epilepsy, familial neonatal- infantile seizures
SCN3A	$Na_v1.3$	2q24	Brain, CNS	Epilepsy, familial hemiplegic migraine, familial autism
SCN4A	$Na_v1.4$	17q23.1–q25.3	Adult skeletal muscle	Muscle sodium channelopathies: hyperkalemic periodic paralysis, paramyotonia congenital, potassium aggravated myotonia
SCN5A	$Na_v1.5$	3p21	Heart muscle, skeletal muscle	Cardiac sodium channelopathies (see text)
SCN6A/SCN7A	Na_x	2q21–q23	PNS, heart muscle, skeletal muscle, uterus	
SCN8A	$Na_v1.6$	12q13	CNS, brain	Cerebellar atrophy, ataxia, mental retardation
SCN9A	$Na_v1.7$	2q24	PNS	Peripheral nerve sodium channelopathies: pain sensitization
SCN10A	$Na_v1.8$	3p24.2–p22	PNS	Peripheral nerve sodium channelopathies
SCN11A	$Na_v1.9$	3p24–p21	PNS	Peripheral nerve sodium channelopathies
SCN1B	$Na_v\beta1$	19q13.1	Brain, heart muscle, skeletal muscle	Brain sodium channelopathies: generalized epilepsy with febrile seizures
SCN4B	$Na_v\beta4$	11q23	Brain, PNS, heart muscle, skeletal muscle	Cardiac sodium channelopathies: long QT syndrome

Abbreviation: PNS, peripheral nerve system.
Data from Koopmann TT, Bezzina CR, Wilde AA. Voltage-gated sodium channels: action players with many faces. Ann Med 2006;38:472–82.

elevated insulin levels, and mechanical compression of the RVOT.

Recently, Meregalli and colleagues[15] presented an alternative "depolarization disorder" theory, providing another possible explanation for the Brugada ECG abnormalities. This model is based on a conduction delay in the RVOT. Because of action potential differences between the RVOT and the rest of the right ventricle, a closed-loop current originates between these two regions and creates an initial ST elevation followed by a negative T wave at the level of the right precordial leads. It is also possible that both of the mechanisms operate in the pathophysiology of the Brugada ECG pattern and the ventricular arrhythmias.

Lev-Lenègre Syndrome

Lev-Lenègre's disease or PCCD is characterized by an age-related alteration of electrical conductance through the His-Purkinje system. This disorder, first described in 1964,[16,17] initially was thought to be degenerative, is caused by selective and progressive fibrosis of the His-Purkinje system. Genetic familial screening of these patients reveals causative gene mutations.

Clinically, PCCD manifests as a progressive blockage of the atrioventricular conduction (requiring pacemaker implantation) or—on an infrahissian level—as a fascicular or bundle branch block. Multiple reports have shown a familial clustering of patients with chronic bundle branch block and various degrees of atrioventricular block (suggesting a genetic origin).[18,19]

In 1995, a South African study group genotyped a large family of 86 members, in which 39 were affected with PCCD.[20] They mapped the first locus to 19q13.2–13.3 in near proximity of the myotonic dystrophy locus, which explained the occurrence of conduction abnormalities in these patients. Another gene locus mapped on 1q32.2–q32.3 was linked to cardiac conduction defects in combination with dilated cardiomyopathy.[21] Probst and colleagues[21] were the first to identify mutations responsible for isolated cardiac conduction defects. They were located on the cardiac sodium channel gene (SCN5A) and segregated in an autosomal dominant fashion. Sequencing the entire SCN5A coding region in a large French family (with 15 affected family members), they identified a T≥C substitution (IVS22 + 2 T≥C) that resulted in an impaired gene product, lacking the voltage sensitive segment of the sodium channel. In a smaller Dutch family, another SCN5A mutation cosegregated with a nonprogressive conduction deficit. A second, thorough, and more complete investigation of the same French pedigree demonstrated that PCCD related to SCN5A mutations is based on the combination of haploinsufficiency of the cardiac sodium channel gene and an additional unknown mechanism (altering cardiac conduction in relation to aging).[22]

Disorders associated with a gain of function of cardiac sodium channels

Long QT3 syndrome In contrast to most long QT-syndrome phenotypes, which are based on mutations that modify the cardiac potassium currents, long QT3 mutations are located on the cardiac sodium channel gene SCN5A. These mutations cause a sustained reopening of sodium channels and result in a small inward current that adds up to the peak upstroke of the ventricular action potential. This additional inward current prolongs cardiac repolarization by selective alteration of phase 1 or the early repolarization phase. The surface ECG manifests a long QT interval with late onset of the T wave. Arrhythmic events occur more commonly during rest or sleep. Beta-blockers are contraindicated in this group because inhibition of the sympathetic activity enhances the risk of arrhythmic events.

POTASSIUM CHANNELOPATHIES

The Cardiac Potassium Channel

Potassium channels, which mediate the outward K^+ currents, play a major role in the formation of the cardiac action potential by enabling repolarization currents to counteract the depolarization front (phases 1 through 4).[23–27] Different expression of voltage-gated potassium channels in the different layers of the cardiac muscle and in different cardiac tissues seems to be responsible for the changes in morphology of the cardiac action potential. The cardiac voltage-gated potassium channel consists of four alpha-subunits ($K_V\alpha$), which together represent a pore-forming unit (see **Fig. 2**). The assembly of a functional tetramer can only occur in the presence of multiple auxiliary units. The slow and fast component of the transient outward current I_{to} is created through the assembly of four α-subunits from the K_v1-K_v4 subfamilies (KCNA to D gene), while joining of the *HERG* (*human ether-a-go-go*–related) gene and K_vLQT1 α-subunits underlie the delayed rectifier current (I_{Kr} and I_{Ks}). Disorders associated with an impaired function of these potassium channels are the long and the short QT syndrome.

Loss of sodium potassium channel function disorders

The long QT syndrome In its idiopathic or congenital form, long QT syndrome refers to a group of genetically transmittable disorders that affect cardiac ion channels in a way that results in slowed ventricular repolarization with prolongation of the QT interval. This can lead to early after-depolarizations and life-threatening torsade de pointes. The incidence of long QT syndrome has been estimated to be approximately 1 per 10,000 without apparent ethnic or geographic predilection. Through the last two decades, eight genotypes (LQT1–8) have been described (with up to 500 mutations and 130 polymorphisms). Each subgroup affects the morphology of the ventricular action potential in a different way and shows minor differences in clinical manifestations. Because most of these repolarization disorders involve the cardiac potassium currents (I_{Ks}, I_{Kr}, I_{Ki}), an overview of the potassium-dependent long QT syndrome subgroups is presented in this section (**Table 2**).

Long QT 1 Long QT 1 syndrome, caused by KCNQ1 mutations, is the most common form of long QT syndrome[27] Mutations in the KCNQ1-gene (α-subunit K_vLQT1) can cause autosomal-dominant Romano-Ward syndrome and autosomal-recessive Jervell and Lange-Nielsen syndrome. KCNQ1 and KCNE1 (minK) form the slowly activating component

Table 2
Long QT-syndrome genotype groups with associated pathophysiologic and clinical features

LQT Subgroup	Gene	Locus	Encoded Protein	Ion Current Affected	Effect of Mutation	Triggers	ECG Findings
LQT1	KvLQT1, KCNQ1	11p15.5	Alpha subunit of potassium channel	I_{Ks}	Loss of function	Exercise, swimming, emotional stress	Broad based T wave, late-onset T wave
LQT2	HERGKCNH2	7q35–36	Alpha subunit of potassium channel	I_{Kr}	Loss of function	Rest, sleep, auditory stimuli, emotional stress, postpartum	Split, notched T wave, low amplitude T wave
LQT3	SCN5A	3p21–24	Alpha subunit of sodium channel	I_{Na}	Gain of function	Rest/sleep	Late onset, peaked, biphasic T wave
LQT4	ANKB, ANK2	4q25–27	Membrane anchoring protein	Na^+, K^+ and Ca^{2+} exchange	Loss of function	Exercise, emotional stress	Inverted or low amplitude T wave, inconsistent QT prolongation, prominent U wave
LQT5	mink,I_sK, KCNE1	21q22.1–2	Beta subunit to KCNQ1	I_{Ks}	Loss of function	Unknown	Unknown
LQT6	MiRP1, KCNE2	21q22.1	Beta subunit to HERG	I_{Kr}	Loss of function	Unknown	Unknown
LQT7	Kir2.1, KCNJ2	17q23	Kir2.1 subunits	I_{KI}	Loss of function	Accompanied by alterations in serum K^+ levels	Prominent U wave, prolonged terminal T downslope
LQT8	CACNA1C	12p13.3	Alpha subunit	$I_{Ca,L}$	Gain of function	Hypoglycemia, sepsis	Severe QT-prolongation, 2:1 atrioventricular block, overt T-wave alternans

Data from Modell SM, Lehmann MH. The long QT syndrome family of cardiac ion channelopathies: a HuGE review. Genet Med 2006;8(3):143–55.

of the delayed rectifier K^+ current (I_{Ks}), which contributes to cardiac repolarization. Functional expression of mutant KCNQ1 α-subunits results in a loss of channel function. More than 100 mutations have been identified and associated with a variety of ion channel dysfunction mechanisms. The net effect of these mutations is a decrease in outward K^+ current during the plateau phase of the cardiac action potential. The channel remains open longer, ventricular repolarization is delayed, and the QT interval is prolonged.[28]

Long QT 2 The second most common cause of congenital long QT syndrome is mutation in the *HERG* (*human-ether-a-go-go–*related*)* gene, which generates the long QT 2 phenotype (35%–45%).[29] Currently, more than 80 mutations, mostly single amino acid substitutions, have been described. *HERG* encodes the voltage-gated potassium channels that produce the rapidly activating rectifier K^+ current (I_{Kr}). Similar as the I_{Ks} in long QT 1, the I_{Kr} plays an important role in controlling the balance of membrane currents during the plateau phase (phase 2) of the cardiac action potential. Long QT 2 is an autosomal-dominant inherited disease in which normal and mutant *HERG* genes are present. Experiments performed by Sanguinetti and Keating[30,31] contributed to our understanding in possible assembly mechanisms of the α-subunits. They concluded that the presence of a single mutant subunit (in a tetramer) conveys a dysfunctional channel phenotype. They called this the "dominant negative effect," which results in a channel function reduction of much more than the expected 50%. Because the *HERG* channel is considered a target for various cardiovascular and noncardiovascular drugs, it is partly responsible for the striking similarities between congenital and acquired or drug-induced forms of long QT syndrome.

Long QT 5 The congenital long QT5 phenotype has been linked to mutations in the minK gene *KCNE1*.[32] MinK is one of the auxiliary units that coassemble with K_v LQT1 to produce the slow delayed rectifier K^+ current I_{Ks}. As in previous long QT groups, the impaired repolarization prolongs the duration of the action potential by influencing phase 2 and, to a lesser degree, phase 3 of the action potential. The function of the regulatory subunit minK may not be restricted to K_vLQT1 alone in its interactions with the voltage-gated potassium channel. Recently, it has been shown to affect the amplitude and gating properties of the *HERG* subunits, raising the possibility that both I_{Ks} and I_{Kr} currents are altered in the long QT 5 syndrome. Currently, only five mutations have been identified.[33]

Long QT 6 Another regulatory protein MiRP1, which is the product of the *KCNE2* gene, is dysfunctional in long QT 6 syndrome.[27] This gene bears many similarities to the *KCNE1* gene, which suggests a common evolutionary origin. Both genes are located next to each other on the same chromosome, and both encode an auxiliary unit of the voltage-gated potassium channel. The *MiRP1* gene product *KCNE2* coassembles as a β-subunit with the *HERG* α-subunits to regulate the I_{Kr} currents. Because it predominantly alters the I_{Kr} currents, it phenotypically mimics the long QT 2 syndrome. The long QT 6 variant is an uncommon variant (<1%) of the disease and is usually associated with minor clinical manifestations (because of its incomplete penetrance).

Long QT 7 The long QT 7 syndrome—or the Andersen-Tawil syndrome—is a skeletal muscle disease associated with periodic paralysis, prolonged QT intervals, and fluctuations in plasma potassium levels.[34] It has been linked to mutations in the *KCNJ2* gene (chromosome 17), encoding for the inward rectifier potassium channel (I_{K1}or Kir2.1). The alterations in action potential morphology occur during phase 3, because the I_{K1} current is predominantly active during late repolarization. Clinically, patients typically present with the triad of periodic paralysis, cardiac arrhythmias, and developmental dysmorphisms. Possible triggers for arrhythmias are hypokalemia and concomitant infections.

Disorders associated with a gain of function of cardiac potassium channels

Short QT syndrome In 2000, Gussak and colleagues[35] first described a clinical syndrome that linked a short QT interval to an increased risk for malignant ventricular arrhythmias. Two years later, Gaita and colleagues[36] reported two families with short QT syndrome and a high incidence of sudden death, providing evidence for a genetic origin. As in long QT syndrome, mutations are located in genes that encode for subunits of the cardiac potassium channel. In contrast to the long QT syndrome, the gain of function of potassium channels results in faster repolarization with shortening of the action potential duration. Currently, three genes have been associated with the syndrome: $KCNH_2$, $KCNQ_l$, and $KCNJ_2$.[37]

$KCNH_2$ gene mutations Brugada and colleagues[38] identified two different missense mutations in the $KCNH_2$ or *HERG* gene in two unrelated families. *HERG* encodes the voltage-gated potassium channels that produce the rapidly activating rectifier K^+ current (I_{Kr}). *HERG* mutations associated with short QT syndrome block the inactivation of the *HERG* channels, which results in an increase in I_{Kr}. Coexpression of the *KCNE₂* gene does not alter these changes. The same group showed that *HERG* mutations cause a selective shortening of the ventricular action potentials that is not present in the Purkinje fibers. These differences in duration of action potentials and refractory periods could possibly create a substrate for re-entry arrhythmias. Because atrial fibrillation is frequently correlated with the same mutations, this heterogeneity probably extends to the atrial tissue.[39] This was demonstrated by identification of another family with short QT syndrome, in which atrial fibrillation was the only clinical manifestation.

$KCNQ_1$ gene mutations To date, only two mutations in the $KCNQ_1$ gene have been identified.[40] The first one exhibited a voltage-dependent character. A gain of function in the outward potassium current (and subsequent shortening of the action potential) could only be demonstrated at more negative potentials. The second mutation was identified in a newborn, who phenotypically showed atrial fibrillation with slowed ventricular response and a short QT interval. A de novo missense mutation revealed a voltage-independent alteration of the potassium currents, which resulted in shortened ventricular repolarization.

$KCNJ_2$ gene mutations Recently, Priori and colleagues[41] described a third form of short QT syndrome linked to mutations in the $KCNJ_2$ gene on chromosome 17, which is encoded for the inward rectifier potassium channel (I_{K1}or Kir2.1). Similarly as in long QT 7, the alterations in action potential morphology occur during phase 3, because the I_{K1} current is predominantly active during late repolarization. This phenotypically manifests as asymmetrical T waves with a rapid terminal phase on the surface ECG. Simulation of the effects of the mutated gene in animal models confirms this selective acceleration of phase 3 of the ventricular action potential.

CALCIUM CHANNELOPATHIES

The Voltage-gated Cardiac Calcium Channel

Cardiac calcium channels play a crucial role in the proper functioning of excitable cardiac cells. The heart expresses different types of voltage-gated $Ca^{2}+$ channels that enable the coupling of electrical signaling to intracellular biochemical changes. In 2000,[42] a new classification model was introduced (**Table 3**) that presented the results of recent genetic, molecular, and biochemical studies. All voltage-gated $Ca^{2}+$ channels are large heteromers that contain a minimum of three core units: $\alpha 1$, $\alpha 2/\delta$, and β. The pore-forming $\alpha 1$ subunits contain the gating machinery required for adequate channel function. A wide spectrum of inherited calcium channelopathies results from mutations in these pore-forming α-subunits.[44]

The most prominent extracellular cardiac calcium channels (located in the cell membrane

Table 3
Ca^{2+}-dependent arrhythmia syndromes

Gene	Locus	Syndrome	Protein	Functional Abnormality
Timothy Syndrome				
CACNA1CA	12p13.3	Timothy syndrome1, autism	$Ca_v1.2\ \alpha_{1C}$	$I_{Ca\text{-}L}\uparrow$
CACNA1C	12p13.3	Timothy syndrome1, autism	$Ca_v1.2\ \alpha_{1C}$	$I_{Ca\text{-}L}\uparrow$
Catecholaminergic polymorphic ventricular tachycardia				
RyR2	1q42	CPVT1, SIDS	RyR2α	SR Ca^{2+} leak ↑
RyR2	1q42–q43	CPVT1, QT prolongation	RyR2α	SR Ca^{2+} leak ↑
RyR2	1q42–q43	CPVT1, ARVC2	RyR2α	SR Ca^{2+} leak ↑
CASQ2	1p13.3	CPVT2	Calsequestrin	SR Ca^{2+} leak ↑
KCNJ2	17q23	CPVT3	Kir2.1α	$I_{K1}\uparrow$
ANK2	4q25	CPVT?	Ankyrin-B	SR Ca^{2+} leak ↑
Dilated cardiomyopathy				
ABCC9	12p12.1	DCM, VT	SUR2Aβ	Ca^{2+} – overload
PLN	6q22.1	DCM, HF, LVH	PLNβ	Ca^{2+} – overload

Abbreviations: ARVC, arrhythmogenic right ventricular dysplasia; CPVT, catecholaminergic polymorphic ventricular tachycardia; DCM, dilated cardiomyopathy; HF, heart failure; LVH, left ventricular hypertrophy; SIDS, sudden infant death syndrome; SR, sarcoplasmatic reticulum; VT, ventricular tachycardia.

Data from Splaswski I, Timothy KW, Sharpe LM, et al. Ca(V)1.2 calcium channel dysfunction causes a multisystem disorder including arrhythmia and autism. Cell 2004;119:19–31.

or in the sarcolemma) are the high voltage–activated $Ca_v1.2/Ca_v1.3$ or slow calcium channels (L-type) (**Fig. 4**), which trigger the release and refilling of calcium in the sarcoplasmatic reticulum (SR). They predominantly affect phase 0 of the action potential in slow fibers (SA and atrioventricular node) or phase 2 in ventricular and atrial muscle cells (fast fibers). The resulting SR- calcium outflow in these cells can induce early after-depolarizations. L-type calcium channels act as a target for various drugs (calcium antagonists) that are aiming for a decrease in excitability of the cardiomyocytes (**Fig. 5**).

The low voltage activated $Ca_v3.1$ and $Ca_v3.2$ fast T-type channels show a relative prominence in pacemaker cells and conductive tissue and activate at more hyperpolarizing potentials. Based on these findings, T channels are presumed to play a vital role in atrial pacemaking.

TIMOTHY SYNDROME

Timothy syndrome is a recently described form of long QT syndrome (long QT 8).[43,45] Extracardiac features of this disease include syndactyly, facial dysmorphy, myopia, immunodeficiency, and generalized cognitive impairment. It results from a de novo, gain-of-function missense mutation in splice exon 8A of CACNA1C that encodes for the pore-forming subunit ($Ca_v1.2$) of the cardiac L-type Ca^{2+}channel. The causative mutation G406R results in loss of voltage-dependent channel inactivation leading to maintained inward Ca^{2+} currents and prolongation of the action potential. Because the combination of neurologic and cardiac phenotypes has been reported in CACNA1-mutations, special interest for neurologic evaluation is indicated in these cases.

The Ryanodine Receptor (or Intracellular Calcium Release Channel)

Activation of the contractile elements of the cardiac muscle is mainly governed by mobilization of calcium out of the sarcoplasmatic reticulum into the cytosol.[46] An increase in intracellular calcium concentration is obtained through complex interaction between different calcium channels (eg,

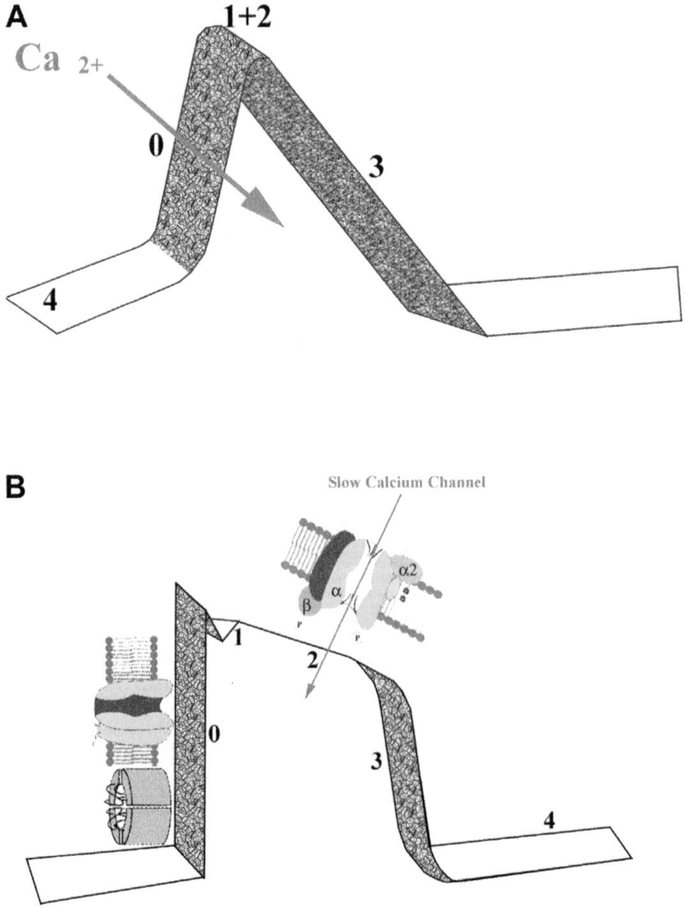

Fig. 4. Calcium channels.

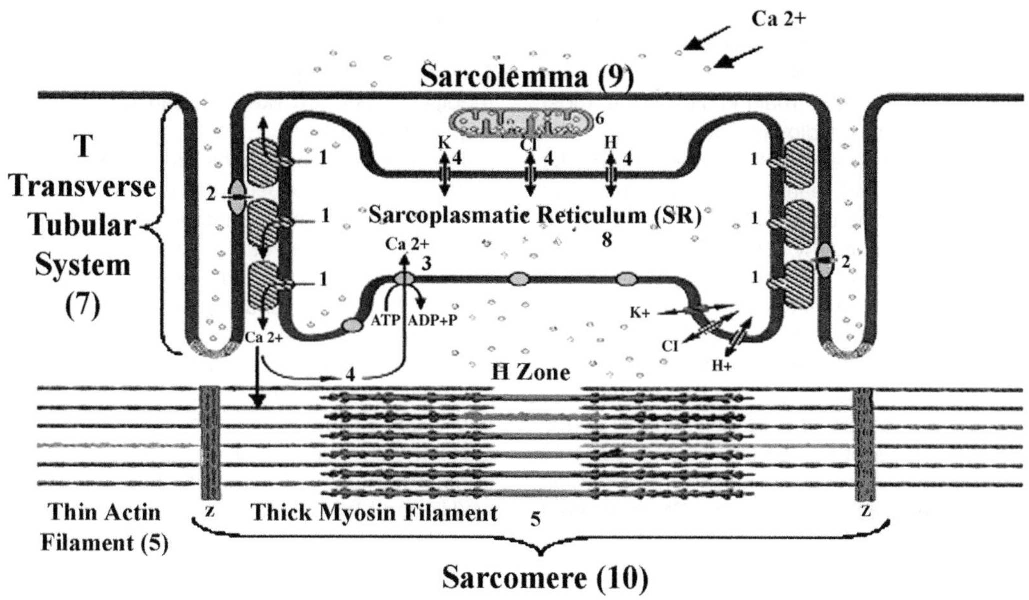

Fig. 5. Outline of cellular activation system.

Ca-ATPase, voltage-gated calcium channels) and auxiliary proteins. The ryanodine receptor (RyR) plays a crucial role in this process and has been identified in the membrane of the sarcoplasmatic reticulum of different excitable cells (RyR1 in skeletal muscle, RyR2 in cardiac muscle, and RyR3 in brain tissue). Depolarization of the cell membrane at the level of the T tubules triggers the voltage-gated L-type calcium channels to release a small amount of calcium. This small rise in intracellular calcium triggers the activation or opening of the RyR2 with subsequent massive release of calcium out of the SR. A cluster of approximately 100 RyR2 channels and 25 L-type calcium channels form a "junction." The systolic contraction of the heart is the result of the simultaneous activation of hundreds of thousands of these junctions.

Cardiac Calsequestrin

Calsequestrin is the most important calcium storage protein in the sarcoplasmatic reticulum. It is able to bind luminal calcium during diastole to prevent Ca^{2+} precipitation and reduce the ionic calcium concentration. In the heart, RyR2 does not act alone but is part of a macromolecular complex that contains several proteins, including calsequestrin, triadin, junctin, and junctophilin, which make up the calcium release unit.

Catecholaminergic Polymorphic Ventricular Tachycardia

Catecholaminergic polymorphic ventricular tachycardia (CPVT) is a familial arrhythmogenic disorder characterized by adrenergically mediated polymorphic or bidirectional ventricular tachycardia.[47] Two genetic variants of CPVT have been identified as an autosomal-dominant trait caused by mutation in the gene encoding for the RyR2 receptor and one recessive form caused by mutations in the cardiac isoform of the calsequestrin gene (*CASQ2*).[48] These findings demonstrate that CPVT is caused by mutations of genes that encode for proteins responsible for the regulation of intracellular calcium. Both genes are located on chromosome one (1q42–Q43 and 1p13–p21). More than 70 RyR2 mutations have been identified so far. All are single base pair substitutions, which are mainly located at the carboxy terminus of the protein. Wehrens and colleagues[49] suggested that the common mechanism by which RyR2 mutations cause CPVT is by reducing the binding affinity of RyR2 for the regulatory protein FKBP12.6 (peptidyl-propyl isomerase). The depressed affinity of mutant RyR2 for FKBP12.6 is present in the resting state and worsens when beta-adrenergic stimulation leads to PKA phosphorylation of RyR2. Another theory, proposed by Jiang and colleagues, claims that CPVT is caused by an increased sensitivity to luminal calcium activation. The exaggerated spontaneous calcium release from the SR facilitates the development of delayed after-depolarizations and triggered arrhythmias.

ARRHYTHMOGENIC CARDIOMYOPATHIES

Hypertrophic Cardiomyopathy

The prevalence of unexplained left ventricular hypertrophy (LVH) in the general population is estimated to be 1 in 500.[50,51] Hypertrophic cardiomyopathy (HCM) is a common autosomal-dominant genetic disorder caused by sarcomere mutations; it may account for up to 60% of unexplained cases of LVH, making HCM the most common genetic cardiovascular disorder.[52–54] This clinical entity was first described in 1958 by a pathologist, Donald Teare, as a "benign muscular hamartoma of the heart."[55] Actually HCM is a well-defined cardiomyopathy characterized macroscopically by LVH, which may be asymmetrical or symmetric. The symmetric form of HCM accounts for more than one third of cases and is characterized by concentric thickening of the left ventricle with a small ventricular cavity dimension. The asymmetrical variant implies thickening of the basal anterior septum, which bulges beneath the aortic valve and causes narrowing of the left ventricular outflow tract; however, HCM may affect any portion of the left ventricle.[56] Another common variant of the asymmetrical form is HCM with apical hypertrophy, which was first described in Japan in 1970 but has been increasingly diagnosed in western populations. The main pathologic hallmark is the triad of myocyte hypertrophy, disarray, and interstitial fibrosis.[57,58]

HCM is caused by dominant mutations in genes that encode constituents of the sarcomere.[59] More than 400 individual mutations have been identified in 11 sarcomere genes, including cardiac α- and β-myosin heavy chains, cardiac troponins T, I, and C, cardiac myosin-binding protein C, α-tropomyosin, actin, titin, and essential and regulatory myosin light chains.[60–62] HCM mutations do not show specific predilections and are unique. Only a few sarcomere mutations have demonstrated a high incidence of premature death or end-stage heart failure, which defines their mutations as potentially "malignant." There are numerous exceptions, however, which indicates the importance of genetic modifiers and the environment on ultimate phenotypic development. Most mutations are single point missense mutations or small deletions or insertions. The most frequent causes of HCM are mutations in cardiac β-myosin heavy chain, cardiac troponin T, cardiac troponin I, and myosin-binding protein C genes.[57]

For each gene, several different mutations have been identified, and specific mutations are associated with different severity and prognosis. For example, mutations in troponin T cause only mild or subclinical hypertrophy associated with a poor prognosis and high risk of sudden death (SD). In contrast, mutations in myosin-binding protein C are associated with mild disease and onset in middle age or late adult life. HCM also exhibits intrafamilial phenotypic variation, whereby affected individuals from the same family with an identical genetic mutation display distinct clinical and morphologic manifestations. This finding suggests that lifestyle factors or modifier genes are likely to influence the hypertrophic response.[57]

The first pathologic gene identified as responsible for HCM has been the gene encoding for β-myosin heavy chain, mapped on chromosome 14q11.[52] Cardiac myosin is formed of two heavy chains, two essential and two regulatory light chains. The heavy chains contain two sites for actin interaction and for ATPase activity, respectively. Each heavy chain is compounded by two isoforms: α and β. The first one is predominantly expressed in the atrium, whereas the β isoform preferentially expresses in the ventricle. The genes that encode the β and α isoforms are MYH7 and MYH6, respectively.[63,64] The identified mutations of the first gene number more than 80 and are responsible for HCM in 30% to 40% of patients. These mutations seem to be associated with a severe form of HCM with early onset, complete penetrance, and increased risk of cardiac sudden death. Mutations of MYH6 are rare; most of these mutations are "missense."[65]

Another gene involved in the pathogenesis of HCM is *MYBPC3*, which encodes cardiac myosin-binding protein C; it is located on chromosome 11q1. More than 50 mutations of *MYBPC3* have been identified; they are responsible for an abnormal protein that is unable to interact with myosin and titin. Mutation of cardiac myosin-binding protein C has been found in 30% to 40% of patients.[66,67]

HCM also could be caused by a mutation of genes that code for the troponin complex. The gene of troponin T (*TNNT2*) contains 17 exons; "missense" mutations have been found in 15% to 20% of patients with HCM.[65] On the other side, the gene that encodes troponin I (*TNNI3*) is a small gene that is compounded by only 6 exons. It is responsible for a rare asymmetrical HCM characterized by a LV apical hypertrophy; actually only 6 missense mutations have been reported.[68]

Mutant essential light chains are responsible for 2% to 3% of HCM; these proteins have a crucial role for calcium linking. *MYL3* is the gene that encodes the isoform light slow ventricular chain (MLC-1 s/v). One single missense mutation (Met 149Val) has been found in this gene causing a form of obstructive HCM.[69] The gene *MYL2* encodes the ventricular isoform regulatory myosin light chain (MLC-2s); 5 different mutations have been reported as causing a phenotype similar to *MYL3* mutation.[69]

Cardiac actin has several isoforms also expressed in the skeletal muscle; its gene is

ACTC. Mutation of this gene causes a mutant product that is not able to interact with β-myosin.[54,70,71] Finally, mutation of gene of α-tropomyosin named *TPM1* is also responsible for 3% of cases of HCM.

Recently genetic studies of familial and sporadic unexplained LVH accompanied by conduction disturbances (progressive atrioventricular block, Wolff-Parkinson-White syndrome, atrial fibrillation) have identified metabolic cardiomyopathies. These genetic forms of hypertrophy reflect mutations in γ2 regulatory subunit (PRKAG2) of AMP-activated protein kinase, an enzyme involved with glucose metabolism, or in the X-linked lysosome-associated membrane protein (LAMP2) gene 22, 23. These clinical entities are distinct from HCM caused by sarcomere protein mutations, despite the shared feature of LVH. A high prevalence of conduction system dysfunction (with the requirement of permanent pacing in 30% of patients) characterizes PRKAG2 mutations. LAMP2 mutations are X linked, which results in male predominance. LAMP2 mutations are associated with early-onset LVH (often in childhood) with rapid progression of heart failure and poor prognosis.

Arrhythmogenic right ventricular dysplasia

Arrhythmogenic right ventricular dysplasia (ARVD) is a disease characterized by the progressive loss of myocytes, and it affects mainly the right ventricular myocardium.[72] It is caused by either massive or partial replacement of myocardium by fatty or fibro-fatty tissue advancing from the epicardium to the endocardium. This infiltration provides a substrate for electrical instability and leads to sustained arrhythmias and sudden death.[73]

There are several current concepts surrounding the pathogenesis of ARVD, including the progressive loss of myocytes by programmed cell death (apoptosis) as a consequence of cardiac injury. In some cases of ARVD, myocarditis has been implicated, and entero- and adenoviruses have been identified as potential etiologic agents.[72] There is a strong familial incidence (approximately 50% of cases) with autosomal-dominant inheritance, variable penetrance, and polymorphic phenotypic expression, which suggests that a genetically determined loss of myocytes may account for many cases of the disease. An autosomal-recessive form of ARVD also has been identified. It is associated with palmoplantar keratoderma and woolly hair (Naxos disease). This type of ARVD is caused by a mutation of the plakoglobin gene, the product of which is a component of desmosomes and adherens junctions.[73] The search for the genes responsible for autosomal-dominant ARVD is still underway, and gene linkage analysis of large pedigree has revealed multiple chromosomal loci involved in the pathogenesis of this cardiomyopathy. According to these gene mutations, several different phenotypes of ARVD have been defined.

Arrhythmogenic right ventricular dysplasia 1 This phenotype is caused by mutation in the transforming growth factor beta-3 gene (TGFβ3) on chromosome 14q23–q24. The coding region encodes for a protein of 849 amino acids with a single transmembrane domain and a short stretch of intracellular domain.[25] Beta-type TGFs are polypeptides that act like hormones and control the proliferation and differentiation of multiple cell types. Rampazzo and colleagues[74] performed linkage studies in two large Italian families, one of which had 19 affected members in four generations. They found that 14q23–q24 locus was frequently involved. They also identified in four affected patients two types of mutations of the TGFβ3 gene: 36 G-A transition in the 5′-UTR and 1723 C-T transition in the 3′ UTR.

Arrhythmogenic right ventricular dysplasia 2 ARVD 2 is an autosomal dominant cardiomyopathy characterized by partial degeneration of right ventricular myocardium, electrical instability, and SD.[75] This disease and catecholaminergic polymorphic ventricular tachycardia (CPVT) can be caused by mutation in the cardiac RyR 2 gene located on chromosome 1q42.1–q43. The channel is a tetramer compounded by 4 RyR2 polypeptides and 4 FK506-binding proteins.[76] In myocardial cells, RyR2 proteins—activated by calcium—induced the release of this ion from the sarcoplasmatic reticulum into the cytosol. Tiso and colleagues[75] have demonstrated that RyR2 mutations provide different effects: ARVD 2-associated mutations increase RyR2-mediated calcium release to the cytoplasm and increase intracellular calcium level. RyR2 is the cardiac counterpart of RyR1, which is located in the skeletal muscle and is involved in malignant hyperthermia susceptibility and in central core disease (CCD).

Studies in a family with a "concealed" form of ARVD demonstrated that affected members did not show any structural heart disease, but they consistently presented effort-induced polymorphic ventricular tachycardias. In this family, however, a linkage to 1q42–q43 was demonstrated. In two other families, linkage to 1q42–q43 and 14q23–q24 (ARVD 1) was excluded, which provided evidence of further genetic heterogeneity.[77]

ARVD 3 The existence of a novel ARVD locus on chromosome 14, in addition to ARVD 1 at 14q23–q24, was suggested by Severini and colleagues[78] that studied the linkage in three small different families. They found linkage to markers on the proximal part of 14q, named 14q12–q22. This locus is mapped on the long arm of chromosome 14; the gene responsible for ARVD is still unknown.

ARVD 4 In studies of three families, Rampazzo and colleagues[79] mapped a novel ARVD locus to 2q32.1–q32.3. Affected members of the three families showed clinical characteristics of ARVD according to the diagnostic criteria. Two episodes of SD in young patients were observed. These families were considered unusual in the finding of localized involvement of the left ventricle with left bundle branch block in some affected members. The gene responsible for ARVD 4 is still unknown.

ARVD 5, 6 By linkage analysis in a large North American family, Ahmad and colleagues[80] identified a novel locus for ARVD on 3p23. Asano and colleagues[81] implicated the laminin receptor-1 gene (LAMR1) as responsible for ARVD. An in vitro study of cardiomyocytes expressing the product of mutated Lamr1 showed early cell death accompanied by alterations of chromatine architecture. Asano found that Lamr1 mapped to 3p21, and its mutant product was able to cause degeneration of cardiomyocytes. This mutation is associated with patients affected by ARVD 5.

After exclusion of the five previously known loci, Li and colleagues[82] identified a novel locus on 10p14–p12; they investigated the involvement of the protein tyrosine phosphatase-like gene in a North American family with early-onset ARVD and high penetrance. Protein tyrosine phosphatases mediate the dephosphorylation of phosphotyrosine and are known to be involved in many signal transduction pathways leading to cell growth, differentiation, and oncogenic transformation. Li and colleagues found a missense mutation in gene encoding for protein tyrosine phosphatases; this is the cause of ARVD6.

ARVD 7 Desmin-related myopathy is another term referring to myofibrillar myopathy in which there are intrasarcoplasmic aggregates of desmin. ARVD 7, which maps to chromosome 10q22.3, is another desmin-related myopathy. This is characterized by skeletal muscle weakness associated with cardiac conduction blocks, arrhythmias, heart failure, and intracytoplasmatic accumulation of desmin-reactive deposits in cardiac and skeletal muscle cells.[83] Approximately one third of desmin-related myopathies are thought to be caused by mutations in the desmin gene. The DES gene encodes desmin, a muscle-specific cytoskeletal protein found in the smooth, cardiac, and heart muscles. Melberg and colleagues[84] identified mutations in the ZASP gene, which is located on 10q22.3; patients affected by this mutation showed myopathy, supraventricular arrhythmias, and bradyarrhythmias. Several patients were found to have dilatation of the right ventricle and showed fibro-fatty replacement of myocardium.

ARVD 8 ARVD 8 is caused by a mutation in the gene encoding desmoplakin, which is the most abundant protein of the desmosomes with two isoforms produced by alternative splicing. The gene mentioned previously is on chromosome 6p24. ARVD 8 seems to be caused by a missense mutation in exon 7 of the desmoplakin gene;[85] another mutation has been identified in exon 23. The first mutation is interesting because a homozygous desmoplakin missense mutation had been reported to cause a dilative cardiomyopathy associated with keratoderma and woolly hair. These data suggest that ARVD 8 results from defects in intercellular connections.

ARVD 9 This form of ARVD is caused by heterozygous mutations in the *PKP2* gene, which encodes plakophilin-2 gene, an essential protein of cardiac desmosome.[86] Desmosomes are a complex of multiprotein structures of the cell membrane and provide structural and functional integrity to adjacent cells. The plakophilins are located in the dense plaque of desmosomes, but they are also found in the nucleus, where they have a role in transcriptional regulation. Gerull and colleagues[87] examined 120 patients with diagnosis of ARVD according the criteria proposed by McKenna. They found a high prevalence of mutation of *PKP2* gene, which was mapped to chromosome 12p11. Gerull and colleagues concluded that lack of plakophilin-2 or incorporation of mutant plakophilin-2 in the cardiac desmosomes impairs cell-cell contacts and provides intrinsic variation in conduction properties that may lead to life-threatening arrhythmias.

ARVD 10 The desmosomal cadherins are cell adhesion molecules, and two classes of desmosomal cadherins are known: the desmogleins and the desmocollins (DSC). The desmogleins gene is mapped to chromosome 18q12.1–q12.2.[88] ARVD 10 is an autosomal-dominant disorder with reduced penetrance characterized by fibrofatty replacement of cardiac myocytes. The more frequent mutation identified is a transition G-to-A at the nucleotide 134 in exon 3. Another mutation, which causes a premature termination of codon, is a 915G-A transition in exon 8.[89]

ARVD 11 This form is caused by a mutation of the *DSC2* gene on chromosome 18q21. Syrris and colleagues[90] identified two different heterozygous mutations in the *DSC2* gene. Both mutations resulted in frame shifts and premature truncation of the DSC protein.

Familial Dilated Cardiomyopathy

Idiopathic dilated cardiomyopathy (DCM) is the most common cause of congestive heart failure and is characterized by an increase in myocardial mass and a reduction in ventricular wall thickness. The heart assumes a globular shape, and there is a pronounced ventricular chamber dilatation and atrial enlargement, often with thrombi in the appendages. It has been estimated that up to 35% of individuals with idiopathic DCM have a familial disease.[59] This estimate has been shown by detailed pedigree analyses of relatives of patients with DCM coupled with the identification of single gene mutations in structural proteins of the myocyte cytoskeleton or sarcolemma.[91] It has been proposed that familial DCM (FDCM) is a form of "cytoskeletalopathy."

The pattern of inheritance of FDCM is variable and includes autosomal-dominant, X-linked, autosomal-recessive, and mitochondrial inheritance.[90] The autosomal form of FDCM is the most frequent and can be further grouped into either a pure CMP phenotype or DCM with cardiac conduction system disease. Major progress has been made in the identification of candidate disease loci and the genes responsible for FDCM, including mutations in the genes that encode cardiac actin, desmin, δ-sarcoglycan, β- sarcoglycan, cardiac troponin T, and α-tropomyosin. Four candidate genetic loci also have been mapped for DCM with cardiac conduction system disease, but to date there has been identification of only one gene, the lamin A/C gene.[91,92] Mutations in the lamin A/C gene also cause autosomal-dominant FDCM with mild skeletal myopathy and autosomal-dominant Emery-Dreifuss muscular dystrophy. Most molecular causes of autosomal DCM are still unknown; linkage analysis allows mapping many mutations in different chromosomes, such as 1p1–1q1, 9q13–q22, and 3p22–p25. The single mutant gene responsible has not been identified, however. Recently, a missense mutation of gene encoding cardiac actin has been localized on 3p22–p25. In these patients a defect of actin-Z band was evidenced.[70]

The X-linked forms of DCM include X-linked DCM and Barth syndrome. The first one is a type of DCM that occurs in boys during adolescence or early adulthood with a rapidly progressive clinical course. Female carriers develop a mild form of DCM with onset in middle age. X-linked DCM is associated with raised concentrations of creatine kinase but without signs of skeletal myopathy and is caused by mutations in the dystrophin gene.[91] Mutations of this gene are also responsible for Duchenne's and Becker's muscular dystrophies. The infantile form of X-linked DCM or Barth syndrome typically affects male infants and is characterized by neutropenia, growth retardation, and mitochondrial dysfunction.[93] One mutant gene, responsible for DCM, is the G4.5, which has been mapped on Xq28. Mutation of this gene causes Barth syndrome, and it seems to be involved in left ventricular noncompaction.[91]

SUMMARY

Sudden cardiac death and its devastating consequences still affect millions of individuals throughout the world. Over the last three decades, a tremendous amount of research has focused on possible contributing pathophysiologic mechanisms. The discovery of inherited primary and secondary electrical disorders caused by alterations in our genetic material opened a whole new era of understanding. The knowledge obtained should be incorporated into our new, contemporary approach to malignant ventricular arrhythmias. In the past, the diagnosis of an idiopathic ventricular arrhythmia (without clear cause) was all too readily made. The search for any other plausible explanations ceased whenever structural heart disease could be excluded. Careful familial screening and genetic analysis should be performed in all of these cases. Cardiac channelopathies represent a group of recently discovered arrhythmogenic disorders in structurally normal hearts. In this field, only a fraction of the causative gene mutations have so far been identified. Prognostic assessment of each member of an affected family calls for an individual approach based on clinical features, family analysis, and genetic results.

REFERENCES

1. Birney E, Stamatoyannopoulos JA, Dutta A, et al. Identification and analysis of functional elements in 1% of the human genome by the ENCODE pilot project. Nature 2007;447(7146):799–816.

2. Towbin JA, Bowles NE. Human molecular genetics and the heart. In: Zipes DP, Jalife J, editors. Cardiac electrophysiology, from cell to bedside. 4th edition. Saunders; 2004. p. 444–61.
3. Noda M, Shimizu S, Tanabe T, et al. Primary structure of electrophorus electricus sodium channel deduced form cDNA sequence. Nature 1984;312:121–7.
4. Marban ET, Yamagisji T, Tomaselli GF. Structure and function of voltage gated sodium channels. J Physiol 1998;508(3):647–57.
5. Balser JR. The cardiac sodium channel: gating function and molecular pharmacology. J Mol Cell Cardiol 2001;33(4):599–613.
6. Grant AO, Carboni MP, Neplioueva V, et al. Long QT-syndrome, Brugada syndrome and conduction disease are linked to a single sodium channel mutation. J Clin Invest 2002;110:1201–9.
7. Brugada P, Brugada J. Right bundle branch block, persistent ST-segment elevation and sudden cardiac death: a distinct clinical and electrocardiographic syndrome. A multicenter report. J Am Coll Cardiol 1992;20:1391–6.
8. Antzelevitch C, Brugada P, Borggrefe M, et al. Brugada syndrome: report of the second consensus conference. Circulation 2005;111:659–70.
9. Chen Q, Kirsch GE, Zhang D, et al. Genetic basis and molecular mechanism for idiopathic ventricular fibrillation. Nature 1998;392:293–6.
10. Weiss R, Barmada MM, Nguyen T, et al. Clinical and molecular heterogeneity in the Brugada syndrome: a novel gene locus on chromosome 3. Circulation 2002;105:707–13.
11. London B, Sanyal S, Michalec M, et al. A mutation in the glycerol-3-phosphate dehydrogenase 1-like gen (GPD1L) causes Brugada syndrome. Circulation 2007;116(20):2260–8.
12. Bezzina CR, Shimizu W, Yang P, et al. Common sodium channel promoter haplotype in Asian subjects underlies variability in cardiac conduction. Circulation 2006;113:338–44.
13. Poelzing S, Forleo C, Samodell M, et al. SCN5A polymorphism restores trafficking of a Brugada syndrome mutation on a separate gene. Circulation 2006;114:368–76.
14. Antzelevitch C. The Brugada syndrome: ionic basis and arrhythmia mechanisms. J Cardiovasc Electrophysiol 2001;12:268–72.
15. Meregallli PG, Wilde AA, Tan HL. Pathophysiological mechanisms of Brugada syndrome: depolarization disorder, repolarization disorder, or more? Cardiovasc Res 2005;67:367–78.
16. Lenègre J, Moreau PH. Le bloc auriculo-ventriculaire chronique: etude anatomique, clinique et histologique. Arch Mal Coeur Vaiss 1963;56:867–88.
17. Lev M. Anatomic basis of atrioventricular block. Am J Cardiol 1964;37:742–8.
18. Combrink JM, Davis WH, Snyman HW, et al. Familial bundle branch block. Am Heart J 1962;64:397–400.
19. Steenkamp WF. Familial trifascicular block. Am Heart J 1972;84:758–60.
20. Brink PA, Ferreira A, Moolman JC, et al. Gene for progressive familial heart block type I maps to chromosome 19q13. Circulation 1995;91:1633–40.
21. Scott JJ, Alshinawi C, Kyndt F, et al. Cardiac conduction defects associate with mutations in SCN5A. Nat Genet 1999;23:20–1.
22. Probst V, Kyndt F, Potet F, et al. Haploinsufficiency in combination with aging causes SCN5A-linked hereditary Lenègre disease. J Am Coll Cardiol 2003;41(4):643–52.
23. Rivolta I, Abriel H, Tateyama M, et al. Inherited Brugada and LQT3-syndrome mutations of a single residue of the cardiac sodium channel confer distinct channel and clinical phenotypes. J Biol Chem 2001;276:30623–30.
24. Deal KK, England SK, Tamkun MM. Molecular physiology of cardiac potassium channels. Physiol Rev 1996;76:49–67.
25. Pongs O, Leicher T, Berger M, et al. Functional and molecular aspects of voltage-gated K-channel B subunits. Ann N Y Acad Sci 1999;868:344–55.
26. Yellen G. The voltage-gated potassium channels and their relatives. Nature 2002;419:36–42.
27. Modell SM, Lehmann MH. The long QT syndrome family of cardiac ion channelopathies: a HuGE review. Genet Med 2006;8(3):143–55.
28. Yoshiyasu A, Kazuo U, Fabiana S, et al. A novel mutation in KCN1 associated with a potent dominant negative effect as the basis for the LQT1 form of the long QT syndrome. J Cardiovasc Electrophysiol 2007;18:972–7.
29. Craig TJ, Qiuming G, Zhou Z, et al. Long QT syndrome: cellular basis and arrhythmia mechanism in LQT2. J Cardiovasc Electrophysiol 2000;11:1413–8.
30. Sanguinetti MC, Keating MT. Role of delayed rectifier potassium channels in cardiac repolarization and arrhythmias. News Physiol Sci 1997;12:152–7.
31. Sanguinetti MC, Jiang C, Curran ME, et al. A mechanistic link between an inherited and an acquired cardiac arrhythmia: HERG encodes the Ikr potassium channel. Cell 1995;81:299–307.
32. Laura B, Zhijun S, Dennis AT, et al. Cellular dysfunction of LQT5-minK mutants: abnormalities of Iks, Ikr and trafficking in long QT syndrome. Hum Mol Genet 1999;8:1499–507.
33. Curran ME, Splawski I, Timothy KW, et al. A molecular basis for cardiac arrhythmias: HERG mutations cause long QT syndrome. Cell 1995;80:795–803.
34. Tsuboi M, Antzelevitch C. Cellular basis for electrocardiographic and arrhythmic manifestations of Andersen-Tawil syndrome (LQT7). Heart Rhythm 2006;3:328–35.

35. Gussak I, Brugada P, Brugada J, et al. Idiopathic short QT-interval: a new clinical syndrome? Cardiology 2000;94:99–102.
36. Gaita F, Cuistetto C, Bianchi F, et al. Short QT-syndrome: a familial cause of sudden death. Circulation 2003;108:965–70.
37. Brugada R, Hong K, Cordeiro JM, et al. Short QT-syndrome. CMAJ 2005;173(II):1349–54.
38. Brugada R, Hong K, Dumaine R, et al. Sudden death associated with short-QT syndrome linked to mutations in HERG. Circulation 2004;109:30–5.
39. Hong K, Bjerregaard P, Gussak I, et al. Short QT-syndrome and atrial fibrillation caused by mutation in KCNH2. J Cardiovasc Electrophysiol 2005;16: 394–6.
40. Hong K, Piper DR, Diaz-Valdecantos A, et al. De novo KCNQ1-mutation responsible for atrial fibrillation and short QT syndrome in utero. Cardiovasc Res 2005;68(3):1310–25.
41. Priori SG, Pandit SV, Rivolta I, et al. A novel form of short QT syndrome (SQT3) is caused by a mutation in the KCNJ2 gene. Circ Res 2005;96:800–7.
42. Ertel EA, Campbell KP, Harpold MM, et al. Nomenclature of voltage-gated calcium channels. Neuron 2000;25:533–5.
43. Splaswski I, Timothy KW, Sharpe LM, et al. Ca(V)1.2 calcium channel dysfunction causes a multisystem disorder including arrhythmia and autism. Cell 2004;119:19–31.
44. Mckeown L, Robinson P, Jones T. Molecular basis of inherited calcium channelopathies: role of mutations in pore forming units. Acta Pharmacol Sin 2006; 27(7):799–812.
45. Lehnart SE, Ackerman MJ, Benson DW, et al. Inherited arrhythmias: a National Heart, Lung, and Blood Institute and Office of Rare Diseases workshop consensus report about the diagnosis, phenotyping, molecular mechanisms, and therapeutic approaches for primary cardiomyopathies of gene mutations affecting ion channel dysfunction. Circulation 2007;116:2325–45.
46. Pitt GS, Dun W, Boyden P. Remodeled cardiac calcium channels. J Mol Cell Cardiol 2006;41:373–88.
47. Mohamed U, Napolitano C, Priori SG. Molecular and electrophysiological bases of catecholaminergic polymorphic ventricular tachycardia. J Cardiovasc Electrophysiol 2007;18:791–7.
48. Liu N, Colombi B, Raytcheva-Buono E, et al. Catecholaminergic polymorphic ventricular tachycardia. Herz 2007;32:212–7.
49. Wehrens XH, Lenhart SE, Huang F, et al. FKBP12.6 deficiency and defective calcium release channel (ryanodine receptor) function linked to exercise induced sudden cardiac death. Cell 2003;113: 829–40.
50. Maron BJ, Gardin JM, Flack JM, et al. Prevalence of hypertrophic cardiomyopathy in a general population of young adults: echocardiographic analysis of 4111 subjects in the CARDIA study. Circulation 1995;92:785–9.
51. Zou Y, Song L, Wang Z, et al. Prevalence of idiopathic hypertrophic cardiomyopathy in China: a population-based analysis of 8080 adults. Am J Med 2004;116:14–8.
52. Van Driest SL, Ellsworth EG, Ommen SR, et al. Prevalence and spectrum of thin filament mutations in outpatient referral population with hypertrophic cardiomyopathy. Circulation 2003;108:445–51.
53. Richard P, Charron P, Carrier L, et al. Hypertrophic cardiomyopathy: distribution of disease genes, spectrum of mutations and implications for a molecular diagnosis strategy. Circulation 2003;107:2227–32.
54. Arad M, Maron BJ, Gorham JM, et al. Glycogen storage diseases presenting as hypertrophic cardiomyopathy. N Engl J Med 2005;352:362–72.
55. Teare D. Asymmetrical hypertrophy of the heart in young adults. Br Heart J 1958;20:1–8.
56. Maron BJ. Sudden death in young athletes. N Engl J Med 2003;349:1064–75.
57. Maron BJ. Hypertrophic cardiomyopathy: a systematic review. JAMA 2002;287:1308–20.
58. Hughes SJ. The pathology of hypertrophic cardiomyopathy. Histopathology 2004;44:412–27.
59. Towbin JA, Bowles NE. The failing heart. Nature 2002;415:227–33.
60. Seidman JG, Seidman C. The genetic basis for cardiomyopathy: from mutation identification to mechanistic paradigms. Cell 2001;104:557–67.
61. Charron P, Heron D, Gargiulo M, et al. Genetic testing and genetic counseling in hypertrophic cardiomyopathy: the French experience. J Med Genet 2002;39:741–6.
62. Geisterfer-Lowrance AA, Kass S, Tanigawa G, et al. A molecular basis for familial hypertrophic cardiomyopathy: a β-myosin heavy chain gene missense mutation. Cell 1990;62(5):999–1006.
63. Jaenicke T, Diederich KW, Haas W, et al. The complete sequence of the human β myosin heavy chain gene and a comparative analysis of its product. Genomics 1990;8:194–7.
64. Liew CC, Sole MJ, Yamauchi-Takihara K, et al. Complete sequence and organization of the human cardiac β myosin heavy chain gene. Nucleic Acids Res 1990;18:3647–52.
65. Watkins H, McKenna WJ, Thierfelder L, et al. Mutations in the genes for cardiac troponin T and α tropomyosin in hypertrophic cardiomyopathy. N Engl J Med 1995;332:1058–63.
66. Nimura H, Bachinski LL, Sangwatanaroj S, et al. Mutations in the gene for cardiac myosin binding protein C and late onset familial hypertrophic cardiomyopathy. N Engl J Med 1998;338:1248–53.
67. Rottbauer W, Gautel M, Zehelein J, et al. Novel splice donor site mutation in the cardiac myosin

binding protein C gene in familial hypertrophic cardiomyopathy: characterization of cardiac transcript and protein. J Clin Invest 1997;100:475–8.
68. Moolman JC, Corfield VA. Sudden death due to troponin T mutations. J Am Coll Cardiol 1997;29: 549–54.
69. Poetter K, Jiang H, Hassanzadeh S, et al. Mutations in either the essential or regulatory light chains of myosin are associated with a rare myopathy in human heart and skeletal muscle. Nat Genet 1996;13:63–6.
70. Olson TM, Michels VV, Thibodeau SN, et al. Actin mutations in dilated cardiomyopathy, a heritable form of heart failure. Science 1998;280:750–2.
71. Blair E, Redwood C, Ashrafian H, et al. Mutations in the gamma(2) subunit of AMP-activated protein kinase cause familial hypertrophic cardiomyopathy: evidence for the central role of energy compromise in disease pathogenesis. Hum Mol Genet 2001;10: 1215–20.
72. Basso C, Thiene G, Corrado D, et al. Arrhythmogenic right ventricular cardiomyopathy: dysplasia, dystrophy or myocarditis? Circulation 1996;94:983–91.
73. Corrado D, Fontine G, Marcus FI, et al. Arrhythmogenic right ventricular dysplasia/cardiomyopathy: need for international registry. Study group on arrhythmogenic right ventricular dysplasia/cardiomyopathy of the working groups of myocardial and pericardial disease and arrhythmias of the European Society of Cardiology and of the Scientific Council of Cardiomyopathies of the World Heart Federation. Circulation 2000;101:E101–6.
74. Rampazzo A, Beggagna G, Nava A, et al. Arrhythmogenic right ventricular cardiomyopathy type 1 (ARVD1): confirmation of locus assignment and mutation screening of four candidate genes. Eur J Hum Genet 2003;11:69–76.
75. Tiso N, Stephan DA, Nava A, et al. Identification of mutations in the cardiac ryanodine receptor gene in family affected by arrhythmogenic right ventricular cardiomyopathy type 2 (ARVD2). Hum Mol Genet 2001;10:189–94.
76. Marx SO, Reiken S, Hisamatsu Y, et al. PKA phosphorylation dissociates FKBP12,6 from the calcium release channel (ryanodine receptor): defective regulation in failing hearts. Cell 2000;101:365–76.
77. Moren A, Ichijo H, Miyazono K. Molecular cloning and characterization of the human and porcine transforming growth factor beta-type III receptors. Biochem Biophys Res Commun 1992;189:356–62.
78. Severini GM, Krajinovic M, Pinamonti B, et al. A new locus for arrhythmogenic right ventricular dysplasia on the long arm of chromosome 14. Genomics 1996;31:193–200.
79. Rampazzo A, Nava A, Miorin M, et al. ARVD4, a new locus for arrhythmogenic right ventricular cardiomyopathy, maps to chromosome 2 long arm. Genomics 1997;45:259–63.
80. Ahmad F, Li D, Karibe A, et al. Localization of a gene responsible for arrhythmogenic right ventricular dysplasia to chromosome 3p23. Circulation 1998; 98:2791–5.
81. Asano Y, Takashima S, Asakura M, et al. Lamr1 functional retroposon causes right ventricular dysplasia in mice. Nat Genet 2004;36:123–30.
82. Li D, Ahmad F, Gardner MJ, et al. The locus of a new gene responsible for arrhythmogenic right ventricular dysplasia characterized by early onset and high penetrance maps to chromosome 10p12-p14. Am J Hum Genet 2000;66:148–56.
83. Ferreiro A, Ceuterick-de Groote C, Marks JJ, et al. Desmin-related myopathy with Mallory body-like inclusions is caused by mutations of the selenoprotein N gene. Ann Neurol 2004;55(5):676–86.
84. Seicen D, Engel AG. Mutations in ZASP define a novel form of muscular dystrophy in humans. Ann Neurol 2005;57:269–76.
85. Rampazzo A, Nava A, Malacrida S, et al. Mutation in human desmoplakin domain binding to plakoglobin causes a dominant form of arrhythmogenic right ventricular dysplasia. Am J Hum Genet 2002;71: 1200–6.
86. Grossmann KS, Grund C, Huelsken J, et al. Requirement of plakophilin 2 for heart morphogenesis and cardiac junction formation. J Cell Biol 2004;167: 149–60.
87. Gerull B, Heuser A, Wichter T, et al. Mutations in the desmosomal protein plakophilin-2 are common in arrhythmogenic right ventricular cardiomyopathy. Nat Genet 2004;36:1162–4.
88. Arnemann J, Spurr NK, Magee AI, et al. The human gene (DSG2) coding for HDGC, a second member of the desmoglein subfamily of the desmosomal cadherins, is like DSG1coding for desmoglein DGI, assigned to chromosome 18. Genomics 1992;13:484–6.
89. Awad MM, Dalal D, Cho E, et al. DSG2 mutations contribute to arrhythmogenic right ventricular dysplasia/cardiomyopathy. Am J Hum Genet 2006; 79:136–42.
90. Syrris P, Ward D, Evans A, et al. Arrhythmogenic right ventricular dysplasia/cardiomyopathy associated with mutations in the desmosomal gene desmocollin-2. Am J Hum Genet 2006;79:978–84.
91. Sinagra G, Di Lenarda A, Brodsky GL, et al. Current perspectives: new insights into the molecular basis of familial dilated cardiomyopathy. Ital Heart J 2001;2:280–6.
92. Kass S, MacRae C, Graber HL, et al. A gene defect that causes conduction system disease and dilated cardiomyopathy maps to chromosome 1p1-1q1. Nat Genet 1994;7:546–51.
93. Bowles NE, Bowles KR, Towbin JA. The "final common pathway" hypothesis and inherited cardiovascular disease. The role of cytoskeletal proteins in dilated cardiomyopathy. Herz 2000;25:168–75.

Index

Note: Page numbers of article titles are in **boldface** type.

Heart Failure Clin 6 (2010) 267–270
doi:10.1016/S1551-7136(10)00010-3

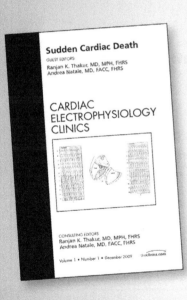